Interferon Methods and Protocols

METHODS IN MOLECULAR MEDICINE™

John M. Walker, SERIES EDITOR

122. **Placenta Research Methods and Protocols:** *Volume 2*, edited by *Michael J. Soares and Joan S. Hunt*, 2005
121. **Placenta Research Methods and Protocols:** *Volume 1*, edited by *Michael J. Soares and Joan S. Hunt*, 2005
120. **Breast Cancer Research Protocols**, edited by *Susan A. Brooks and Adrian Harris*, 2005
119. **Human Papilloma Viruses:** *Methods and Protocols*, edited by *Clare Davy and John Doorbar*, 2005
118. **Antifungal Agents:** *Methods and Protocols*, edited by *Erika J. Ernst and P. David Rogers*, 2005
117. **Fibrosis Research:** *Methods and Protocols*, edited by *John Varga, David A. Brenner, and Sem H. Phan*, 2005
116. **Inteferon Methods and Protocols**, edited by *Daniel J. J. Carr*, 2005
115. **Lymphoma:** *Methods and Protocols*, edited by *Timothy Illidge and Peter W. M. Johnson*, 2005
114. **Microarrays in Clinical Diagnostics**, edited by *Thomas Joos and Paolo Fortina*, 2005
113. **Multiple Myeloma:** *Methods and Protocols*, edited by *Ross D. Brown and P. Joy Ho*, 2005
112. **Molecular Cardiology:** *Methods and Protocols*, edited by *Zhongjie Sun*, 2005
111. **Chemosensitivity:** *Volume 2, In Vivo Models, Imaging, and Molecular Regulators*, edited by *Rosalyn D. Blumethal*, 2005
110. **Chemosensitivity:** *Volume 1, In Vitro Assays*, edited by *Rosalyn D. Blumethal*, 2005
109. **Adoptive Immunotherapy:** *Methods and Protocols*, edited by *Burkhard Ludewig and Matthias W. Hoffman*, 2005
108. **Hypertension:** *Methods and Protocols*, edited by *Jérôme P. Fennell and Andrew H. Baker*, 2005
107. **Human Cell Culture Protocols,** *Second Edition*, edited by *Joanna Picot*, 2005
106. **Antisense Therapeutics,** *Second Edition*, edited by *M. Ian Phillips*, 2005
105. **Developmental Hematopoiesis:** *Methods and Protocols*, edited by *Margaret H. Baron*, 2005
104. **Stroke Genomics:** *Methods and Reviews*, edited by *Simon J. Read and David Virley*, 2004
103. **Pancreatic Cancer:** *Methods and Protocols*, edited by *Gloria H. Su*, 2004

102. **Autoimmunity:** *Methods and Protocols*, edited by *Andras Perl*, 2004
101. **Cartilage and Osteoarthritis:** *Volume 2, Structure and In Vivo Analysis*, edited by *Frédéric De Ceuninck, Massimo Sabatini, and Philippe Pastoureau*, 2004
100. **Cartilage and Osteoarthritis:** *Volume 1, Cellular and Molecular Tools*, edited by *Massimo Sabatini, Philippe Pastoureau, and Frédéric De Ceuninck*, 2004
99. **Pain Research:** *Methods and Protocols*, edited by *David Z. Luo*, 2004
98. **Tumor Necrosis Factor:** *Methods and Protocols*, edited by *Angelo Corti and Pietro Ghezzi*, 2004
97. **Molecular Diagnosis of Cancer:** *Methods and Protocols, Second Edition*, edited by *Joseph E. Roulston and John M. S. Bartlett*, 2004
96. **Hepatitis B and D Protocols:** *Volume 2, Immunology, Model Systems, and Clinical Studies*, edited by *Robert K. Hamatake and Johnson Y. N. Lau*, 2004
95. **Hepatitis B and D Protocols:** *Volume 1, Detection, Genotypes, and Characterization*, edited by *Robert K. Hamatake and Johnson Y. N. Lau*, 2004
94. **Molecular Diagnosis of Infectious Diseases,** *Second Edition*, edited by *Jochen Decker and Udo Reischl*, 2004
93. **Anticoagulants, Antiplatelets, and Thrombolytics,** edited by *Shaker A. Mousa*, 2004
92. **Molecular Diagnosis of Genetic Diseases,** *Second Edition*, edited by *Rob Elles and Roger Mountford*, 2004
91. **Pediatric Hematology:** *Methods and Protocols*, edited by *Nicholas J. Goulden and Colin G. Steward*, 2003
90. **Suicide Gene Therapy:** *Methods and Reviews*, edited by *Caroline J. Springer*, 2004
89. **The Blood–Brain Barrier:** *Biology and Research Protocols*, edited by *Sukriti Nag*, 2003
88. **Cancer Cell Culture:** *Methods and Protocols*, edited by *Simon P. Langdon*, 2003
87. **Vaccine Protocols,** *Second Edition*, edited by *Andrew Robinson, Michael J. Hudson, and Martin P. Cranage*, 2003
86. **Renal Disease:** *Techniques and Protocols*, edited by *Michael S. Goligorsky*, 2003

METHODS IN MOLECULAR MEDICINE™

Interferon Methods and Protocols

Edited by

Daniel J. J. Carr

Department of Ophthalmology, The University of Oklahoma Health and Sciences Center, Oklahoma City, OK

HUMANA PRESS ✳ TOTOWA, NEW JERSEY

© 2005 Humana Press Inc.
999 Riverview Drive, Suite 208
Totowa, New Jersey 07512

www.humanapress.com

All rights reserved.

No part of this book may be reproduced, stored in a retrieval system, or transmitted in any form or by any means, electronic, mechanical, photocopying, microfilming, recording, or otherwise without written permission from the Publisher. Methods in Molecular Medicine™ is a trademark of The Humana Press Inc.

All papers, comments, opinions, conclusions, or recommendations are those of the author(s), and do not necessarily reflect the views of the publisher.

This publication is printed on acid-free paper. ∞
ANSI Z39.48-1984 (American Standards Institute) Permanence of Paper for Printed Library Materials.

Production Editor: C. Tirpak

Cover design by Patricia F. Cleary

Cover Illustration: From Fig. 2, Chapter 14, "Interferon Subtype Gene Therapy for Regulating Cytomegalovirus Disease," by Cassandra M. James, Emmalene J. Bartlett, Josephine P. Mansfield, and Vanessa S. Cull.

For additional copies, pricing for bulk purchases, and/or information about other Humana titles, contact Humana at the above address or at any of the following numbers: Tel: 973-256-1699; Fax: 973-256-8341; E-mail: orders@humanapr.com; or visit our Website: www.humanapress.com

Photocopy Authorization Policy:
Authorization to photocopy items for internal or personal use, or the internal or personal use of specific clients, is granted by Humana Press Inc., provided that the base fee of US $30.00 per copy is paid directly to the Copyright Clearance Center at 222 Rosewood Drive, Danvers, MA 01923. For those organizations that have been granted a photocopy license from the CCC, a separate system of payment has been arranged and is acceptable to Humana Press Inc. The fee code for users of the Transactional Reporting Service is: [1-58829-418-8/05 $30.00].

e-ISBN:1-59259-939-7

ISSN: 1543-1894

Printed in the United States of America. 10 9 8 7 6 5 4 3 2 1

Library of Congress Cataloging-in-Publication Data

Interferon methods and protocols / edited by Daniel J.J. Carr.
  p. ; cm. -- (Methods in molecular medicine ; 116)
Includes bibliographical references and index.
ISBN 1-58829-418-8 (alk. paper)
1. Interferon--Laboratory manuals.
[DNLM: 1. Interferons. QW 800 I615 2005] I. Carr, Daniel J. J. II. Series.
QR187.5.I57184 2005
616.07'95--dc22

2005006203

Preface

Observation of the phenomenon of virus interference, by which one virus blocks the growth of another virus when both try to infect the same target cell, led the way in the development of the field of interferon research. Originally described as early as 1935, the research team of Werner and Gertrude Henle published a sentinel paper in 1943 suggesting that the interference phenomenon could be induced by inactivated virus, which further suggested that perhaps a component of the inactivated virus somehow modified the cell to become insensitive to subsequent viral infection. However, it was not until the research team of Alick Isaacs and Jean Lindenmann published their article in 1957 showing that the interference had nothing to do with the virus particle but, rather, stemmed from an unknown factor liberated from the cells in response to the virus did the scientific community begin to appreciate the potential impact that such a factor might have in medicine and biomedical research. This interference factor was termed "interferon" and so, a field was born.

Today, interferons (IFNs) composed of type I and type II IFN species are approved for therapeutic use for a number of conditions including selective malignancies, multiple sclerosis, and certain types of viral infections (e.g., hepatitis B virus). The IFN cytokines are prescribed in more than 80 countries with annual sales well over US$1 billion annually. The success in their application stems from the antiviral, antiproliferative, and immunoregulatory properties associated with the activation of multiple IFN-stimulatory genes and pathways. With the advent of gene array techniques, we now have identified more than 300 IFN-stimulatory genes, many of which have unknown functions. It is the task of current and future researchers in this field to ascertain the functions of the IFN-stimulatory gene products in the hopes of identifying additional pathways that will facilitate our understanding of the many biological events influenced by IFNs.

Interferon Methods and Protocols, a volume in the *Methods in Molecular Medicine* series embarks on illustrating some of the current techniques developed to study specific aspects of IFN-elicited events. Unique to this series, the first two chapters are devoted to adding a historical perspective to the field in general discussing the successes and failures of past and present day technology as well as consideration to future endeavors. The remainder of the volume includes a compilation of contributions that, although not exhaustive, represents a field that has expanded exponentially since its origin nearly 50 years ago. It is anticipated that this volume will be essential to all those who work on interferon research, as well as quite useful to investigators across such overlapping disciplines as immunology, virology, biochemistry, and molecular biology.

I am indebted to Professor John Walker who had the foresight to initiate this endeavor and allow us to organize this volume. It is worthwhile to note that many of the authors have made a significant impact in our understanding of IFN biology. I am grateful to all the authors for their willingness to contribute, in a succinct and timely manner, their experience in the form of the methods (some of which are very unique and sophisticated) included in this volume.

Daniel J. J. Carr

Contents

Preface v
Contributors xi

1. Biological and Clinical Basis for Molecular Studies of Interferons
   *Katie R. Pang, Jashin J. Wu, David B. Huang, Stephen K. Tyring,
   and Samuel Baron* 1
2. Interferon Research: *A Brief History*
   Myriam S. Kunzi and Paula M. Pitha 25
3. Virus Infection and the Interferon Response: *A Global View
   Through Functional Genomics*
   *Marcus J. Korth, John C. Kash, Jeffrey C. Furlong,
   and Michael G. Katze* 37
4. Genomic DNA Affinity Chromatography: *A Technique to Isolate
   Interferon-Inducible DNA Binding Factors*
   Jyothi Kumaran and Eleanor N. Fish 57
5. Protein Engineering of Interferon Alphas
   Renqiu Hu, Ke-jian Lei, Joseph Bekisz, and Kathryn C. Zoon 69
6. Assays for the Interferon-Induced Enzyme 2',5'
   Oligoadenylate Synthetases
   Saumendra N. Sarkar, Mitali Pandey, and Ganes C. Sen 81
7. A Convenient and Sensitive Fluorescence Resonance Energy
   Transfer Assay for RNase L and 2',5' Oligoadenylates
   *Chandar S. Thakur, Zan Xu, Zhengfu Wang, Zachary Novince,
   and Robert H. Silverman* 103
8. Regulation of Murine Interferon Regulatory Factor
   Gene Expression in the Central Nervous System Determined
   by Multiprobe RNase Protection Assay
   Shalina S. Ousman and Iain L. Campbell 115
9. Mitogen-Activated Protein Kinase Pathways
   in Interferon Signaling
   Antonella Sassano, Amit Verma, and Leonidas C. Platanias 135
10. Development of an Interferon-Based Cancer Vaccine Protocol:
    Application to Several Types of Murine Cancers
    W. Robert Fleischmann, Jr. and Tzu G. Wu 151

11. Type I Interferons as Regulators of the Differentiation/
    Activation of Human Dendritic Cells: *Methods
    for the Evaluation of IFN-Induced Effects*
    Stefano M. Santini, Caterina Lapenta, and Filippo Belardelli *167*
12. Flow Cytometric Techniques for Studying Plasmacytoid Dendritic
    Cells in Mixed Populations
    Stacey L. Olshalsky and Patricia Fitzgerald-Bocarsly *183*
13. Analysis of Anti-Interferon Properties of the Herpes Simplex
    Virus Type I ICP0 Protein
    Karen Mossman *195*
14. Interferon Subtype Gene Therapy for Regulating
    Cytomegalovirus Disease
    **Cassandra M. James, Emmalene J. Bartlett,
    Josephine P. Mansfield, and Vanessa S. Cull** *207*
15. Transfection of Müller Cells With Type I Interferon Transgenes:
    Resistance to HSV-1 Infection
    Benitta John-Philip and Daniel J. J. Carr *221*

Index 233

Contributors

SAMUEL BARON • *Departments of Microbiology and Immunology, and Internal Medicine, University of Texas Medical Branch, Galveston, TX*
EMMALENE J. BARTLETT • *Division of Health Sciences, Murdoch University, Western Australia, Australia*
JOSEPH BEKISZ • *Division of Intramural Research, National Institute of Allergy and Infectious Diseases, National Institutes of Health, Bethesda, MD*
FILIPPO BELARDELLI • *Department of Cell Biology and Neurosciences, Istituto Superiore di Sanità, Rome, Italy*
IAIN L. CAMPBELL • *School of Molecular and Microbial Biosciences, The University of Sydney, New South Wales, Australia*
DANIEL J. J. CARR • *Department of Ophthalmology, The University of Oklahoma Health Sciences Center, Oklahoma City, OK*
VANESSA S. CULL • *Division of Health Sciences, Murdoch University, Murdoch, Western Australia, Australia*
ELEANOR N. FISH • *Department of Immunology, University of Toronto, Toronto, ON, Canada*
PATRICIA FITZGERALD-BOCARSLY • *University of Medicine and Dentistry of New Jersey, Department of Pathology and Laboratory Medicine, Newark, NJ*
W. ROBERT FLEISCHMANN, JR. • *Department of Urologic Surgery, University of Minnesota Medical School, Minneapolis, MN*
JEFFREY C. FURLONG • *Department of Microbiology and Washington National Primate Research Center, University of Washington, Seattle, WA*
RENQIU HU • *Division of Intramural Research, National Institute of Allergy and Infectious Diseases, National Institutes of Health, Bethesda, MD*
DAVID B. HUANG • *Division of Infectious Diseases, Department of Medicine, Baylor College of Medicine, Houston, TX; University of Texas School of Public Health, Division of Infectious Diseases, Department of Medicine, University of Texas Health Science Center at Houston, TX*
CASSANDRA M. JAMES • *Division of Health Sciences, Murdoch University, Murdoch, Western Australia, Australia*
BENITTA JOHN-PHILIP • *Department of Ophthalmology, The University of Oklahoma Health Sciences Center, Oklahoma City, OK*
JOHN C. KASH • *Department of Microbiology and Washington National Primate Research Center, University of Washington, Seattle, WA*

MICHAEL G. KATZE • *Department of Microbiology and Washington National Primate Research Center, University of Washington, Seattle, WA*
MARCUS J. KORTH • *Department of Microbiology and Washington National Primate Research Center, University of Washington, Seattle, WA*
JYOTHI KUMARAN • *Department of Immunology, University of Toronto Medical Sciences Bldg., Toronto, ON, Canada*
MYRIAM S. KUNZI • *The Sydney Kimmel Comprehensive Cancer Center, The Johns Hopkins University, Baltimore, MD*
CATERINA LAPENTA • *Department of Cell Biology and Neurosciences, Istituto Superiore di Sanità, Rome, Italy*
KE-JIAN LEI • *Oral Infection of Immunity Branch, National Institute of Dental and Craniofacial Research, National Institutes of Health, Bethesda, MD*
JOSEPHINE P. MANSFIELD • *Division of Health Sciences, Murdoch University, Murdoch, Western Australia, Australia*
KAREN MOSSMAN • *Center for Gene Therapeutics, Department of Pathology and Molecular Medicine, McMaster University, Hamilton, ON, Canada*
ZACHARY NOVINCE • *Department of Biological, Geological, and Environmental Sciences, Cleveland State University, and Department of Cancer Biology, Cleveland Clinic Foundation, Cleveland, OH*
STACEY L. OLSHALSKY • *University of Medicine and Dentistry of New Jersey, Department of Pathology and Laboratory Medicine, Newark, NJ*
SHALINA S. OUSMAN • *Department of Neurology and Neurological Sciences, Stanford University, Stanford, CT*
MITALI PANDEY • *Department of Molecular Biology, The Lerner Research Institute, Cleaveland Clinic Foundation, Cleveland, OH*
KATIE R. PANG • *Center for Clinical Studies, Houston, TX*
PAULA M. PITHA • *The Sidney Kimmel Comprehensive Cancer Center, The Johns Hopkins University, Baltimore, MD*
LEONIDAS C. PLATANIAS • *Robert H. Lurie Comprehensive Cancer Center and Division of Hematology-Oncology, Northwestern University Medical School, Chicago, IL*
STEFANO M. SANTINI • *Department of Cell Biology and Neurosciences, Istituto Superiore di Sanità, Rome, Italy*
SAUMENDRA N. SARKAR • *Department of Molecular Biology, The Lerner Research Institute, Cleaveland Clinic Foundation, Cleveland, OH*
ANTONELLA SASSANO • *Robert H. Lurie Comprehensive Cancer Center and Division of Hematology-Oncology, Northwestern University Medical School, Chicago, IL*
GANES C. SEN • *Department of Molecular Biology, The Lerner Research Institute, Cleaveland Clinic Foundation, Cleveland, OH*

Contributors

ROBERT H. SILVERMAN • *Department of Cancer Biology, Cleveland Clinic Foundation, Cleveland, OH*
CHANDAR S. THAKUR • *Department of Chemistry, Cleveland State University, Department of Cancer Biology, Cleveland Clinic Foundation, Cleveland, OH*
STEPHEN K. TYRING • *Department of Dermatology, University of Texas Health Science Center at Houston; and Center for Clinical Studies, Houston, TX*
AMIT VERMA • *Robert H. Lurie Comprehensive Cancer Center and Division of Hematology-Oncology, Northwestern University Medical School, Chicago, IL*
ZHENGFU WANG • *Department of Cancer Biology, Cleveland Clinic Foundation, Cleveland, OH*
TZU G. WU • *Department of Urologic Surgery, University of Minnesota Medical School, Minneapolis, MN*
JASHIN J. WU • *Department of Dermatology, University of California, Irvine, CA*
ZAN XU • *Ridgeway Biosystems Inc., Cleveland, OH*
KATHRYN C. ZOON • *Division of Intramural Research, National Institute of Allergy and Infectious Diseases, National Institutes of Health, Bethesda, MD*

1

Biological and Clinical Basis for Molecular Studies of Interferons

Katie R. Pang, Jashin J. Wu, David B. Huang, Stephen K. Tyring, and Samuel Baron

Summary

The cytokine family of interferons (IFNs) has multiple functions, including antiviral, antitumor, and immunomodulatory effects and regulation of cell differentiation. The multiple functions of the IFN system are thought to be an innate defense against microbes and foreign substances. The IFN system consists first of cells that produce IFNs in response to viral infection or other foreign stimuli and second of cells that establish the antiviral state in response to IFNs. This process of innate immunity involves multiple signaling mechanisms and activation of various host genes. Viruses have evolved to develop mechanisms that circumvent this system. IFNs have also been used clinically in the treatment of viral diseases. Improved treatments will be possible with better understanding of the IFN system and its interactions with viral factors. In addition, IFNs have direct and indirect effects on tumor cell proliferation, effector leukocytes and on apoptosis and have been used in the treatment of some cancers. Improved knowledge of how IFNs affect tumors and the mechanisms that lead to a lack of response to IFNs would help the development of better IFN treatments for malignancies.

Key Words: Antibacterial mechanisms; anti-tumor mechanisms; antiviral mechanisms; apoptosis; biological mechanisms; circulating interferon; clinical application; cytokines; effector proteins; evasive mechanisms; immunomodulation; interferon; medical indications; receptors; response genes; signaling mechanisms.

1. Introduction

Almost 50 yr ago, interferons (IFNs) were discovered to be a natural defense system in the human body because of their antiviral activity *(1)*. This family of cytokines functions to regulate antiviral, anti-tumor, and immune responses and cell differentiation *(2–11)*. The IFN system consists of cells that produce and secrete IFNs as a response to viral infection or other foreign stimuli and cells that respond to IFNs by creating an antiviral state. An overview of the IFN system at the cellular level is diagrammed in **Fig. 1**. Foreign nucleic acids,

From: *Methods in Molecular Medicine, Vol. 116: Interferon Methods and Protocols*
Edited by: D. J. J. Carr © Humana Press Inc., Totowa, NJ

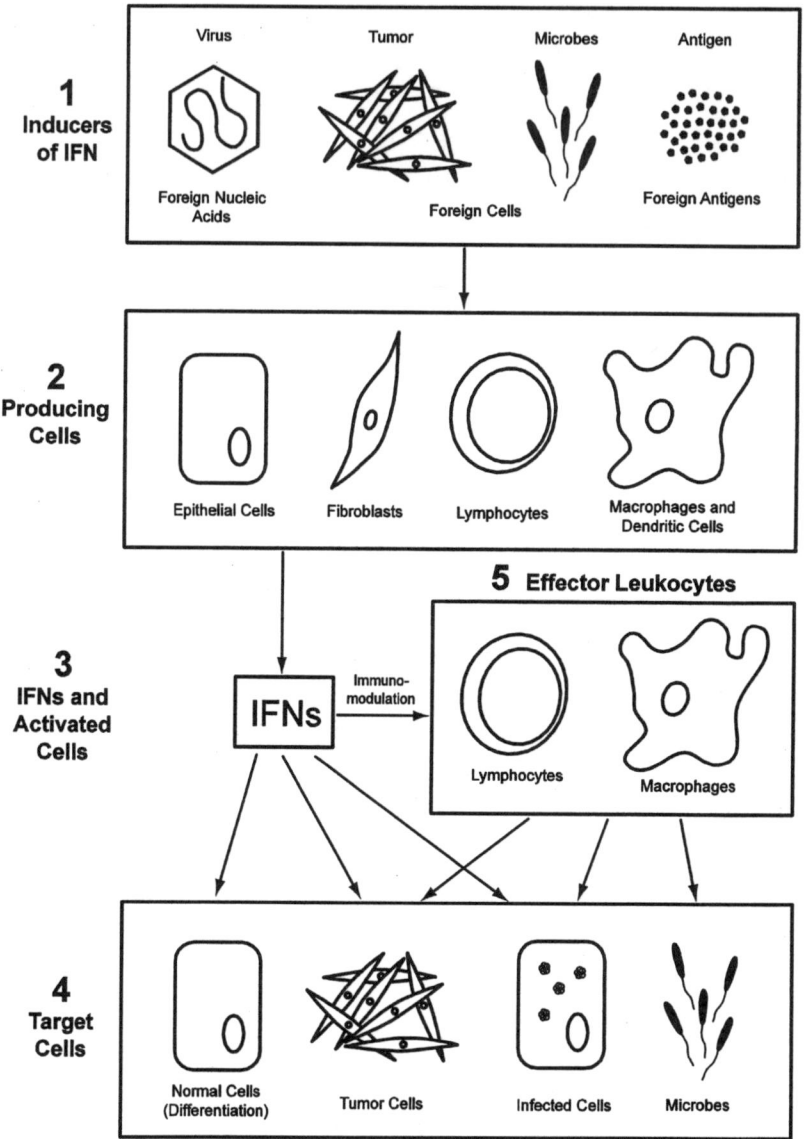

Fig. 1. Overview of the cellular events in the induction, production, and action of IFN foreign substances (**1**) induce a variety of cell types; (**2**) to produce and secrete IFN (**3**). The secreted IFN (α, β, or γ) acts directly on target cells (**4**) and also acts indirectly against target cells by activating effector lymphocytes or macrophages (**5**).

Table 1
Induction of IFN-α, -β, and -γ by Foreign Cells, Foreign Nucleic Acids, and Foreign Antigens

Inducer	IFN-producing cell	IFN produced
Foreign cells Eukaryotic, xenogenic, tumor, virus-infected, prokaryotic.	Dendritic cells Macrophages	α
Foreign nucleic acids Viral Other	Epithelial cells Fibroblasts	β
Foreign antigens and mitogens	T lymphocytes (sensitized) NK lymphocytes	γ

antigens, and also mitogens newly induce host cell proteins designated as the interferons. Secreted interferon binds to cells and induces them to produce effector proteins that block various stages of viral replication. IFN also (1) inhibits multiplication of some normal and tumor cells, bacteria, and some intracellular parasites, such as rickettsiae and protozoa; (2) modulates the immune response; and (3) affects cell differentiation.

There are two main types of interferon: α- and β-interferons classified as type I and γ-interferon classified as type II (**Table 1**). α-Interferon mainly is produced by certain leukocytes (dendritic cells and macrophages), β-Interferon by epithelial cells and fibroblasts, and γ-interferon by T- and natural killer cells. An overview of the IFN system at a more molecular level is shown in **Fig. 2**.

Viruses have established different mechanisms to circumvent these host responses *(12)*. Some of the many signaling mechanisms and host genes activated by viral infection and the adaptations that viruses use to defend against the IFN response have been characterized in molecular biology studies. IFNs also have been studied clinically and were the first cytokines to be used in clinical therapy, including the treatment of viral infections and malignancies (**Table 2 *[13]***).

2. IFN As a Natural Defense Against Viruses

The important role played by IFN as a defense mechanism against viruses is supported by three types of findings: (1) for many viral infections, a strong correlation has been established between IFN production and natural recovery; (2) inhibition of IFN production or action enhances the severity of infection; and (3) treatment with IFN protects against infection. In addition, the IFN system is one of the initial mechanisms of the known host defenses, becoming

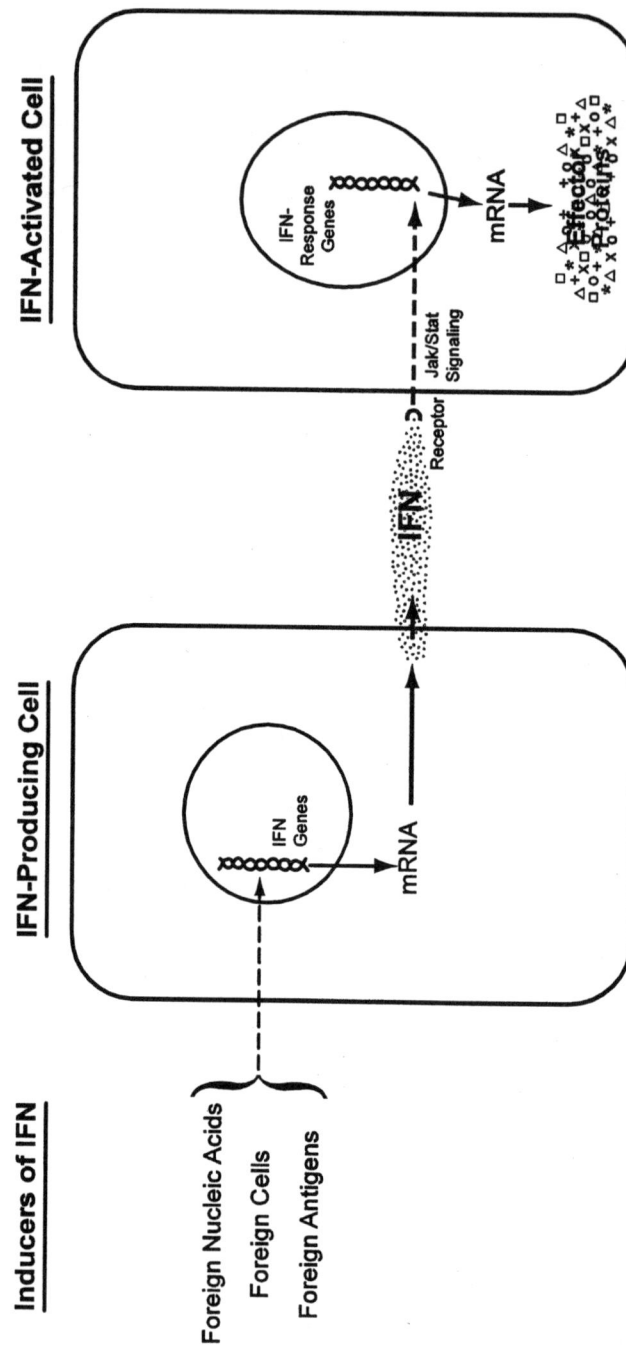

Fig. 2. Overview of the molecular events in the induction, production, and action of IFN. Inducers of IFN react with cells to newly induce the messenger RNA (mRNA) for interferon, which is translated into the interferon protein, which is then secreted extracellularly. The extracellular interferon binds to the IFN receptors on the membrane of surrounding (or the producing) cells to initiate a JAK/STAT signaling cascade. Those signals activate the IFN-response genes to produce mRNA for the IFN-effector proteins. The effector proteins mediate the antiviral, anti-tumor, immunomodulatory, and all differentiation effects of the IFN system as described in the text.

Table 2
FDA-Approved Uses of Interferons

Interferon α-2α (Roferon®)
    Hairy cell leukemia
    AIDS-related KS
    Chronic hepatitis C[a]
    Chronic phase, Philadelphia chromosome (Ph)-positive CML patients with CML who are minimally pretreated (within 1 yr)
Pegylated IFN-α-2α (PEGASYS®)
    Chronic hepatitis C[a]
IFN-α-2β
    Genital warts
    Chronic hepatitis B
    Chronic hepatitis C[a]
    Hairy cell leukemia
    AIDS-related KS
    Adjuvant therapy for malignant melanoma
    In combination with chemotherapy for non-Hodgkin's lymphoma (follicular lymphoma)
Pegylated IFN-α-2β (PEG-Intron®)
    Chronic hepatitis C[a]
IFN-α-n3 (Alferon®)
    Condylomata acuminata
IFN-alfacon-1 (Infergen®)
    Chronic hepatitis C
IFN-β-1α (Avonex®, Rebif®)
    Relapsing forms of multiple sclerosis
IFN-β-1β (Betaseron®)
    Relapsing-remitting multiple sclerosis
IFN-γ (Actimmune®)
    Chronic granulomatous disease
    Malignant osteopetrosis

[a]In the treatment of chronic hepatitis C, unpegylated and pegylated IFN-α-2α and α-2β are given in combination with oral ribavirin except if ribavirin is contraindicated

operative within hours of infection. **Figure 3** compares the early production of IFN and innate immunity with the later production of antibody and adaptive immunity during experimental infection of humans with influenza virus. IFN and its inducers also play an important role in protection against many viruses, including hepatitis B and C viruses, poxvirus, coronaviruses, papovaviruses, rhinoviruses, and herpes simplex virus.

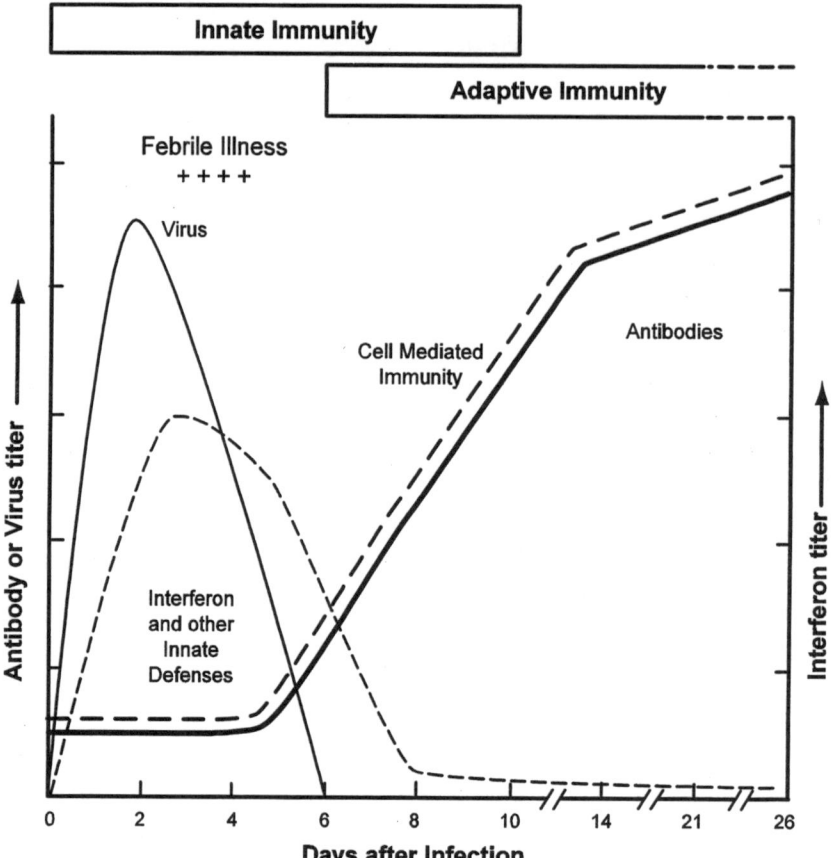

Fig. 3. The roles of innate and adaptive immunity during acute influenza virus infection of humans. During virus infection, the earliest defenses are innate. They include interferon, anatomic barriers, nonspecific inhibitors, phagocytosis, fever, and inflammation. The innate defenses begin within hours and continue until virus is eliminated. The adaptive defenses are specific antibody and cell-mediated immunity. They begin within 5 to 7 d of infection and persist for months after virus is eliminated. Virus levels initially increase rapidly, begin to decline in the presence of the innate defenses, and virus is eliminated after the development of the adaptive defenses. Adapted from **ref. 4**.

3. Host Antiviral Response

IFNs act as one of the first lines of defense against viral infection by creating an intracellular milieu that restricts viral replication and alerts the adaptive branch of the immune system to the presence of a viral pathogen. After virus infection, early events in the interferon production response (overviewed in **Fig. 2**) include the posttranslational activation by phosphorylation of inactive transcription factor families, including nuclear factor (NF)-κB, ATF-2/c-Jun, and interferon regulatory factors (IRFs), which activate immediate early genes, like genes that encode type I IFNs IFN-α, IFN-β, and IFN-γ *(14)*. IFNs tend to be species-specific in their activation of cells. This process occurs with the activation of multiple signal transduction cascades like the NF-κB/inhibitory factor κB (IκB) kinase complex and stress-activated mitogen-activated protein kinase pathways, which converge in the nucleus to turn on a variety of immunoregulatory genes and proteins that together establish the antiviral state. Specifically, after IFN-α and IFN-β are transcribed and translated, they activate gene expression in adjacent cells by binding to cell surface IFN receptors (**Fig. 1**), which trigger activation of the Janus kinase (Jak)/signal transducer and activator of transcription (STAT) signaling pathways *(15)*. This allows heterodimers of STAT-1/2 to combine with IRF-9 to create IFN-stimulated gene (ISG) factor (ISGF)-3, which binds to IFN-stimulated response elements (ISREs), which are found in different IFN-induced antiviral genes *(15)*, including IRF-7, which adds to the amplification of the transcriptional response by starting a second wave of IFN gene expression, including other IFN-α genes that were not induced during the early events after viral infection *(16,17)*. The IRF, STAT, and NF-κB transcription factors then translocate to the nucleus and work together to activate a network of antiviral genes like double-stranded ribonucleic acid (RNA)-activated protein kinase (PKR), 2'-5'-oligoadenylate synthase, and the Mx proteins, which interfere with viral transcription and translation *(5,15)*.

The type II IFN, IFN-γ, acts similarly to the type I IFNs to stimulate the Jak/STAT-signaling pathways. The activated STAT-1 homodimers translocate to the nucleus to bind the IFN-γ activated sequence family of enhancers, which induces genes, including IRF-1 and IFP-53.

4. Viral Evasion of the IFN System

Viruses have developed mechanisms to defend against the antiviral activities of the IFN system. These mechanisms can occur on different levels, including interference with the signaling pathways initiated by interferons, disturbance of the protein–protein interactions necessary for production of interferons, and disturbance of the function of antiviral proteins *(18)*. During infection, poxviruses and herpesviruses encode IFN receptor homologs, which prevent interferon signaling *(15)*. The products of various viruses, including C protein of paramyxoviruses, large T antigen of murine polyoma virus, and E6 of human papillomavirus (HPV), can inhibit the signaling capacity of the Jak family of tyrosine kinases *(15)*. STAT proteins also can be compromised, for example, through STAT-mediated degradation and inhibition of STAT synthesis by paramyxoviruses *(19)*. Direct inhibition by the E7 protein of HPV and inhibition after herpesviruses infection can affect the actions of IRF-9 *(12)*.

An IκBα inhibitor encoded by the African swine fever virus can block NF-κB, and after infection with this virus, the NF-κB p65 subunit also can be downregulated *(20)*. An RNA-binding protein, the NS1 protein of influenza A, can inhibit virus-induced and double-stranded RNA-induced NF-κB and IRF-3 actions *(21)*. Adenoviruses, herpesviruses, and retroviruses can inhibit PKR activity through small viral RNA products that bind to PKR but can not activate its serine kinase activity *(22)*. Us11, an RNA-binding protein that is encoded by herpes simplex virus-1, can bind intracellular double-stranded RNA and directly inhibit activation of PKR *(23)*. MC159L, a protein encoded by molluscum contagiosum virus, can inhibit PKR-induced activation of NF-κB *(24)*.

IFN-α has been approved by the US Food and Drug Administration (FDA) in the therapy of chronic hepatitis B and C, Kaposi's sarcoma (KS), and condyloma acuminatum, but other HPV-associated diseases have been treated using IFN, with inconsistent results *(25)*. In theory, treatment with IFNs should eliminate visible HPV lesions and the virus itself. Some studies have shown that type I IFN-α is less effective than type I IFN-β in treating HPV infection, perhaps related to the higher diffusibility of IFN-α. Compared with type I IFNs, type II IFN-γ is more effective *(26)*. The differences in response may be explained by several factors, including varied levels of expression of HPV oncogenes, interactions between viral proteins and cellular factors that influence viral and host gene expression and function, and mutations found in infected cells that may decrease the IFN response. Proteins of high-risk but not low-risk HPV, like HPV-16 E6, can bind to IRF-3 to inactivate its transactivating function and can inhibit the expression of IFN-inducible genes by the decreasing IFN-β gene expression *(27)*. Also, the expression of high-risk HPV-18 E6 inhibits the Jak-STAT activation in response to IFN-α *(28)*.

It has been shown that HPV has enhancer elements, such as the HPV-interferon responsive element-1 of HPV 16 that is located in the upstream regulatory region and from which transcription of E6 and E7 genes are initiated, can bind IRF-1 during treatment with IFN-γ and stimulate transcription in a dose-dependent and cell type-specific manner; also, mutations in HPV-interferon responsive element-1 decrease its ability to bind IFN-α-induced proteins *(29)*.

Interestingly, virus evasion in vitro may not always occur in vivo. In vitro poxviruses are relatively resistant to IFNs (**Tables 3** and **4**). However, in vivo, poxviruses are susceptible to IFNs and their inducers (**Fig. 4** *[30,31]*). **Figure 4** shows strong protection of mice against a virulent vaccinia virus infection *(31,32)*.

Table 3
Comparative Sensitivity to Murine IFN of Vaccinia (Ihd-E) and Vesicular Stomatitis Viruses on Murine L929 Cells

IFN	IFN titer, U/ML		Fold lower vaccinia
	Vaccinia virus	Vs virus	
α standard[a]	70	1000	14
β standard[a]	30	2000	67
γ standard[a]	20	200	10
rα[b]	1×10^5	3×10^7	300
rβ[b]	1×10^5	2×10^7	200
α/β[c]	20	7000	350

[a]Reference standards from NIH.
[b]PBL Laboratories.
[c]Cytimmune Laboratories.

Table 4
Comparative Sensitivity to Human IFN of Vaccinia (IHD-E) and Sindbis Viruses on Human Wish Cells

IFN	IFN titer, U/ML		Fold Lower Vaccinia
	Vaccinia virus	Sindbis virus	
α standard[a]	<3	250	>83
rα 001[b]	630	3×10^6	5000
rα 012[b]	450	1×10^6	2000
rα 015[b]	1000	2×10^6	2000
rα B2[b]	<100	1×10^4	>100
rα H2[b]	2500	3×10^6	1000
rα 2a[b]	150	2×10^6	10,000
rα A/D[c]	75	2×10^5	2000^3
β standard1[a]	<3	200	>67
rβ2	125,000	5×10^6	40
γ standard[a]	50	325	6
rγ-1b[d]	<3	37	>13

[a]Reference standards from NIH.
[b]PBL Laboratories.
[c]Cytimmune Laboratories.
[d]Actimmune, InterMune Pharmaceuticals, Inc.

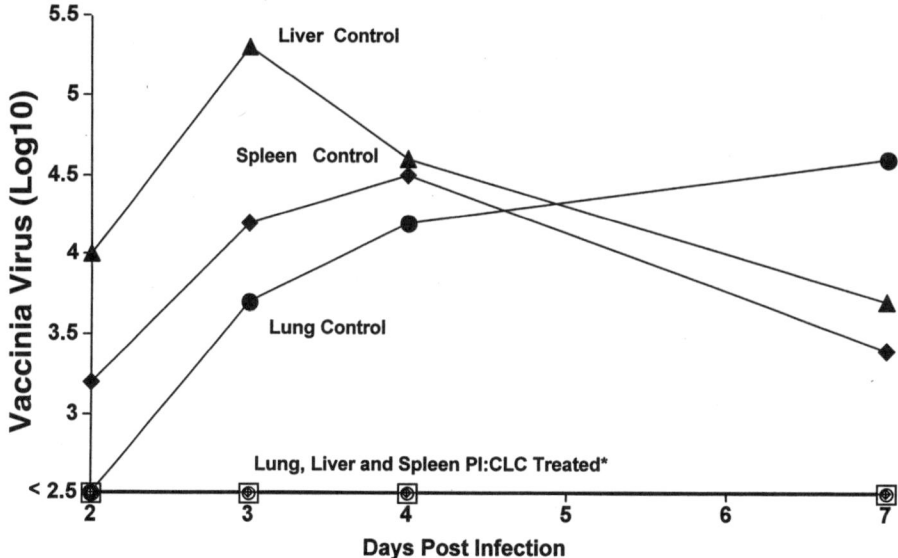

Fig. 4. Effect of 100 µg of poly I:CLC given intramuscularly on virus multiplication in mouse organs after intraperitoneal infection with vaccinia virus strain Ihd-E.

5. Clinical Use of IFNs for Viral Diseases
5.1. Hepatitis B Virus (HBV)

IFN α-2b was approved by the FDA for the treatment of chronic HBV infection in 1992, with $5–10 \times 10^6$ IU given three times a week for at least 3 mo. The goals of IFN therapy are long-term suppression of HBV replication and viremia, improvement of liver function, and prevention of end-stage liver disease. Because they have an increased risk of progression to chronic active hepatitis and cirrhosis and of hepatocellular carcinoma, patients who test positive for hepatitis Be antigen (HBeAg) are offered therapy *(33,34)*. The benefits of IFN therapy in those patients who are asymptomatic HBeAg-negative chronic carriers with viral loads less than 10^5 genomes/mL and normal liver function test values are less clear and under investigation. Markers of effectiveness include the loss of HBeAg with seroconversion to anti-HBe positive status, decrease in viral load, and improvement in liver function tests, and this effectiveness is achieved in 30 to 46% of patients who tolerate IFN therapy *(35)*. Seroconversion usually is correlated to improved histological findings in the liver and is normally maintained long term *(36)*. In patients with cirrhosis, IFN-α treatment also is associated with reduced risk of hepatocellular carcinoma and reduction in mortality from decompensated cirrhosis *(37)*. Loss of hepatitis B surface antigen (HBsAg) and undetectable virus load after treatment, or true cure, is observed only in 1 to 5% of patients. However, true cures may increase over time after treatment.

5.2. Hepatitis C Virus (HCV)

The current standard of care for HCV infection is combination therapy with a pegylated IFN-α and ribavirin *(38)*. Combination therapy is more effective than monotherapy in all patient groups and especially in patients with characteristics that are associated with low virologic response rates, such as HCV genotype 1 infection, viremia greater than 800,000 IU/mL, increased quasi-species heterogeneity, mutation within the NS5A protein, previous nonresponse to IFN therapy, African-American ethnicity, older age, obesity, and renal impairment *(39)*. The standard measure of favorable response to IFN therapy is sustained virologic response (SVR), or the absence of detectable serum HCV RNA by PCR (<50 IU/mL) 24 wk after completion of therapy, which is correlated with long-term histological improvement and clinical outcome *(40)*. Treatment with pegylated IFN, which has a polyethylene glycol (PEG) moiety covalently bonded to an IFN backbone that increases IFN's half-life and improves its biological activity, has yielded increased rates of SVR compared with IFN therapy *(41)*. In multicenter, international, randomized, controlled studies of pegylated IFN α-2b and of pegylated IFN α-2a, combination therapy with pegylated IFN and ribavirin for 48 wk increased SVR from 43% to 54–56% *(42–44)*. These trials also showed that those patients with baseline levels of HCV RNA less than 2×10^6 copies/mL or 600,000 IU/mL, with less advanced fibrosis seen on pretreatment biopsy, with body weight of less than 75 kg, and with genotypes 2 and 3 were more likely to achieve SVR. Even though they are less likely to achieve SVR, patients with chronic hepatitis C who are at a higher risk for progression to cirrhosis also are encouraged to receive IFN treatment, including those patients with detectable serum HCV RNA, increased liver function test values, and moderate or greater inflammation of portal fibrosis on liver biopsy *(45)*. The benefit of treatment for patients that do not meet the recommended criteria is less clear and should be considered on an individual basis. Also, patients who currently abuse alcohol or other substances or have severe psychiatric illness or co-morbidities, such as autoimmune or renal disease, are not candidates for IFN therapy *(46)*.

6. Apoptosis

Apoptosis has multiple significant functions for the cells, such as in cellular differentiation, preventing viral replication by eliminating virus-infected cells, and eradication of cells that undergo uncontrolled cellular proliferation or sustain genetic damage *(47)*. Inhibition of apoptosis can lead to resistance to therapy and malignancy. Advances in molecular genetics have clearly shown that malignant cells usually have defects in cell death control and apoptosis *(47)*.

6.1. Direct Apoptotic Effects of Interferons

6.1.1. Apoptotic Effects

Independent of cell cycle arrest, p53, or expression of Bcl2 family members, IFNs can be cytotoxic for some malignant cells. In vitro studies show that the IFN-induced apoptosis is IFN-species specific and dependent on cell histology. IFN-α and IFN-β can stimulate apoptosis in hematopoietic cells, such as chronic myelogenous leukemia and multiple myeloma *(48)*. IFN-β alone stimulated apoptosis in melanoma *(49)*, multiple myeloma *(50)*, and ovarian carcinoma *(51)*. However, for all cell types, stimulation of apoptosis by all IFN subtypes has involved fas- associated death domain (FADD)/caspase-8 signaling, launch of the caspase cascade, release of cytochrome c from mitochondria, interference of mitochondrial potential, changes in plasma membrane symmetry, and deoxyribonucleic acid (DNA) fragmentation *(50)*. Inhibitors of caspase-3, caspase-8, or dominant negative mutants of FADD in general can prevent IFN-induced cell death *(52)*. IFN-induced apoptosis occurs relatively late (after 48 h of treatment), which suggests the involvement of genes activated by IFNs or intermediate cellular effectors.

6.1.2. Antiproliferative Effects

An acquired defect in one or more proteins that act as check points for normal cell cycle progression often is a requirement for proliferation of cancer cells. Both IFN-α and IFN-β can influence all stages of the cell cycle, typically with a block in G1 or sometimes by lengthening of all phases (G1, G2, and S *[53]*). IFN-α modulates the retinoblastoma protein (pRb), which is a cell cycle inhibitor by binding to various transcription factors like E2F. In late G1, cyclin-cdk complexes phosphorylates pRb, and the hyperphosphorylated form releases E2F, which activates genes for DNA replication. Treatment of cells with IFN-α results in inhibition of cell cycle kinases and cyclins such as cyclin D3, cyclin E, cyclin A, and cdc25A. These actions suppress pRb phosphorylation and thus slow progression into S phase *(53,54)*. The additive prolongation of the cell cycle could result in cytostasis, increase in cell size and, eventually, apoptosis *(55)*.

6.1.3. Pro-Apoptotic IFN-Stimulated Genes

IFN also stimulates multiple genes that create a pro-apoptotic environment. Gene microarray studies have found more than 15 presumed IFN-stimulated genes with pro-apoptotic functions, which include caspase-4 and caspase-8, DAP kinases, galectin-9, TRAIL/Apo2L, Fas/CD95, XAF-1, phospholipid scramblase, RIDs, PKR, and 2',5'-oligoadenylate synthetase *(55,56)*. Although none of these IFN-stimulated genes alone are likely sufficient to induce apoptosis, their additive effects with or without other stimuli may result in apoptosis.

6.2. Indirect Mechanisms That Promote Apoptosis

6.2.1. Angiogenesis Inhibition

Another mechanism of the anti-tumor effect of IFN is the inhibition of angiogenesis. IFN-α inhibits basic fibroblast growth factor *(57)*. Tumors produce basic fibroblast growth factor and other cytokines to promote local neovascularization. Endothelial cells of tumors show microvascular injury and necrosis after treatment with IFN. In athymic mice, IFN-β-gene therapy using adenoviral IFN-β (Ad-hIFN-β and Ad-mIFN-β) constructs inhibited tumorigenesis and metastasis of a human transitional cell carcinoma cell line *(58)*. Ad-mIFN-β therapy of tumors increased tumor cell apoptosis (terminal deoxynucleotidyl transferase-mediated deoxyuridine triphosphate-digoxigenin nick end labeling positivity), heavy infiltration of macrophages, inducible nitric oxide synthase expression, and decreased proliferation marker PCNA. As seen by anti-CD31 immunohistochemistry, tumor-induced angiogenesis microvessel density was significantly reduced within tumors treated with Ad-mIFN-β. Tumors treated with Ad-hIFN-β gene therapy had significant tumor cell and endothelial cell apoptosis, as demonstrated by double staining immunofluorescence (terminal deoxynucleotidyl transferase-mediated deoxyuridine triphosphate-digoxigenin nick end labeling and CD-31 *[58]*).

6.2.2. Immunomodulation

IFNs modulate the antibody response, positively or negatively, depending on timing, dose, and type of IFN *(59)*. Protection against antibody-mediated myasthenia gravis in a murine model occurs by downregulation of antibody against the acetylcholine receptor *(60)* and may be the mechanism by which IFN benefits patients with multiple sclerosis. IFNs also exert antitumor effects by enhancing the functions of cytotoxic T cells, dendritic cells, monocytes (Baron, S., Hernandez, J., and Zoon, K., et al., personal communication, 2004) and natural killer (NK) cells *(4,5)*. In vitro studies demonstrated that IFN-α, IFN-β, and IFN-γ stimulated dendritic cells expressing Tumor necrosis factor-related apoptosis-inducing ligand (TRAIL) and induced apoptosis of target cells by activation of caspase-3 and NF-κB. Apoptosis of the target tumor cells results in ensuing uptake and processing of apoptotic bodies and presentation of antigenic peptides to CD8+ cytotoxic lymphocytes. IFNs amplify T-cell and NK-cell cytotoxicity by increasing cell surface expression of TRAIL *(61)* or Fas ligands and release of perforin from NK cells. IFN-augmented T cells and NK cells have active Fas- and TRAIL-mediated cytotoxic pathways, implying that IFNs also may induce tumor cell apoptosis by activating immune effector cells.

7. Clinical Uses of IFNs for Malignancies

7.1. Basal Cell Carcinoma and Squamous Cell Carcinoma

Since the 1980s, multiple reports have demonstrated the safety and efficacy of IFN-α for treatment of basal cell carcinomas (BCCs *[62]*) and squamous cell carcinomas (SCCs *[63]*). The total amount of IFN-α-2b needed to treat a tumor, length of period necessary for the IFNα-2b to stimulate the immune system for cure, and the number of injections required are not fully established. Evidence exists that 1.5×10^6 IU of IFN-2b three times a week for 3 wk is adequate therapy for most BCCs and SCCs; however, larger and more aggressive tumors probably need a higher total and/or individual dose to cure the malignancy *(64)*. IFN-α-2b treatment for nonmelanoma skin cancers often is not used because several arguments have been established against its use as first-line treatment. The cure rates are much less than the cure rates for established surgical modalities, such as Mohs micrographic surgery. The need for frequent visits and the cost of multiple injections may be more burdensome for the patient than are electrodesiccation and curettage or surgical modalities. The advantages of IFN-α-2b include minimal invasiveness and scarring, and it may be preferable to surgery in patients with systemic disease or poor circulation, those on anti-coagulants, and those with a higher risk of poor wound healing, such as diabetics and the elderly. It may be an important alternative to consider for BCCs and SCCs in which surgery would be deforming or would destroy function and for treatment of positive margins after surgical excision *(64)*.

Imiquimod is an immune response modifier that stimulates monocytes/macrophages and dendritic cells to produce IFN-α and other cytokines that are important in stimulating cell-mediated immunity. When applied topically, it is effective against BCCs (although its use is pending approval by the FDA *[65]*), actinic keratosis *(66)*, Bowen's disease and SCCs *(67)*, and genital warts (the use of which has been approved by the FDA *[68]*).

7.2. Melanoma

In 1996, the FDA approved high-dose IFN-α-2b for stage IIB–III melanoma as a postsurgical adjuvant therapy. It has become the standard of care and was widely adopted in the medical community. However, the results of both early and subsequent trials have not been clear, and its use in melanoma treatment remains controversial. The low-dose regimen consists of 2 to 3 mU administered two to three times each week for 1 to 3 yr. Early results suggested that there may be some effectiveness with the low-dose regimens *(69)*, but later trials have demonstrated no benefit to survival *(70)*.

The high-dose regimen in the landmark E1684 trial (IFN-α-2b 2.0×10^7 IU IV 5 d/wk for 4 wk followed by a maintenance phase of 1.0×10^7 IU SC 3 d/wk for the rest of the year) showed a clear improvement in survival *(71)*. In four major randomized trials examining a high-dose regimen, all four demonstrated improvement in relapse-free survival, and three of the four demonstrated increases in overall survival *(72)*. The E1684 trial showed the cost-effectiveness of IFN as adjuvant therapy based on both disease-free and overall survival rates. Another reason to consider the use of IFN as postsurgical adjuvant therapy is that no large randomized trial of adjuvant chemotherapy, radiation therapy, or vaccine therapy has shown an advantage for high-risk melanoma patients *(72)*.

7.3. Kaposi's Sarcoma

With its antiangiogenic and anti-human herpesvirus 8 properties, IFN-α has been used successfully to treat vascular tumors such as AIDS-related KS. Since 1981, IFN has been used in the treatment of HIV-associated KS. Early treatment regimens used doses in the 2.0×10^7 IU/d range, which were associated with significant response rates but also elevated levels of toxicity *(73)*. In later studies, it was found that the response rate was correlated with CD4 count. Patients with CD4 counts greater than 400/mm^3 responded, whereas none of those with CD4 counts of less than 150/mm^3 had a response *(73)*. Lower dosages of IFN-α combined with zidovudine (i.e., AZT) were found to be effective in treating HIV-associated KS, including those with lower CD4 counts, but with dose-limiting hematological adverse events. However, it was reported that granulocyte-macrophage colony-stimulating factor as an adjunct to combination IFN-α/AZT therapy resulted in an increased end-of-study absolute neutrophil count *(74)*.

7.4. Other Malignancies

Other cancers such as hairy cell leukemia, chronic myelogenous leukemia (CML), cutaneous T-cell lymphoma and Sezary syndrome, bladder and renal cell carcinomas, follicular lymphoma, and multiple myeloma have all responded to IFNs *(55)*. IFN-α-induced apoptosis of nonadherent hairy cells by increasing the secretion of tumor necrosis factor (TNF)-α and the sensitization of hairy cells to the pro-apoptotic effect of TNF-α. In hairy cell leukemia, IFN-α induces partial responses in most patients but complete responses in only the minority of patients *(75)*. IFN-α is beneficial for those in whom purine analog therapy has failed and those with active infections and are unable to undergo purine nucleoside analog therapy because of the resultant T-cell immunosuppression. IFN-α-2a is administered at a dose of 3.0×10^6 IU SQ QD for 6 mo and then reduced to three times a week for an additional 6 mo. IFN-α-2b is administered at a dose of 2.0×10^6 IU SQ three times a week for 12 mo.

One of the most important advances in the treatment of CML has been IFNs. Complete and partial hematological remission rates after recombinant IFN-α therapy combined with other therapies are reported in approx 70 and 10% of patients, respectively. Recombinant IFN-α-2a or recombinant IFN-α-2b combined with chemotherapy with either cytarabine or hydroxyurea can prolong life in patients with CML *(76)*. Only when combined with cytarabine or hydroxyurea does IFN prolong survival compared with busulfan and hydroxyurea. For all patients treated with recombinant IFN-α, the 5-yr survival is 57% compared with 43% for patients treated with hydroxyurea.

8. Adverse Events Associated With IFN Treatment

In the treatment of HBV, IFN-α can cause a flare of liver injury, usually just before or during loss of HBeAg. This may be a reflection of the immunomodulatory activity of IFN-α, which can upregulate major histocompatability complex class I antigens on hepatocytes and increase the recognition of HCV infected cells by cytotoxic T lymphocytes. The flares are inherent to treatment with IFN-α and usually foretell a successful outcome as a marker of increased immune responsiveness to HBV. However, the possibility of IFN-α-induced flares that precipitate liver failure means that IFN-α is contraindicated in advanced cirrhosis. Also, IFN-α may exacerbate cytopenias present in patients with advanced liver disease and splenomegaly. To increase rates of SVR, close adherence to combination therapy with pegylated IFN and ribavirin is essential, which is especially true in patients with HCV genotype 1 and other factors usually associated with low SVR rates *(77)*. In the management of adverse events, it is preferred to adjust doses rather than temporarily interrupt or prematurely discontinue treatment. Patient education about possible adverse events and regular follow-up visits are important to detect side effects early and to encourage compliance to therapy.

Adverse events associated with IFN and ribavirin combination therapy include flu-like symptoms, neuropsychiatric symptoms, and hematological abnormalities. Treatment with pegylated IFN combinations yielded small increases in the rates of mild injection site reactions, dose reductions caused by cytopenias, and influenza-like symptoms when compared with standard IFN combination therapy *(43,44)*. In as many as one third of patients, depression occurs during IFN therapy, and many patients are prescribed therapeutic or prophylactic treatment with selective serotonin reuptake inhibitors. Approximately 80% of patients with HCV infection that experienced depression induced by IFN therapy completed their course of treatment when given paroxetine concomitantly in a prospective trial *(78)*. Hematopoietic growth factors have been used in patients with significant therapy-related cytopenias to prevent dose reductions of IFN and ribavirin and encourage completion of therapy. Patients with HCV who developed ribavirin-induced anemia were given epoetin alpha in a prospective study and were found to have increased hemoglobin levels and were able to maintain ribavirin dosing compared with those who received placebo *(79)*. In another study of patients with HCV who were treated with IFN, those patients who received adjunctive epoetin alpha had improved quality-of-life scores compared with patients who received placebo *(80)*. However, there is no evidence that growth factors improve rates of SVR.

At doses used to treat cutaneous cancers, adverse events of IFNs are dose dependent and are usually mild to moderate. They include flu-like symptoms, such as fever, chills, fatigue, malaise, anorexia, headache, arthralgias, and myalgias. These symptoms diminish with repeated exposure and can be easily controlled with acetaminophen. Some infrequent neurological short-term adverse events include confusion, dizziness, dysarthria, motor weakness, paresthesia, and short-term memory loss. At higher doses, such as those used for treatment of HBV and HCV, depression and transiently elevated liver enzymes, which normalize within 2 to 5 d after therapy, are noted. This treatment modality has dose-related bone marrow suppression, which is reversible upon discontinuation.

In the E1684 trial (high-dose regimen) for adjuvant treatment for melanoma, treatment delays and dosage reductions were required during the study, including half of patients during the induction period and 48% of patients during the maintenance phase *(71)*. Grade 3 toxicities were reported in 67% of all treated patients, whereas 9% had grade 4 toxicities. Adverse events at higher doses include nausea and vomiting, flu-like symptoms, liver function abnormalities, neutropenia, and psychiatric symptoms, including depression.

9. Conclusions

IFNs are the first line of defense against viruses. However, viruses have evolved mechanisms to evade host surveillance by inhibiting the production and activity of IFNs. The molecular pathways of the IFN system are numerous. The interpretation of the significance of each pathway probably should consider its frequency, magnitude, interactions, occurrence in different cell types, and its effect in vivo. Prophylaxis of viral infections with IFNs generally is more effective than therapy *(5)*. Clinically, many ongoing viral infections and diseases inconsistently respond to IFN therapy and frequently recur after IFN treatment is stopped. However, the development of pegylated IFN for use in HCV infection has improved response rates in that disease. Molecular studies on IFN signaling pathways and viral effects on IFN responses help to elucidate viral pathogenesis and the interactions between the host factors that establish innate immunity. This increased understanding will allow the development of improved antiviral treatments, such as molecules that inhibit the evasive interactions and restore the IFN response.

Despite the beneficial effects of IFNs in some cancers, a substantial percentage of patients still fail to respond. However, the use of IFN-α inducers like imiquimod has increased response rates in the treatment of condyloma acuminatum, SCCs, and BCCs. Improved knowledge of the mechanisms of how IFN affects tumors and the factors that are responsible for a lack of response to IFNs would lead to an improved use of IFN in malignancies, including decreased toxicity with IFN therapy.

Acknowledgments

The authors thank Rhonda Peake for her excellent editorial assistance and Dr. Ferdinando Dianzani for his insightful review of the manuscript.

References

1. Isaacs, A. and Lindenmann, J. (1957) Virus interference. I. The interferon. *Proc. R. Soc. Lond. B. Biol. Sci.* **174,** 258.
2. Isaacs, A. (1963) Interferon, in *Advances in Virus Research* (Smith, K. M., Lauffer, M. A., eds). Academic Press, Inc., New York, pp. 1–35.
3. Baron, S. (1963) Mechanism of recovery from viral infection, in *Advances in Virus Research* (Smith, K. M., Lauffer, M. A., eds). Academic Press, Inc., New York, pp. 39–64.
4. Dianzani, F. and Baron, S. (1996) Nonspecific defenses, in *Medical Microbiology* (Baron, S., ed.). The University of Texas Medical Branch at Galveston, Galveston, TX, pp. 1–624.
5. Baron, S., Coppenhaver, D. H., Dianzani, F., et al. (1992) *Interferon: Principles and Medical Applications.* The University of Texas Medical Branch, Galveston, TX, p. 624.
6. Bekisz, J., Schmeisser, H., Pontzer, C., and Zoon, K. C. (2003) Interferons: Alpha, beta, omega, and tau, in *Encyclopedia of Hormones and Related Cell Regulators.* (Henry H., and Norman, A., eds.). Academic Press, New York, pp. 397–405.
7. Finter, N. B. (1966) Interferons, in *Frontiers of Biology.* (Neuberger, A., and Tatum, E. L., eds.). North-Holland Publishing Company, Amsterdam, p. 340.
8. Pestka, S. (2000) The human interferon alpha species and receptors. *Biopolymers* **55,** 254–287.
9. Taniguchi, T. and Takaoka, A. (2001) A weak signal for strong responses: interferon-α/β revisited. *Nat. Rev. Mol. Cell Biol.* **2,** 378–386.
10. Stark, G. R., Kerr, I. M., Williams, B. R., Silverman, R. H., and Schreiber, R. D. (1998) How cells respond to interferon. *Ann. Rev. Biochem.* **67,** 227–264.
11. Baron, S., Tyring, S. K., Fleischmann, W. R., Jr., et al. (1991) The Interferons. Mechanisms of action and clinical applications. *JAMA* **266,** 1375–1383.
12. Miller, D. M., Zhang, Y., Rahill, B. M., and et al. (1999) Human cytomegalovirus inhibits IFN-alpha-stimulated antiviral and immunoregulatory responses by blocking multiple levels of IFN-alpha signal transduction. *J. Immunol.* **162,** 6107–6113.

13. Borden, E. C., Lindner, D., Dreicer, R., Hussein, M., and Peereboom, D. (2000) Second-generation interferons for cancer: clinical targets. *Semin. Cancer Biol.* **10,** 125–144.
14. Lin, R., Heylbroeck, C., Pitha, P. M., and Hiscott, J. (1998) Virus-dependent phosphorylation of the IRF-3 transcription factor regulates nuclear translocation, transactivation potential, and proteasome-mediated degradation. *Mol. Cell Biol.* **18,** 2986–2996.
15. Samuel, C. E. (2001) Antiviral actions of interferons. *Clin. Microbiol. Rev.* **14,** 778–809.
16. Sato, M., Suemori, H., Hata, N., et al. (2000) Distinct and essential roles of transcription factors IRF-3 and IRF-7 in response to viruses for IFN-alpha/beta gene induction. *Immunity* **13,** 539–548.
17. Hughes, T. K. and Baron, S. (1987) A large component of the antiviral activity of mouse interferon-gamma may be due to its induction of interferon-alpha. *J. Biol. Regul. Homeostatic Agents* **1,** 29–32.
18. Yuan, W. and Krug, R. M. (2001) Influenza B virus NS1 protein inhibits conjugation of the interferon (IFN)-induced ubiquitin-like ISG15 protein. *EMBO J* **20,** 362–371.
19. Garcin, D., Curran, J., Itoh, M., and Kolakofsky, D. (2001) Longer and shorter forms of Sendai virus C proteins play different roles in modulating the cellular antiviral response. *J. Virol.* **75,** 6800–6807.
20. Hiscott, J., Kwon, J., and Genin, P. (2001) Hostile takeovers: viral appropriation of the NF-kappaB pathway. *J. Clin. Invest.* **197,** 143–151.
21. Wang, X., Li, M., Zheng, H., and et al. (2000) Influenza A virus NS1 protein prevents activation of NF-kappaB and induction of alpha/beta interferon. *J. Virol.* **74,** 11566–11573.
22. Sen, G. C. (2001) Viruses and interferons. *Annu. Rev. Microbiol.* **55,** 255–281.
23. Poppers, J., Mulvey, M., Khoo, D., and Mohr, I. (2000) Inhibition of PKR activation by the proline-rich RNA binding domain of the herpes simplex virus type 1 Us11 protein. *J. Virol.* **74,** 11215–11221.
24. Gil, J., Rullas, J., Alcami, J., and Esteban, M. (2001) MC159L protein from the poxvirus molluscum contagiousum virus inhibits NF-kappaB activation and apoptosis induced by PKR. *J. Gen. Virol.* **82,** 3027–3034.
25. Kim, K. Y., Blatt, L., and Taylor, M. W. (2000) The effects of interferon on the expression of human papillomavirus oncogenes. *J. Gen. Virol.* **81(Part 3):** 695–700.
26. Koromilas, A. E., Li, S., and Matlashewski, G. (2001) Control of interferon signaling in human papillomavirus infection. *Cytokine Growth Factor Rev.* **12,** 157–170.
27. Ronco, L. V., Karpova, A. Y., Vidal, M., and Howley, P. M. (1998) Human papillomavirus 16 E6 oncoprotein binds to interferon regulatory factor-3 and inhibits its transcriptional activity. *Genes Dev.* **12,** 2061–2072.
28. Li, S., Labrecque, S., Gauzzi, M. C., et al. (1999) The human papilloma virus (HPV)-18 E6 oncoprotein physically associates with Tyk2 and impairs Jak-STAT activation by interferon-alpha. *Oncogene* **18,** 5727–5737.

29. Arany, I., Grattendick, K. J., Whitehead, W. E., Ember, I. A., and Tyring, S. K. (2003) A functional interferon regulatory factor-1 (IRF-1)-binding site in the upstream regulatory region (URR) of human papillomavirus type 16. *Virology* **310,** 280–286.
30. Baron, S., Salazar, A., Pestka, S., and Poast, J. (2002) Smallpox: prevention by IFN and an IFN inducer. *J. Interferon Cytokine Res.* **22,** 86.
31. Baron, S., Salazar, A., Pestka, S., Poast, J., and Clark, W. (2003) Smallpox model: Should IFN or an inducer be given along with vaccination during an epidemic? iIn *Cytokines, Signaling and Diseases: Annual Meeting of the ISICR in Conjunction With the Society for Cytokines, Inflammation and Leukocytes*, (Liebert, M. A. I., ed.), Cairns, Australia.
32. Baron, S., Pan, J., and Poast, J. (2003) Frequency of revaccination against smallplox. *Emerg. Infect. Dis.* **9,** 1489–1490.
33. Liaw, Y. F., Tai, D. I., Chu, C. M., and Chen, T. J. (1988) Development of cirrhosis in patients with chronic type B hepatitis: a prospective study. *Hepatology* **8,** 493–496.
34. Yang, H. I., Lu, S. N., Liaw, Y. F., et al. (2002) Hepatitis B e antigen and the risk of hepatocellular carcinoma. *N. Engl. J. Med.* **347,** 168–174.
35. Wong, D. K., Cheung, A., O'Rourke, K., et al. (1993) Effect of alpha-interferon in patients with hepatitis B e antigen-positive chronic hepatitis B: a meta-analysis. *Ann. Intern. Med.* **119,** 312–323.
36. Niederau, C., Heintges, T., Lange, S., et al. (1996) Long-term follow-up of HBeAg-positive patients treated with interferon alfa for chronic hepatitis, B. *N. Engl. J. Med.* **334,** 1422–1427.
37. Lok, A. S., Heathcote, E. J., and Hoofnagle, J. H. (2001) Management of hepatitis B: 2000—a summary of a workshop. *Gastroenterology* **120,** 1828–1853.
38. National Institutes of Health. (2002) NIH consensus statement on management of hepatitis C: 2002. *NIH Consensus Statements* **19,** 1–46.
39. Hadziyannis, S. J., Sette, H. Jr., Morgan, T. R., et al. (2004) Peginterferon-[alpha]2a and ribavirin combination therapy in chronic hepatitis C. A randomized study of treatment duration and ribavirin dose. *Ann. Intern. Med.* **140,** 346–355.
40. Lau, D. T., Kleiner, D. E., Ghany, M. G., et al. (1998) Ten year follow-up after interferon-alpha therapy for chronic hepatitis C. *Hepatology* **28,** 1121–1127.
41. Shiffman, M. L. (2001) Pegylated interferons: what role will they play in the treatment of chronic hepatitis C? *Curr. Gastroenterol. Rep.* **3,** 30–37.
42. Poynard, T., Marcellin, P., Lee, S. S., et al. (1998) Randomized trial of interferon alfa-2b plus ribavirin for 48 weeks or for 24 weeks versus interferon alfa-2b plus placebo for 48 weeks for treatment of chronic infection with hepatitis C virus. International Interventional Therapy Group. *Lancet* **352,** 1426–1432.
43. Manns, M. P., McHutchinson, J. G., Gordon, S. C., et al. (2001) Peginterferon alfa-2b plus ribavirin compared with interferon alfa-2b plus ribavirin for initial treatment of chronic hepatitis C: a randomized trial. *Lancet* **358,** 958–965.
44. Fried, M. W., Shiffman, M. L., Reddy, R., et al. (2002) Peg interferon alpha-2a plus ribavirin for chronic hepatitis C. *N. Engl. J. Med.* **347,** 975–982.

45. Fontaine, H., Nalpas, B., Poulet, B., et al. (2001) Hepatitis activity is a key factor in determining the natural history of chronic hepatitis, B. *Hum. Pathol.* **32,** 904–909.
46. Muir, A. J. and Provenzale, D. (2002) A descriptive evaluation of eligibility for therapy among veterans with chronic hepatitis C virus infection. *J. Clin. Gastroenterol.* **34,** 268–271.
47. Raff, M. (1998) Cell suicide for beginners. *Nature* **39,** 119–122.
48. Sangfelt, O., Erickson, S., Castro, J., Heiden,T., Einhorn, S., and Grander, D. (1997) Induction of apoptosis and inhibition of cell growth are independent responses to interferon-alpha in hematopoietic cell lines. *Cell Growth Differ.* **8,** 343–352.
49. Chawla-Sarkar, M., Leaman, D. W., and Borden, E. C. (2001) Preferential induction of apoptosis by interferon (IFN)-β compared with IFN-a2, Correlation with TRAIL/Apo2L induction in melanoma cell lines. *Clin. Cancer Res.* **7,** 1821–1831.
50. Chen, Q., Gong, B., Mahmoud-Ahmed, A. S., et al. (2001) Apo2L/TRAIL and Bcl-2-related proteins regulate type I interferon-induced apoptosis in multiple myeloma. *Blood* **98,** 2183–2192.
51. Morrison, B. H., Bauer, J. A., Kalvakolanu, D. V., and Lindner, D. J. (2001) Inositol hexakisphosphate kinase 2 mediates growth suppressive and apoptotic effects of interferon-beta in ovarian carcinoma cells. *J. Biol. Chem.* **276,** 24965–24970.
52. Balachandran, S., Roberts, P. C., Kipperman, T., et al. (2000) Alpha/beta interferons potentiate virus-induced apoptosis through activation of the FADD/Caspase-8 death signaling pathway. *J. Virol.* **74,** 1513–1523.
53. Balkwill, F. and Taylor-Papadinitriou, J. (1978) Interferon affects both G1 and S+G2 in cells stimulated from quiescence to growth. *Nature* **274,** 798–800.
54. Subramaniam, P. S., Cruz, P. E., Hobeika, A. C., and Johnson, H. M. (1998) Type I interferon induction of the Cdk-inhibitor p21 WAF1 is accompanied by order G1 arrest, differentiation and apoptosis of the Daudi B-cell line. *Oncogene* **16,** 1885–1890.
55. Chawla-Sarkar, M., Lindner, D. J., Liu, Y. F., et al. (2003) Apoptosis and interferons: role of interferon-stimulated genes as mediators of apoptosis. *Apoptosis* **8,** 237–249.
56. de Veer, M. J., Holko, M., Frevel, M., et al. (2001) Functional classification of interferon-stimulated genes identified using microarrays. . *Leukoc. Biol.* **69,** 912–920.
57. Folkman, J. (1995) Clinical applications of research on angiogenesis. *N. Engl. J. Med.* **333,** 1757–1763.
58. Izawa, J. I., Sweeney, P., Perrotte, P., et al. (2002) Inhibition of tumorigenicity and metastasis of human bladder cancer growing in athymic mice by interferon-beta gene therapy results partially from various antiangiogenic effects including endothelial cell apoptosis. *Clin. Cancer Res.* **8,** 1258–1270.
59. Johnson, H. M. and Baron, S. (1976) The nature of the suppressive effect of interferon and interferon inducers on the in vitro immune response. *Cell Immunol.* **25,** 106–115.
60. Deng, C. , Goluszko, E. , Baron, S. , Wu, B., and Christadoss, P. (1996) IFN-alpha therapy is effective in suppressing the clinical experimental myasthenia gravis. *J. Immunol.* **157,** 5675–5682.

61. Sato, K., Hida, S., Takayanagi, H., et al. (2001) Antiviral response by natural killer cells through TRAIL gene induction by IFN-alpha/beta. *Eur. J. Immunol.* **31**, 3138–3146.
62. Greenway, H. T., Cornell, R. C., Tanner, D. J., Peets, E., Bordin, G. M., and Nagi, C. (1986) Treatment of basal cell carcinoma with intralesional interferon. *J. Am. Acad. Dermatol.* **15**, 437–443.
63. Edwards, L., Berman, B., Rapini, R. P., et al. (1992) Treatment of cutaneous squamous cell carcinomas by intralesional interferon alfa-2b therapy. *Arch. Dermatol.* **128**, 1486–1489.
64. Kim, K. H., Yavel, R. M., Gross, V. L., and Brody, N. (2004) Intralesional interferon alpha-2b in the treatment of basal cell carcinoma and squamous cell carcinoma: revisited. *Dermatol. Surg.* **30**, 116–120.
65. Geisse, J., Caro, I., Lindholm, J., Golitz, L., Stampone, P., and Owens, M. (2004) Imiquimod 5% cream for the treatment of superficial basal cell carcinoma: results from two phase III, randomized, vehicle-controlled studies. *J. Am. Acad. Dermatol.* **50**, 722–733.
66. Lebwohl, M., Dinehart, S., Whiting, D., et al. (2004) Imiquimod 5% cream for the treatment of actinic keratosis: results from two phase III, randomized, double-blind, parallel group, vehicle-controlled trials. *J. Am. Acad. Dermatol.* **50**, 714–721.
67. Nouri, K., O'Connell, C., and Rivas, M. P. (2003) Imiquimod for the treatment of Bowen's disease and invasive squamous cell carcinoma. *J. Drugs Dermatol.* **2**, 669–673.
68. Carrasco, D., vander Straten, M., and Tyring, S. K. (2002) Treatment of anogenital warts with imiquimod 5% cream followed by surgical excision of residual lesions. *J. Am. Acad. Dermatol.* **47**, S212–S216.
69. Kokoschka, E. M., Trautinger, F., Knobler, R. M., Pohl-Markl, H., and Micksche, M. (1990) Long-term adjuvant therapy of high-risk malignant melanoma with interferon alpha 2b. *J. Invest. Dermatol.* **95**, 193S–197S.
70. Rusciani, L., Petraglia, S., Alotto, M., Calvieri, S., and Vezzoni, G. (1997) Postsurgical adjuvant therapy for melanoma. Evaluation of a 3-year randomized trial with recombinant interferon-alpha after 3 and 5 years of follow-up. *Cancer* **79**, 2354–2360.
71. Kirkwood, J. M., Strawderman, M. H., Ernstoff, M. S., Smith, T. J., Borden, E. C., and Blum, R. H. (1996) Interferon alfa-2b adjuvant therapy of high-risk resected cutaneous melanoma: the Eastern Cooperative Oncology Group Trial EST 1684. *J. Clin. Oncol.* **14**, 7–17.
72. Sabel, M. S., and Sondak, V. K. (2003) Pros and cons of adjuvant interferon in the treatment of melanoma. *Oncologist* **8**, 451–458.
73. Jonasch, E. and Haluska, F. G. (2001) Interferon in oncological practice: review of interferon biology, clinical applications, and toxicities. *Oncologist* **6**, 34–55.
74. Scadden, D. T., Bering, H. A., Levine, J. D., et al. (1991) Granulocyte-macrophage colony-stimulating factor mitigates the neutropenia of combined interferon alfa and zidovudine treatment of acquired immune deficiency syndrome-associated Kaposi's sarcoma. *J. Clin. Oncol.* **9**, 802–808.

75. Goodman, G. R., Bethel, K. J., and Saven, A. (2003) Hairy cell leukemia: an update. *Curr. Opin. Hematol.* **10,** 258–266.
76. Silver, R. T. (2003) Chronic myeloid leukemia. *Hematol. Oncol. Clin. North Am.* **17,** 1159–1173.
77. McHutchinson, J. G., Manns, M., Patel, K., et al. (2002) Adherence to combination therapy enhances sustained response in genotype-1-infected patients with chronic hepatitis C. *Gastroenterology* **123,** 1061–1069.
78. Kraus, M. R., Am, S. , Faller, H., et al. (2002) Paroxetine for the treatment of interferon-alfa-induced depression in chronic hepatitis C. *Aliment Pharmacol. Ther.* **16,** 1091–1099.
79. Dieterich, D. T., Wasserman, R., Brau, N., et al. (2003) Once-weekly epoetin alfa improves anemia and facilitates maintenance of ribavirin dosing in hepatitis C virus-infected patients receiving ribavirin and interferon alfa. *Am. J. Gastroenterol.* **98,** 2491–2499.
80. Afdhal, N. H., Goon, B., Smith, K., et al. (2003) Epoetin-alfa improves and maintains health-related quality of life in anemic HCV-infected patients receiving interferon/ribavirin: HRQL from the Proactive Study. *Hepatology* **38(suppl 1),** 302A–303A.

2

Interferon Research
A Brief History

Myriam S. Kunzi and Paula M. Pitha

Summary

Interferons are the antiviral early inflammatory proteins produced in the cells in response to the infectious agents. The characterization of the interferon genes, their expression, and their function was advanced with the development of novel techniques in molecular and cellular biology. Using genetically modified mice revealed the critical role of the interferons in innate and acquired immune response. The critical steps and discovery that lead to the understanding of the interferon system and its role in the antiviral immune response are summarized in this chapter.

Key Words: Innate immunity; interferon; genes; receptors; clinical use; Toll receptors; viruses.

1. Introduction

Interferon (IFN) was described in 1957 by Isaacs and Lindenmann (*1*) as an antiviral protein synthesized by the cell in response to viral infection. The characterization of this protein, its expression, and its function has been closely linked to the availability of new methods and advances in cellular and molecular biology. Indeed, the isolation and detection of antiviral proteins synthesized by infected cells was dependent on the development of techniques enabling the cultivation of eukaryotic cells and the ability to use them for in vitro viral replication. Later, the availability of specific antibodies and molecular biology techniques made it possible to recognize that IFN is represented by a family of closely related, but distinct genes, to characterized IFN genes and to purify IFNs, as well as produce sufficient amounts for clinical studies.

From the onset, researchers held the hope that IFNs could be used as a general antiviral agent in the fight against viral infections, much like antibiotics are used to control bacterial infections, thanks to their ability to inhibit a variety of ribonucleic acid (RNA) and deoxyribonucleic acid (DNA) viruses. Unfortunately, the broad antiviral application has gone largely unfulfilled, mostly because of the pleiotropic effects that IFNs exert on the cells. Nevertheless, the critical role of IFNs in the antiviral immune response and cancer editing is just emerging from studies using the genetically modified mice, and IFNs have been used in the clinic for the treatment of selective viral infections and malignancies.

2. Purification and Characterization of IFNs

IFNs were initially identified as a group of proteins secreted by cells upon viral infection and able to inhibit the growth of a wide range of unrelated viruses. Whereas IFN did not appear to be virus-specific, it was recognized to be species-specific. Human white blood cells were shown to produce IFN upon infection, and they were regarded as a possible source of IFN for clinical purposes. A number of experiments using actinomycin D at doses that inhibited cell RNA synthesis, but not viral replication, demonstrated that IFN was a product of the cell genome. The use of protein synthesis inhibitors further suggested that IFN exerted its antiviral effect via the synthesis of one or more proteins, which were the actual antiviral effectors. Quickly, it was recognized as well that IFNs had properties able to regulate both cell growth and function. IFN preparations available at that time, however, contained a number of impurities, and the purification of small quantities of highly active IFN proved difficult. It was not until the advent of IFN-specific antibodies *(2)*, which permitted the isolation of IFN to near purity by column chromatography, that the cell antigrowth effects of IFN could be confirmed.

The development of molecular biology techniques led to the detection messenger RNA (mRNA) and genomic DNA in cells. The translation of interferon mRNA in eukaryotic cell such as *Xenopus oocytes* and the high specific activity of IFN allowed for the detection of interferon proteins by their antiviral activity in cell cultures *(3)*.

3. Identification and Cloning of the IFN Genes

Once a standard assay for IFN mRNAs was established, several laboratories nearly simultaneously cloned the IFN genes. The cloning of the IFN genes brought two unexpected findings. First, it became clear that IFN is represented by large number of cellular genes. These genes known as type I IFN, are represented by a family of 13 IFNA genes expressed in cells of lymphoid origin and one IFNB gene expressed in a majority of infected cells *(4–6)*. Although it was believed for some time that there was at least one more IFN-β protein, IFN-β-2, this protein was shown to be identical to IL-6. A single IFNW gene *(7)*, with sequence homology to IFNA, was found to be expressed in leucocytes, and recently one IFNk gene, with sequence homology to both IFNA and IFNB, was found to be expressed in keratinocytes and dendritic cells *(8)*. Second, it was found that all type I IFN genes are nonspliced genes, and although their expression shows cell specificity, all the genes are localized on the short arm of chromosome 9 in human cells and on chromosome 4 in the mouse. All type I IFNs are secreted proteins, although secretion of IFN-κ seems to be very inefficient. IFN-β is modified by glycosylation, whereas the majority of IFN-α are unglycosylated *(9)*.

Finally, IFN-γ, or type II IFN, is encoded by a spliced gene localized on chromosome 12 and has been shown to be synthesized selectively in cells of the immune system, such as natural killer cells, CD4 Th-1 cells, and CD8 suppressor cells *(10,11)*. The ability to express IFN genes in bacterial expression systems, coupled with affinity purification, provided sufficient amounts of IFN proteins to study their specificity and ultimately provided sufficient amounts for clinical studies

4. IFN Gene Regulation

The optimization of DNA transfection into eukaryotic cells has facilitated the identification of the regulatory regions of the IFN genes. In this method, genomic fragments localized at the 5' or 3' end of an IFN gene are cloned in front of a reporter gene encoding an easily detectable protein, transfected into cultured cells, and then their ability to induce expression of the reporter gene in infected and uninfected cells is analyzed. These studies have identified a virus-regulated element (VRE) in the promoter region of IFNA and IFNB, which alone confer responsiveness to virus infection *(12–14)*.

Studies of the molecular mechanism involved in the virus-mediated activation of type I IFN genes has brought about the discovery of IFN regulatory factors (IRFs), a new group of transcriptional factors *(15)*. The IRFs play a critical role in the induction of type I IFN genes; chemokine genes; and genes mediating antiviral, antibacterial, and inflammatory responses. Three of these IRFs, IRF-3, IRF-5, and IRF-7, function as direct transducers of virus-mediated signaling *(16–18)*. In uninfected cells, these IRFs are expressed in the cytoplasm, whereas in infected cells, they are activated by a C' terminal serine phosphorylation, which results in their translocation from cytoplasm to nucleus *(19)*. Recently, an IKK kinase, TBK-1, was shown to be responsible for the phosphorylation and activation of IRF-3 and IRF-7 in infected cells, as well as cells treated with double-stranded RNA (dsRNA)-polyIC *(20,21)*. The target of TBK-1 phosphorylation is a cluster of 4 serines in the carboxy terminus of the IRF-3 polypeptide *(22)*. In infected cells, the ubiquitously expressed IRF-3 mediates the induction of IFNB *(23,24)*. Activation of this gene involves co-operative assembly of several transcription factors: nuclear factor (NF)κB, ATF-2/c-june, IRF-3, and IRF-7 on the VRE of the IFNB promoter *(25)*. This complex-enhanceosome recruits two coactivators, acetyltransferase CBP/P300 and holoenzyme polII *(26)*, whereas in the uninfected cells the IFNB promoter is under a negative control *(27)*. Most of the promoters of IFNA genes do not contain an NFκB site, and their activation depends not only on IRF-3 but also on IRF-5 or IRF-7, both of which were shown to be components of the IFNA enhanceosome assembled on the VRE of IFNA genes *(19,28)*. The chromatin precipitation assay has permitted the detection of these enhanceosomes in living cells. IRF-5 or IRF-7 expression in infected cells, unable to express IFNA genes, restored the expression of a number of IFNA genes and IFN-α synthesis *(18,29)*. In most of the cells, expression of IRF-7 can be induced by interferon induced transcriptional factor ISGF3 *(30)*. Type I IFN genes can be therefore generally divided into two groups: immediate-response genes, represented by IFNB, which requires only IRF-3 for its induction and is therefore rapidly induced in most infected cells, and late IFNA genes, which require IFN-activated IRF-5 or IRF-7. The fact that IFNB-null mice are unable to synthesize IFN-α supports the dependence of IFNA expression on IFNB and the hypothesis of a positive feedback operation in interferon mediated antiviral response *(31,32)*. However, the recently developed quantitative RT-PCR analysis of RNA transcripts, as well as the sensitive detection of proteins by intracellular immune staining, have shown that the high IFN-α-producing pDC2 cells, considered to be natural IFN-producing cells, express high levels of IRF-7 constitutively in the absence of IFN synthesis *(33)*. Thus the requirement for IFN-β synthesis may not apply to these cells.

The discovery of toll receptors (TLRs) and their role in the innate immune response has brought further unexpected findings. Three of these TLRs, TLR-3, TLR-7, and TLR-9, are intracellular and double stranded RNA (dsRNA), single-stranded RNA (ssRNA), and CpGDNA, respectively, are their ligands. Furthermore, binding of the dsRNA to TLR-3 activates TBK-1 and results in phosphorylation of IRF-3 and IRF-7 and the induction of type I IFNs. In contrast, TLR7 and TLR9 activate IRF-5 and IRF-7 but not IRF-3 *(60,61)*.

It is noteworthy that synthesis of IFN-β also can be induced by the binding of lipopolysaccharide to TLR-4 and that the induction proceeds through activation of TBK-1, and activation of IRF-3 and IRF-7 *(34)*. These results indicate that although the initial recognition of the infectious entity may be distinct, the cellular response to bacterial or viral infection shows profound similarities. However, none of these mechanisms could have been unambiguously established, without the availability of genetically modified null mice with various components of the TLR-mediated signaling pathway deleted.

Experiments with genetically modified mice have also indicated a role for the members of the IRF family in the antiviral immune response. Thus, targeted disruption of IRF-1 results in an increased sensitivity to viral infection, a defect in the development of TH-1 responses and a resistance to apoptosis.

IRF-4-null mice have a defect in both T- and B-cell maturation and, consequently, defective immune functions *(35)*. IRF-8-null mice show an increased sensitivity to viral infection and a defect in the development of myeloid cells and pDC2 subtype of dendritic cells that are high IFN-producing cells *(36,37)*. IRF-5-null mice show a profound defect in CPG DNA mediated responses *(62)*. Furthermore, because that the IRF-5 is a component of the p53-mediated growth inhibitory and pro-apoptotic pathway *(38)* and, thus, a recently observed antiviral activity of p53 may be mediated by IRF-5 *(39)*.

5. IFN Receptors

Cellular receptors for type I IFNs and IFN-γ belong to the class 2 cytokine receptor subfamily. In recent years, these receptors and the signaling pathways they induce have been elucidated *(40–42)*.

With varying degrees of avidity, all type I IFNs bind to the same receptor made of two subunits, IFNAR1 and IFNAR2, of which there are a short and a long variant, the result of differential mRNA splicing. IFN-α or INF-β induces the association of IFNAR1 with the long variant of IFNAR2 and initiate a signaling pathway involving the tyrosine kinases Tyk2, Jak1, and the ultimate migration of activated transcription activators signal transducer and activator of transcription (STAT)-1 and STAT-2 to the nucleus, where they bind together with IRF-9 to a specific sequences (i.e., IFN-stimulated response elements) within the promoters of IFN-stimulated genes (ISGs) and initiate their transcriptional activation *(43,44)*. The IFN-γ receptor also comprises two subunits and the signaling pathway with which it is associated, involves Jak1, Jak2, and STAT-1. Activated STAT-1 homodimers translocate to the nucleus and bind to the γ-IFN activation sequence, culminating in the transcriptional activation of specific genes *(11)*.

Infection of genetically modified mice in which type I IFNR or IFNgR receptor or critical component of the IFN signaling pathways had been deleted has shown a central but not redundant role for type I and II IFNs in the host response to infection. Thus, elimination of type I IFNR increases sensitivity to infection by number of RNA viruses, whereas these mice are still resistant to some bacterial infections *(45,46)*. However, IFNGR-null mice show increased sensitivity to microbial infections, as well as infection with some DNA viruses such as HSV-1 and vaccinia *(47)*.

6. IFN-Stimulated Genes

Although IFNs were initially identified by their antiviral properties, it was recognized early on that the actual effector was not IFN itself, but one or several proteins induced by IFN. Recently, microarray analysis of the cellular transcripts induced in cells treated with IFN has estimated that IFN stimulates more than 300 ISGs with homology to genes involved in signaling, host defense, immune modulation, transcription, translation, apoptosis, cell adhesion, antiviral and inflammatory responses, ubiquitination, and antigen processing *(48,49)*.

Not surprisingly, the most studied ISGs have been those with antiviral properties. The enzymes of the 2,5-oligosynthetase family (OAS-1 and OAS-2) catalyze the synthesis of short oligoadenylates, which binds and activate RNAseL, an enzyme that cleaves viral and cellular RNAs, thus inhibiting protein synthesis *(50)*. DsRNA-activated protein kinase (PKR) phosphorylates the translation initiation factor eIF2a, also resulting in the inhibition of viral and cellular protein syntheses *(51)*. More recently, PKR also was found to be required for the activation of the transcription factor NFκB, a central actor in inflammatory cytokine induction, immune modulation, and apoptosis *(52)*. Mx proteins are GTPases and this intrinsic activity is required for antiviral effect *(53)*. Mx proteins inhibit the replication of RNA viruses by either preventing transport of viral particles within the cell, or transcription of viral RNA *(54)*. Another very interesting ISG is the RNA-editing adenosine deaminase that converts adenosine to inosine, thus causing hypermutation of viral RNA genomes, such as those of VSV and measles virus *(55,56)*.

A number of ISGs encode chemokines such as interleukin-8 and monokine induced by IFN-γ (Mig), which are involved in lymphocyte recruitment to the site of infection and inflammation and the expression of genes encoding adhesion molecules, such as ICAM-1 and CD-47, which are crucial for the ability of leukocytes to adhere to, infected cells. Other ISGs encode transcription factors, most of them activators of transcription. ISG-15 is an ubiquitin-like protein, conjugated to cellular proteins and has been shown to target Jak-1, STAT-1, and extracellular signal-regulated kinase-1 *(57,58)*.

7. Clinical Uses of IFN

Recombinant IFN-α (rIFN-α; Roferon A; Intron A) and recently its pegylated form (Pegasys), either alone or in combination with an antiviral agent, are used in the treatment of chronic hepatitis C virus infection. Because a number of ISGs are shown to have pro-apoptotic characteristics, there is also a renewed interest in using IFN in the clinic to control malignancies. In the past, Roeferon A–rIFNα has been used in the treatment of malignant melanomas, Kaposi's sarcoma, genital warts, and hairy cell leukemia *(59)*. Avonex (IFN-β), produced in hamster cells, remains an essential element in the treatment of multiple sclerosis (MS). Peripheral blood mononuclear cells isolated from patients with active MS show decreased sensitivity to type I IFNs, decreased ISG expression, and hypophosphorylation of STAT-1. In vitro treatment of these cells with IFN-β overcomes these defects, thus suggesting that IFN-β therapy may serve to restore normal levels of ISG expression in active MS.

One should be mindful to remember however, that IFN therapy is accompanied with burdensome side effects, presumably because of the large scope of biological processes influenced by IFN and that, at best, it has been able so far to only forestall but not halt the progression of the diseases mentioned here.

8. Conclusion

IFNs were the first early inflammatory proteins recognized to be produce in cells in the response to viral infection. The characterization of IFN genes, their regulation and functions, facilitated by the newly emerging techniques of molecular biology, opened a new insight into our understanding of the basic mechanisms involved in the virus cells interaction and in the innate antiviral response. The availability of genetically modified mice allowed them to study in vivo the role of the IFN system in the antiviral response. These studies have revealed the importance of the IFN system not only for the innate, but also for the acquired immunity and pointed out to the existence of the cross talk between interferon system and other cytokines. Furthermore, it has become obvious that the role of IFN is not limited to the antiviral response, but that the IFN system plays an important role in the regulation of cell growth, apoptosis, and maturation of lymphoid cells. Understanding the mechanisms of the cellular effects of IFNs and their interaction with other cytokines may also provide more realistic approach to the clinical use of IFNs.

References

1. Isaacs, A. and Lindenmann, J. (1957) Virus interference. I. The interferon. *Proc. R. Soc. Lond. B. Biol. Sci.* **147,** 258–267.
2. Paucker, K. and Cantell, K. (1962) Neutralization of interferon by specific antibody. *Virology* **18,** 145–147.
3. Reynolds, F. H., Jr., Premkumar, E., and Pitha, P. M. (1975) Interferon activity produced by translation of human interferon messenger RNA in cell-free ribosomal systems and in Xenopus oocytes. *Proc. Natl. Acad. Sci. USA* **72,** 4881–4885.
4. Derynck, R., Content, J., DeClercq, E., Volckaert, G., Tavernier, J., Devos, R., and Fiers, W. (1980) Isolation and structure of a human fibroblast interferon gene. *Nature* **285,** 542–547.
5. Kelley, K. A. and Pitha, P. M. (1985) Characterization of a mouse interferon gene locus II. Differential expression of alpha-interferon genes. *Nucleic Acids Res.* **13,** 825–839.
6. Nagata, S., Mantei, N., and Weissmann, C. (1980) The structure of one of the eight or more distinct chromosomal genes for human interferon-alpha. *Nature* **287,** 401–408.
7. Hauptmann, R. and Swetly, P. (1985) A novel class of human type I interferons. *Nucleic Acids Res.* **13,** 4739–4749.

8. LaFleur, D. W., Nardelli, B., Tsareva, T., Mather, D., Feng, P., Semenuk, M., et al. (2001) Interferon-kappa, a novel type I interferon expressed in human keratinocytes. *J. Biol. Chem.* **276,** 39765–39771.
9. Samuel, C. E. (1991) Antiviral actions of interferon. Interferon-regulated cellular proteins and their surprisingly selective antiviral activities. *Virology* **183,** 1–11.
10. Gessani, S. and Belardelli, F. (1998) IFN-gamma expression in macrophages and its possible biological significance. *Cytokine Growth Factor Rev.* **9,** 117–123.
11. Schroder, K., Hertzog, P. J., Ravasi, T., and Hume, D. A. (2004) Interferon-gamma: an overview of signals, mechanisms and functions. *J. Leukoc. Biol.* **75,** 163–189.
12. Goodbourn, S., Zinn, K., and Maniatis, T. (1985) Human beta-interferon gene expression is regulated by an inducible enhancer element. *Cell* **41,** 509–520.
13. Raj, N. B. K., Engelhardt, J., Au, W.-C., Levy, D. E., and Pitha, P. M. (1989) Virus infection and interferon can activate gene expression through a single synthetic element, but endogenous genes shown distinct regulation. *J. Biol. Chem.*, **264,** 16658–16666.
14. Ryals, J., Dierks, P., Ragg, H., and Weissmann, C. (1985) A 46-nucleotide promoter segment from an IFN-alpha gene renders an unrelated promoter inducible by virus. *Cell* **41,** 497–507.
15. Nguyen, H., Hiscott, J., and Pitha, P. M. (1997) The growing family of interferon regulatory factors. *Cytokine Growth Factor Rev.* **8,** 293–312.
16. Au, W.-C., Moore, P. A., Lowther, W., Juang, Y.-T., and Pitha, P. M. (1995) Identification of a member of the interferon regulatory factor family that binds to the interferon-stimulated response element and activates expression of interferon-induced genes. *Proc. Natl. Acad. Sci. USA.* **92,** 11657–11661.
17. Au, W. C., Moore, P. A., LaFleur, D. W., Tombal, B., and Pitha, P. M. (1998) Characterization of the interferon regulatory factor-7 and its potential role in the transcription activation of interferon A genes. *J. Biol. Chem.* **273,** 29210–29217.
18. Barnes, B. J., Moore, P. A., and Pitha, P. M. (2001) Virus-specific activation of a novel interferon regulatory factor, IRF-5, results in the induction of distinct interferon alpha genes. *J. Biol. Chem.* **276,** 23382–23390.
19. Barnes, B., Lubyova, B., and Pitha, P. M. (2002) On the role of IRF in host defense. *J. Interferon Cytokine Res.* **22,** 59–71.
20. Fitzgerald, K. A., McWhirter, S. M., Faia, K. L., Rowe, D. C., Latz, E., Golenbock, D. T., et al. (2003) IKKepsilon and TBK1 are essential components of the IRF3 signaling pathway. *Nat. Immunol.* **4,** 491–496.
21. Sharma, S., tenOever, B. R., Grandvaux, N., Zhou, G. P., Lin, R., and Hiscott, J. (2003) Triggering the interferon antiviral response through an IKK-related pathway. *Science* **300,** 1148–1151.
22. McWhirter, S. M., Fitzgerald, K. A., Rosains, J., Rowe, D. C., Golenbock, D. T., and Maniatis, T. (2004) IFN-regulatory factor 3-dependent gene expression is defective in Tbk1-deficient mouse embryonic fibroblasts. *Proc. Natl. Acad. Sci. USA* **101,** 233–238.

23. Jhang, Y. T., Lowther, W., Kellum, M., et al. (1998) Primary activation of interferon A and interferon B gene transcription by interferon regulatory factor 3. *Proc. Natl. Acad. Sci.* **95,** 9837–9842.
24. Schafer, S. L., Lin, R., Moore, P. A., Hiscott, J., and Pitha, P. M. (1998) Regulation of type I interferon gene expression by interferon regulatory factor-3. *J. Biol. Chem.* **273,** 2714–2720.
25. Wathelet, M. G., Lin, C. H., Parekh, B. S., Ronco, L. V., Howley, P. M., and Maniatis, T. (1998) Virus infection induces the assembly of coordinately activated transcription factors on the IFN-beta enhancer in vivo. *Mol. Cell* **1,** 507–518.
26. Yie, J., Senger, K., and Thanos, D. (1999) Mechanism by which the IFN-beta enhanceosome activates transcription. *Proc. Natl. Acad. Sci. USA* **96,** 13108–13113.
27. Ren, B., Chee, K. J., Kim, T. H., and Maniatis, T. (1999) PRDI-BF1/Blimp-1 repression is mediated by corepressors of the Groucho family of proteins. *Genes Dev.* **13,** 125–137.
28. Au, W. C. and Pitha, P. M. (2001) Recruitment of multiple interferon regulatory factors and histone acetyltransferase to the transcriptionally active interferon a promoters. *J. Biol. Chem.* **276,** 41629–41637.
29. Yeow, W. S., Au, W. C., Juang, Y. T., Fields, C. D., Dent, C. L., Gewert, D. R., et al. (2000) Reconstitution of virus-mediated expression of interferon alpha genes in human fibroblast cells by ectopic interferon regulatory factor-7. *J. Biol. Chem.* **275,** 6313–6320.
30. Lu, R., Au, W. C., Yeow, W. S., Hageman, N., and Pitha, P. M. (2000) Regulation of the promoter activity of interferon regulatory factor-7 gene. Activation by interferon and silencing by hypermethylation. *J. Biol. Chem.* **275,** 31805–31812.
31. Marie, I., Durbin, J. E., and Levy, D. E. (1998) Diffential viral induction of distinct interferon-α genes by positive feedback through interferon regulatory factor 7. *EMBO J* **17,** 6660–6668.
32. Taniguchi, T. and Takaoka, A. (2001) A weak signal for strong responses: interferon-alpha/beta revisited. *Nat. Rev. Mol. Cell Biol.* **2,** 378–386.
33. Izaguirre, A., Barnes, B. J., Amrute, S., Yeow, W. S., Megjugorac, N., Dai, J., et al. (2003) Comparative analysis of IRF and IFN-alpha expression in human plasmacytoid and monocyte-derived dendritic cells. *J. Leukoc. Biol.* **74,** 1125–1138.
34. Fitzgerald, K. A., Rowe, D. C., Barnes, B. J., Caffrey, D. R., Visintin, A., Latz, E., et al. (2003) LPS-TLR4 signaling to IRF-3/7 and NF-kappaB involves the toll adapters TRAM and TRIF. *J. Exp. Med.* **198,** 1043–1055.
35. Mittrucker, H. W., Matsuyama, T., Grossman, A., Kundig, T. M., Potter, J., Shahinian, A., et al. (1997) Requirement for the transcription factor LSIRF/IRF4 for mature B and T lymphocyte function. *Science* **275,** 540–543.
36. Schiavoni, G., Mattei, F., Sestili, P., Borghi, P., Venditti, M., Morse, H. C., 3rd, et al. (2002) ICSBP is essential for the development of mouse type I interferon-producing cells and for the generation and activation of CD8alpha(+) dendritic cells. *J. Exp. Med.* **196,** 1415–1425.
37. Tamura, T. and Ozato, K. (2002) ICSBP/IRF-8, its regulatory roles in the development of myeloid cells. *J. Interferon Cytokine Res.* **22,** 145–152.

38. Barnes, B. J., Kellum, M. J., Pinder, K. E., Frisancho, J. A., and Pitha, P. M. (2003) Interferon regulatory factor 5, a novel mediator of cell cycle arrest and cell death. *Cancer Res.* **63,** 6424–6431.
39. Takaoka, A., Hayakawa, S., Yanai, H., Stoiber, D., Negishi, H., Kikuchi, H., et al. (2003) Integration of interferon-alpha/beta signalling to p53 responses in tumour suppression and antiviral defence. *Nature* **424,** 516–523.
40. Bach, E. A., Aguet, M., and Schreiber, R. D. (1997) The IFN gamma receptor: a paradigm for cytokine receptor signaling. *Annu. Rev. Immunol.* **15,** 563–591.
41. Brierley, M. M. and Fish, E. N. (2002) Review: IFN-alpha/beta receptor interactions to biologic outcomes: understanding the circuitry. *J. Interferon. Cytokine Res.* **22,** 835–845.
42. Mogensen, K. E., Lewerenz, M., Reboul, J., Lutfalla, G., and Uze, G. (1999) The type I interferon receptor: structure, function, and evolution of a family business. *J. Interferon Cytokine Res.* **19,** 1069–1098.
43. Darnell, J. E. J., Kerr, I. M., and Stark, G. R. (1994) Jak-STAT pathways and transcriptional activation in response to IFNs and other extracellular signaling proteins. [Review]. *Science* **264,** 1415–1421.
44. Pestka, S., Langer, J. A., Zoon, K. C., and Samuel, C. E. (1987) Interferons and their actions. *Annu. Rev. Biochem.* **56,** 727–777.
45. Grieder, F. B. and Vogel, S. N. (1999) Role of interferon and interferon regulatory factors in early protection against Venezuelan equine encephalitis virus infection. *Virology* **257,** 106–118.
46. Muller, U., Steinhoff, U., Reis, L. F., Hemmi, S., Pavlovic, J., Zinkernagel, R. M., et al. (1994) Functional role of type I and type II interferons in antiviral defense. *Science* **264,** 1918–1921.
47. Huang, S., Hendriks, W., Althage, A., Hemmi, S., Bluethmann, H., Kamijo, R., et al. (1993) Immune response in mice that lack the interferon-gamma receptor. *Science* **259,** 1742–1745.
48. de Veer, M. J., Holko, M., Frevel, M., Walker, E., Der, S., Paranjape, J. M., et al. (2001) Functional classification of interferon-stimulated genes identified using microarrays. *J Leukoc Biol*, **69,** 912–920.
49. Der, S. D., Zhou, A., Williams, B. R., and Silverman, R. H. (1998) Identification of genes differentially regulated by interferon alpha, beta, or gamma using oligonucleotide arrays. *Proc. Natl. Acad. Sci. USA* **95,** 15623–15628, 1998.
50. Rebouillat, D., Hovnanian, A., David, G., Hovanessian, A. G., and Williams, B. R. (2000) Characterization of the gene encoding the 100-kDa form of human 2',5' oligoadenylate synthetase. *Genomics* **70,** 232–240.
51. Samuel, C. E. (2001) Antiviral actions of interferons. *Clin. Microbiol. Rev.* **14,** 778–809.
52. Williams, B. R. (1999) PKR; a sentinel kinase for cellular stress. *Oncogene* **18,** 6112–6120.
53. Pitossi, F., Blank, A., Schroder, A., Schwarz, A., Hussi, P., Schwemmle, M., et al. (1993) A functional GTP-binding motif is necessary for antiviral activity of Mx proteins. *J. Virol.* **67,** 6726–6732.

54. Pavlovic, J., Arzet, H. A., Hefti, H. P., Frese, M., Rost, D., Ernst, B., et al. (1995) Enhanced virus resistance of transgenic mice expressing the human MxA protein. *J. Virol.* **69,** 4506–4510.
55. Cattaneo, R. (1994) Biased (A{rarrow}I) hypermutation of animal RNA virus genomes. *Curr. Opin. Genet. Dev.* **4,** 895–900.
56. O'Hara, P. J., Nichol, S. T., Horodyski, F. M., and Holland, J. J. (1984) Vesicular stomatitis virus defective interfering particles can contain extensive genomic sequence rearrangements and base substitutions. *Cell* **36,** 915–924.
57. Haas, A. L., Ahrens, P., Bright, P. M., and Ankel, H. (1987) Interferon induces a 15-kilodalton protein exhibiting marked homology to ubiquitin. *J. Biol. Chem.* **262,** 11315–11323.
58. Malakhova, O. A., Yan, M., Malakhov, M. P., Yuan, Y., Ritchie, K. J., Kim, K. I., et al. (2003) Protein ISGylation modulates the JAK-STAT signaling pathway. *Genes Dev.* **17,** 455–460.
59. Masci, P., Bukowski, R. M., Patten, P. A., Osborn, B. L., and Borden, E. C. (2003) New and modified interferon alfas: preclinical and clinical data. *Curr. Oncol. Rep.* **5,** 108–113.
60. Kawai, T., Sato, S., Ishii, K. J., Coban, C., Hemmi, H., Yamamoto, M., et al. (2004) Interferon-α induction through Toll-like receptors involves a direct interaction of IRF7 with MyD88 and TRAF6. *Nat. Immun.* **5,** 1061–1068.
61. Schoenemeyer, A., Barnes, B. J., Mancl, M. E., Latz, E., Goutagny, N., Pitha, P. M., et al. (2005) The interferon regulatory factor, IRF5, is a central mediator of TLR7 signaling. *J. Biol. Chem.* Jan 28 (in press).
62. Takaoka, A., Yanai, H., Kondo, S., Duncan, G., Negishi, H., Mizutani, T., et al. (2005) Integral role of IRF-5 in the gene induction programme activated by Toll-like receptors. *Nature* **434,** 243–249.

3

Virus Infection and the Interferon Response

A Global View Through Functional Genomics

Marcus J. Korth, John C. Kash, Jeffrey C. Furlong, and Michael G. Katze

Summary

The primary focus of this chapter is on providing an overview of how we use the tools of functional genomics to study virus infection, the interferon response, and the mechanisms by which viruses attenuate or evade this response to ensure successful replication. We provide examples of the types of analyses we perform, experimental design considerations, and the tools and techniques we use for data processing and mining. We have not attempted to provide detailed protocols for performing microarray or proteomics experiments because even individual components of such analyses, for example, techniques for the isolation and amplification of ribonucleic acid, could easily be the subject of an entire chapter. Rather, our goal is to show how data obtained from global gene expression and protein profiling can be used to gain new insights into virus–host interactions, with particular emphasis on the interferon response and its modulation by virus infection.

Key Words: Bioinformatics; genomics; hepatitis C virus; influenza virus; interferon; proteomics.

1. Introduction

High-throughput technologies for profiling global gene expression or protein levels are prime tools for studying complex signaling pathways such as the cellular interferon (IFN) response. Indeed, a number of laboratories have reported on the use of deoxyribonucleic (DNA) microarrays to explore IFN-mediated changes in gene expression using a variety of experimental systems *(1–6)*. These studies have revealed an ever-increasing list of IFN-regulated genes (now numbering more than 300), the products of which function in antiviral, antiproliferative, or immunomodulatory pathways. Our interests in virus–host interactions have led us to use genomic technologies to provide a global picture of the cellular response to infection. In particular, we are interested in the innate antiviral response and the strategies used by viruses to evade the antiviral effects of IFN. These strategies vary depending upon the virus and may include the disruption of IFN signaling or the inactivation of IFN-induced gene products *(7–9)*. We therefore use a variety of methods to tailor our experiments and data analyses to provide information on the nature of the IFN response and the impact of virus infection on IFN-regulated gene expression. Because an in-depth description of microarray and proteomic methodologies is beyond the scope of this chapter, our goal is to provide an overview of our approach to using genomic technologies and the methods and tools we use for analyzing large amounts of gene expression and proteomic data. An outline of the topics covered in this chapter is provided in **Fig. 1**.

2. Materials

The technologies of functional genomics are becoming ever more accessible. It is now possible to purchase DNA microarrays from a number of sources, and a variety of data analysis tools are freely available. However, because of the tremendous amount of data generated by these technologies, laboratories that wish to use microarrays or proteomics on a large scale and on an ongoing basis must make a substantial investment in equipment, software, and infrastructure. In particular, data storage and analysis systems are essential for managing, integrating, and mining large amounts of gene expression, clinical, and proteomic data. In the following sections, we provide a brief description of the primary tools we use for our analyses.

2.1. Expression Array Manager

Researchers venturing into microarray experiments are immediately faced with the problem of how to store and analyze the enormous amounts of information generated from this technology. Sample annotation, feature annotation, raw images, raw analysis results, and experimental design annotation are all examples of what needs to be captured for a microarray experiment to be useful immediately and to the scientific community in the future *(10)*. Many microarray analysis packages are available commercially but most place emphasis on higher order analysis and do not address the basic laboratory information management requirements associated with microarray experiments. To fill this void, and to provide a cost-free method for the dissemination of the raw results of our experiments to the scientific community, we have developed an in-house gene expression database application called Expression Array Manager (EAM).

The development of EAM has been driven specifically by the need for managing related image analysis, experimental design annotation, and sample annotation in an environment where researchers use DNA microarrays and proteomics to study the virus–host interactions of a variety of different viruses,

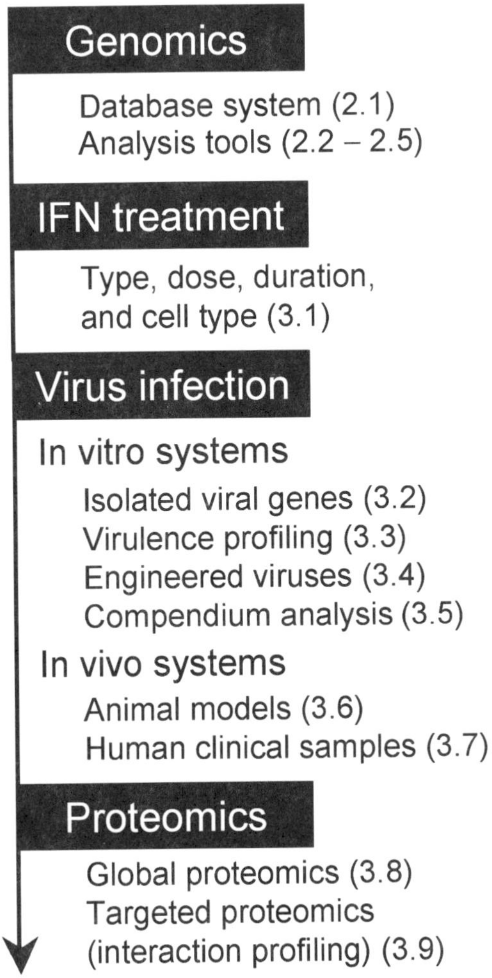

Genomic Analysis of the Interferon Response

Genomics
- Database system (2.1)
- Analysis tools (2.2 – 2.5)

IFN treatment
- Type, dose, duration, and cell type (3.1)

Virus infection
- In vitro systems
  - Isolated viral genes (3.2)
  - Virulence profiling (3.3)
  - Engineered viruses (3.4)
  - Compendium analysis (3.5)
- In vivo systems
  - Animal models (3.6)
  - Human clinical samples (3.7)

Proteomics
- Global proteomics (3.8)
- Targeted proteomics (interaction profiling) (3.9)

Fig. 1. Overview of experimental approaches and systems for studying virus infection and the IFN response. The numbers to the right refer to the corresponding section of the text.

tissues, and animal models. Numerous benefits have resulted from building EAM in our own environment. Foremost among these is the freedom from commercial database applications. Microarrays are a young technology, and analysis techniques are still changing. This freedom allows us to examine our results through different analysis packages and maintain pace with newly emerging analysis techniques. We are able to do this because the raw data are always available in EAM in their original format. The general requirements for EAM were as follows:

1. Act as a central repository for storing expression array data in an organized, generalized, and consistent fashion.
2. Provide export tools for translating EAM data into formats understood by other expression array analysis applications (e.g., Resolver and SpotFire DecisionSite).
3. Provide the ability for users to publish raw data to the world research community.
4. Streamline the microarray processing and analysis pipeline to facilitate higher throughput.
5. Integrate various types of image analysis packages (e.g., Agilent Feature Extraction).
6. Associate feature annotation data in a way that allows for continual updating and the ability to associate proteomic data with microarray data.
7. Provide a mechanism for associating clinical data to experimental results.
8. Provide application user interface availability at all desktop workstations.

EAM was built using Java, Oracle, and Java-based technologies, including WebMacro, TOPLink, Java Advanced Imaging, and Tomcat Servlet engine. These technologies were chosen so that the architecture would be as flexible as possible, allowing EAM to accommodate the many changes that continue to occur with changes in microarray protocol, platforms, and analysis. Currently, EAM integrates with Resolver (Rosetta Biosoftware, Seattle, WA) and SpotFire DecisionSite (SpotFire, Inc., Somerville, MA) analysis platforms, and it contains a series of basic analysis tools. EAM provides Web-based access for public dissemination of the data in GEML, MAGE-ML and tab-delimited formats. A basic model of EAM architecture and workflow can be seen in **Fig. 2**.

2.2. Gene Expression Analysis Software

Most of our data analysis functions are performed using Resolver, a software and database package designed for managing and analyzing large amounts of gene expression data. Resolver supports a variety of unsupervised clustering algorithms, including agglomerative, divisive, K-means, K-medians, and self-organizing maps; principal component analysis; and supervised clustering algo-

---

Fig. 2. *(opposite page)* Software architecture and workflow of EAM. (**A**) The core of EAM uses Java Servlet technology and is deployed in a Jakarta-Tomcat Servlet container. The Servlets leverage two other technologies, Oracle's TOPLink for object-relational mapping, and WebMacro for HTML rendering. The relational database underneath EAM was developed in Oracle. (**B**) Microarray analysis workflow. EAM is the central point for all basic microarray data processing. Raw image analysis data is exported from EAM to Resolver and SpotFire for higher order analysis.

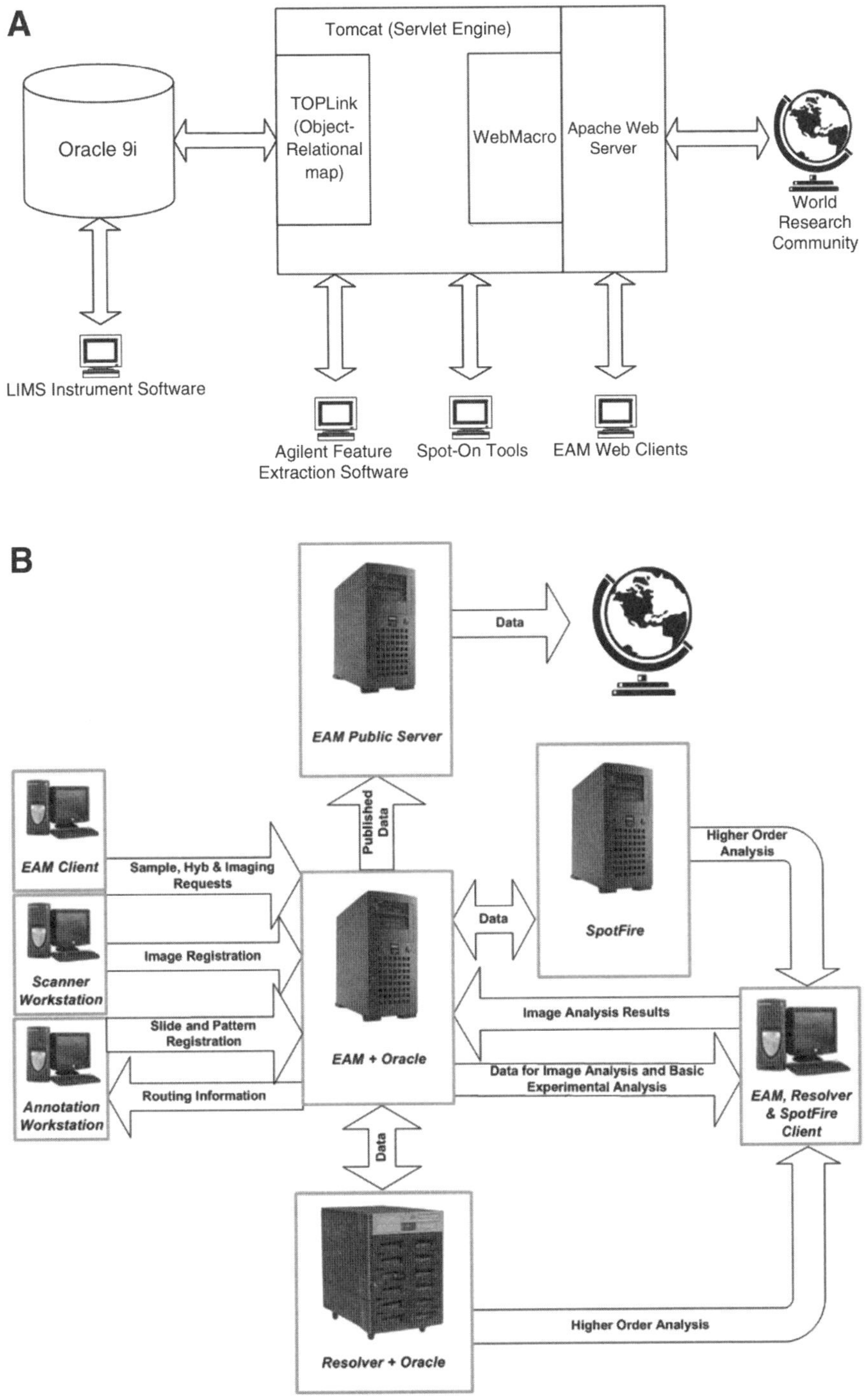

Genomic Analysis of the Interferon Response

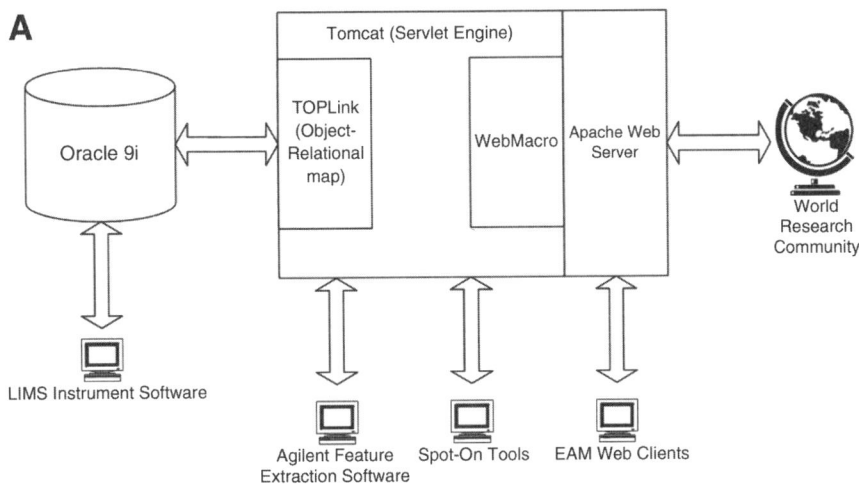

rithms that allow previous knowledge of a data set to be applied to the characterization of new data sets. Other tools include a similarity search engine, which provides a list of genes or experiments that are correlated or anti-correlated with a query item; analysis of variance; and pathway analysis tools for integrating gene expression data with publicly available pathways such as GenMAPP (http://www.genmapp.org). Users can also create and store biosets, which can be applied to future analyses (described in more detail in **Subheading 2.5.**). Importantly, Resolver uses technology-specific statistical error modeling and calculates p-values and error bars for every gene expression measurement, and this error modeling is carried throughout the system's analysis tools.

In addition to Resolver, we have also recently added Spotfire DecisionSite for Functional Genomics to our data analysis capabilities. SpotFire also provides a suite of analytic tools, including a variety of clustering algorithms and expression profile searching tools, and a number of unique visualization tools that are very good at displaying gene expression data. Using Spotfire we have built custom guides (scripts within SpotFire) that allow us to process microarray data directly from the EAM database. We are able to import data into SpotFire both directly and through the custom guides. This allows us to use SpotFire as a tool for combining and visualizing data specific to our projects (e.g., combining clinical data with microarray and proteomic results).

2.3. Computing Hardware Infrastructure

Although a complete description of our computing hardware infrastructure is beyond the scope of this chapter, the subject deserves some mention since a significant amount of computing hardware is required for the analysis tools and databases that we use. A large amount of disk storage is needed to house the databases and raw data, and manipulating the data is very computationally intensive. Building our hardware infrastructure has been an iterative process. We have had to continue upgrading servers and storage devices to accommodate our growing databases and to keep up with increasing throughput. A diagram of our current core computing infrastructure is shown in **Fig. 3**.

2.4. Gene Annotation Resources

A key component to rigorous and meaningful gene expression analysis is up to date, flexible, and accurate gene annotation within the laboratory database. This is important with both complimentary DNA (cDNA) and oligonucleotide arrays because many different sequences can represent one gene with different sequence identifiers. Further stressing the importance of flexible annotation is the necessity of comparing expression data derived from different array platforms, the continual improvements in array chemistry and production, and the

Genomic Analysis of the Interferon Response 43

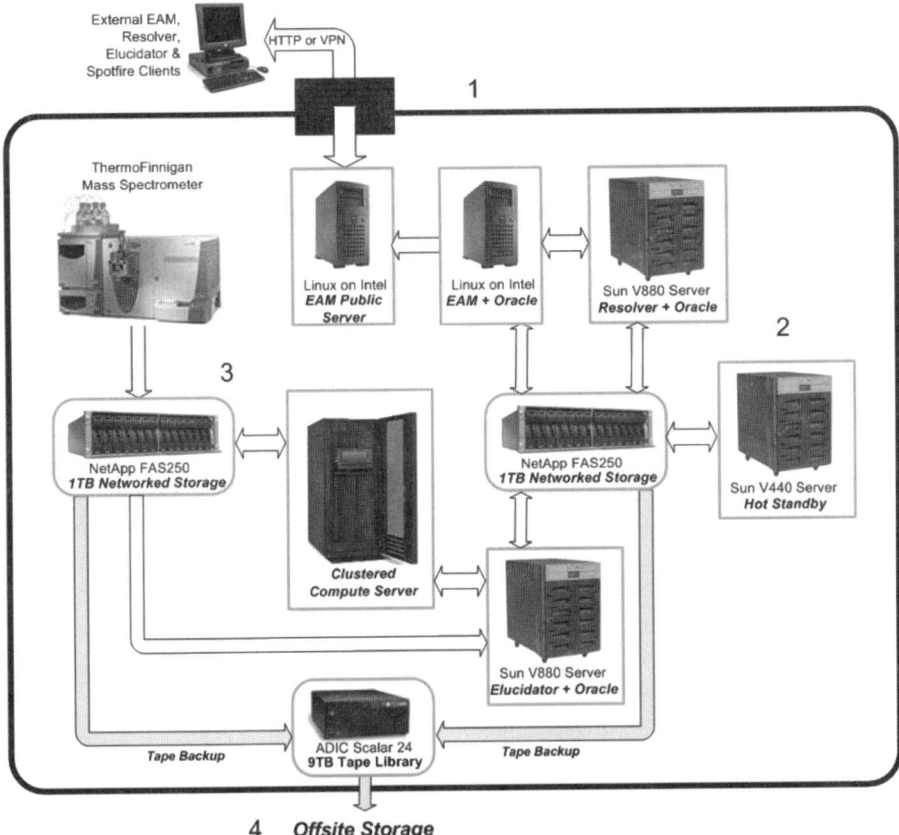

Fig. 3. Core computing infrastructure. Our server backbone network is isolated behind a firewall (**1**). The public Internet and private intranet instances of EAM are each deployed on Linux servers. Resolver and Elucidator, a proteomics analysis database application currently being developed at Rosetta Biosoftware, are both deployed on Sun V880 servers. A Sun V440 acts as a hot standby in case either V880 server fails (**2**). Two NetApp FAS250 Filers provide network-attached storage to heterogeneous systems (**3**). Backups are routinely sent to off-site vaulted storage (**4**).

increasingly broad coverage of the human genome. The National Center for Biotechnology Information has helped develop and made public many useful databases and search tools to aid the research community in the dissemination and use of up-to-date gene annotation. Principal among these is the Entrez Gene site (http://www.ncbi.nlm.nih.gov/entrez/), which serves as a central repository of information and links for gene-specific information from a broad variety of organisms. Another useful resource is the MatchMiner program from the National Cancer Institute (http://discover.nci.nih.gov/matchminer/), which is a set of tools that translations disparate identifiers for the same gene using data from a variety of sources, including University of California Santa Cruz, LocusLink (replaced by Entrez Gene), and Unigene databases.

2.5. Venn Diagram and Bioset Tools

For our studies, we use a combination of undirected and directed analyses to interpret functional genomic data. Both types of analysis can identify important gene expression events associated with virus infection and the IFN response. When performing undirected analyses, the investigator makes decisions regarding the array data based solely on a comparison of expression profiles across a prespecified group of samples or series of experiments. Typically, one or more clustering algorithms can be used to generate and visualize these comparisons *(11,12)*. To further facilitate undirected analyses, we have engineered a simple software tool to perform set analysis on differentially regulated genes and create Venn diagrams. Combined with sound experimental design, set analysis can be extremely useful for interpreting functional genomic data by showing common and restricted gene expression changes across a series of experiments. However, because set analysis is performed using some static, investigator-defined feature (such as fold change), it is critical to export the gene lists created from Venn diagrams and compare them to the raw data to identify genes that show true differences in gene expression.

For directed analyses of gene expression data, we frequently employ user-defined lists of genes, referred to as biosets. Biosets are constructed to contain all genes related to a particular biological pathway (e.g., IFN-responsive genes) and are typically generated from prior experimental data and review of the scientific literature. In this way, we are able to quickly monitor and compare gene expression changes associated with specified sets of genes across a variety of experiments. Biosets can be stored for future analyses and shared with other investigators through Resolver.

3. Methods

The following sections provide details and examples of how we design experiments and use our data analysis tools to mine and extract biological meaning from gene expression and proteomic data. We will provide information on IFN treatment, in vitro and in vivo experimental systems, and a brief discussion of how we are using proteomics to provide a more comprehensive understanding of the IFN response. The examples provided demonstrate the flexibility of using functional genomic analyses to study the cellular IFN response and the impact of virus infection on IFN-regulated gene expression.

3.1. IFN Treatment

A first step in understanding the interplay between virus infection and the IFN response is to profile the cellular gene expression changes that occur in response to IFN treatment. When performing such experiments, a number of variables must be taken into consideration, including the type and dose of IFN, the duration of treatment, and the cell type examined. For the majority of our experiments, we treat cells with IFN-α/β (Hayashibara Biochemical Laboratories) or Intron-A (recombinant IFN-α_{2b}; Schering-Plough) at a dose of 10 to 400 IU/mL. Cells are then harvested at multiple time points after treatment (e.g., 2, 4, 6, 8, 16, and 24 h) to identify early, late, or sustained changes in gene expression, as well as trends across time points or the coordinated expression of multiple genes. Later time points may also reveal secondary effects of IFN treatment. In addition, a time series allows identification of the time point at which the maximum number of gene expression changes can be identified. We often choose this time point for use in subsequent experiments aimed at examining the effects of virus infection, or the expression of individual viral genes, on IFN-regulated changes in gene expression.

Cell type-specific responses to IFN treatment must also be taken into consideration. For example, we recently profiled IFN-induced changes in gene expression using several types of human cells, including HeLa cells, liver cell lines, and primary fetal hepatocytes *(13)*. We found that in response to IFN, at least 50 genes were consistently induced in each of these cell types and another 60 were induced in a cell type-specific manner. In general, gene expression profiles for cells of liver origin were more similar to one another than they were to those of HeLa cells, and primary fetal hepatocytes were the most responsive to IFN treatment. These differences highlight the importance of considering cell type as a variable when comparing results obtained from multiple experimental systems.

Functional genomics also has the extended ability to identify novel IFN-responsive genes. For example, our expression array analyses of human liver (Huh7) cells treated with IFN-α (100 IU/mL for 24 h) revealed a greater than twofold ($p < 0.05$, $n = 4$) induction of approx 173 genes and a greater than twofold repression of approx 97 genes *(13)*. Many of the genes identified as upregulated by IFN treatment were known beforehand to be IFN-regulated genes, but this analysis also identified genes that were not previously recognized as being responsive to IFN. However, care must be taken when interpreting these data, since the relative measurement of steady-state messenger ribonucleic acid (mRNA) concentrations obtained from microarray experiments does not provide a direct causal relationship between IFN-receptor stimulation and mRNA expression. Accordingly, the identification of putative novel IFN-regulated genes requires further examination using both computational (such as promoter/enhancer prediction algorithms) and experimental systems (such as reporter-gene promoter analysis) to demonstrate a link between IFN treatment and alterations in gene expression *(13)*. Unfortunately, the rather large variations in IFN-responsive *cis*-element consensus sequences, such as the IFN-stimulated response element, can make their detection by prediction algorithms difficult. Still, the identification of putative novel IFN-regulated genes by expression analysis is an important component in furthering our understanding of the complexity and expanse of the cellular IFN response.

3.2. Expression of Isolated Viral Genes

We use a variety of experimental systems to examine the interplay between virus infection and the IFN response. These systems include the transient or stable expression of individual viral genes, infection of cell lines with wild-type or engineered viruses, and the examination of tissue samples from experimental animal models or human clinical biopsies. Each of these systems will be discussed in the following sections.

The ability of a virus to attenuate or evade the IFN response is essential to its ability to establish a successful infection, and there is increasing evidence that many viruses encode one or more proteins that function as IFN antagonists (reviewed in **ref. *14***). The mechanisms by which these proteins perform their function, however, are in general poorly understood. One approach to examining the role of individual viral genes in evading the IFN response is to express viral genes in cell culture and monitor their effects on cellular gene expression. For example, as part of our studies to gain insight into the molecular basis of HCV resistance to IFN, we used microarrays to determine whether expression of the HCV NS5A protein has an effect on IFN-regulated gene expression *(13)*. An analysis of IFN-treated HeLa cells expressing NS5A (under the control of an inducible promoter) revealed that NS5A partially blocks the IFN-mediated induction of at least 14 IFN-stimulated genes. NS5A-mediated attenuation of IFN-stimulated gene expression may therefore be one mechanism by which HCV resists the antiviral effects of IFN. In contrast, when we analyzed Huh7 cells containing an HCV subgenomic replicon (which encodes NS5A as well as other viral nonstructural proteins), we found that the replicon had very little effect on IFN-regulated gene expression *(13)*. This may be related to the IFN-sensitive phenotype of the replicon *(15,16)*, or to the presence of other HCV proteins that may alter the functions of NS5A. As these experiments reveal, results obtained by studying viral genes in isolation can provide valuable insights. However, because of the artificial nature of this experimental system, such results must be interpreted with caution.

3.3. Virulence Profiling

A more biologically relevant approach is to examine the changes in cellular gene expression that occur in cell lines (or primary cells) infected with wild-type viruses that display known differences in virulence, an approach we have termed "virulence profiling." We have used this approach extensively to study the cellular response to influenza virus infection and have found that the response varies significantly depending upon the strain of infecting virus *(17,18)*. For example, infection of human A549 lung epithelial cells with influenza virus strain A/PR/8/34 results in a significant induction of genes involved in the IFN pathway, whereas IFN-stimulated gene expression is not observed in cells infected with influenza virus strain A/WSN/33 *(18)*. This observation suggests that A/WSN/33 encodes a mechanism to efficiently attenuate the IFN response, which may in part be responsible for its high virulence in mouse infection models.

In another example of this approach, we are studying (in collaboration with Drs. Elke Mühlberger and Hans-Dieter Klenk at Philipps University, Marburg, Germany) the changes in gene expression profiles elicited after the infection of human hepatocytes with Ebola or Marburg viruses. In the analysis shown in **Fig. 4A**, we compared the expression of genes that were regulated twofold or greater ($p \leq 0.05$, $n = 4$) in Huh7 cells after treatment with IFNα (100 IU/mL for 24 h) with their expression in response to infection with Ebola Zaire or Marburg viruses. This analysis clearly indicated the profound ability of Ebola and Marburg viruses to antagonize the type-I IFN response by shutting off the expression of IFN-stimulated genes. Another intriguing observation is that Ebola and Marburg virus infection induced the upregulation of several genes whose expression was repressed by IFN treatment in mock-infected cells.

3.4. Engineered Viruses

Although studying different wild-type viruses can reveal differences in the cellular response to infection, the use of engineered viruses can help to determine the contribution of specific viral genes to the host response. Our work with influenza virus again provides an example of this approach. Given the evidence that the influenza virus NS1 protein functions as an IFN antagonist *(19–21)*, we have examined engineered strains of the virus that contain a deletion in the NS1 gene, or which contain a heterotypic NS1 gene such as that from the highly pathogenic 1918 pandemic strain *(18)*. These studies revealed that in cells infected with influenza virus lacking the NS1 gene, there are an increased number of differentially expressed cellular genes, including many implicated in IFN, nuclear factor-κB, and other antiviral pathways. This observation suggests that at least one means by which NS1 functions as an IFN

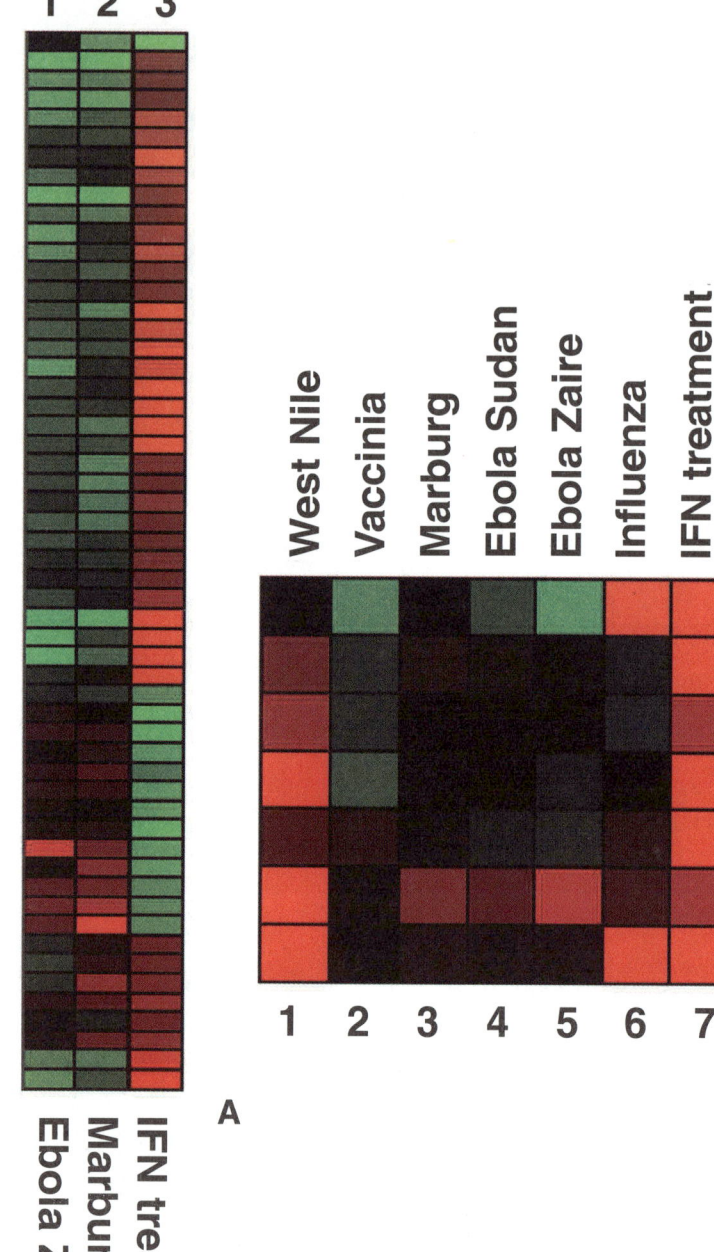

antagonist may be through an attenuation of IFN-regulated gene expression. In contrast, we found that an engineered virus containing the NS1 gene from the 1918 pandemic strain was more efficient at blocking the expression of IFN-regulated genes than the parental virus. This finding suggests that the extreme virulence of the 1918 virus may have been due in part to the ability of its NS1 protein to act as a particularly efficient IFN antagonist.

3.5. Compendium Analysis

These analyses also can be extended to compare gene expression changes associated with infection by unrelated viruses, an approach we have termed "viral compendium" analysis. An example of this approach is shown in **Fig. 4B**, where we have compared the expression of IFN-stimulated genes (using Unigene identifications) in cells infected with West Nile virus, vaccinia virus, Marburg virus, Ebola Sudan virus, Ebola Zaire virus, or type A influenza virus. The data from this analysis suggest that the highly virulent viruses, such vaccinia, Ebola Zaire, and influenza, may be more efficient at preventing the expression of ISGs than a less pathogenic virus, such as West Nile virus. Again, one must be cautious with this type of analysis, because gene expression changes in response to virus infection can be greatly influenced by differences in cell lineage or the peculiarities of a given cell line. Additional experimental approaches are therefore required to explore differences and similarities revealed by these types of analyses. Not withstanding the need for prudent interpretation of viral compendium analysis, we believe that identifying similarities and differences in cellular gene expression induced by a wide range of viruses will lead to a better understanding of viral pathogenesis and the methods used by different viruses to evade or modulate the IFN response.

Fig. 4. *(opposite page)* Viral antagonism of the type I IFN response. **(A)** Hierarchical cluster diagram of IFN-regulated genes that showed a twofold or greater ($p < 0.05$; $n = 4$) change in expression in human liver (Huh7) cells infected for 24 h (multiplicity of infection = 0.1 plaque forming unit) with Ebola Zaire virus (column 1), Marburg virus (column 2), or treated with IFN-α (100 IU/mL) for 24 h (column 3). Genes shown in red indicate up-regulation, genes in green indicate downregulation, and genes in black indicate no change in expression relative to mock-infected or treated controls. **(B)** Hierarchical cluster diagram of IFN-regulated genes afterinfection of 293 cells with West Nile virus (column 1); HeLa cells infected with vaccinia virus (column 2); Huh7 cells infected with Marburg, Ebola Sudan, or Ebola Zaire viruses (columns 3–5), A549 cells infected with A/WSN/33 influenza virus (column 6); or treatment of Huh7 cells with IFNα (100 IU/mL; column 7). Genes shown in red indicate upregulation, genes in green indicate downregulation, and genes in black indicate no change in expression relative to mock-infected or treated controls.

3.6. Animal Models

Applying a functional genomics approach to in vivo systems, such as experimental animal infection models, provides a number of benefits over in vitro systems. Most importantly, by examining cells or tissues from experimentally infected animals, it is possible to obtain a picture of the gene expression changes that occur in a whole animal in response to a bona fide infection. Moreover, it is possible to correlate gene expression changes with clinical data, and by obtaining samples at various times post infection, one can gain insights into disease progression. However, the challenges associated with analyzing in vivo systems are many. Tissue samples may contain many cell types, each of which may have their own gene expression program. The percentage of infected cells in a tissue may be quite low, and gene expression may change in direct response to virus infection, in response to the release of cytokines from virus-infected cells (which may vary depending upon cell type, such as epithelial cells, macrophages, or dendritic cells), or in response to cytokines secreted by lymphocytes attracted to the site of infection.

Despite these challenges, we believe that applying genomic technologies to complex in vivo systems provides the best opportunities to decipher and understand the intricacies of virus–host interactions, including early events such as the innate immune response. As an example, we recently combined histopathology and gene expression profiling to evaluate lung tissue from mice experimentally infected with wild-type or engineered strains of influenza virus *(22)*. Mice infected with highly lethal influenza viruses displayed severe lung pathology and the marked upregulated expression of genes associated with interferon and inflammatory responses, including immune cell activation, chemotaxis, and necrosis. These findings were consistent with the increased recruitment and accumulation of phagocytes (macrophages and neutrophils) observed by histopathology. Thus, we were able to obtain a coordinated picture of gene expression and physiological changes in response to both attenuated and highly virulent influenza virus infection and build an experimental model describing the relationship between gene expression and the severity of pulmonary disease. We have also recently performed similar types of analyses using a macaque model of influenza virus infection *(23)*.

3.7. Human Clinical Samples

Finally, clinical samples from human infections provide the most physiologically relevant material for studying gene expression or protein changes. As with samples from experimental animal infections, clinical samples may contain many cell types and the percentage of infected cells in a tissue may be quite low. In addition, investigators typically have little (if any) control over experimental parameters. Thus, analyzing data obtained from clinical samples presents many challenges. However, the physiological relevance of such

Genomic Analysis of the Interferon Response 51

samples, together with the opportunity to correlate gene expression changes with clinical data, makes their study highly worthwhile.

Much of our work using human samples is focused on profiling gene expression changes that occur in liver tissue owing to HCV-associated disease. These studies have led to the identification of marker genes, the expression patterns of which are correlated with cirrhosis or hepatocellular carcinoma *(24,25)*. We also are profiling gene expression changes in serial liver biopsies from patients with recurrent HCV after liver transplantation. These samples provide an unusual opportunity to obtain a dynamic picture of gene expression changes over time, rather than only looking at end-stage disease, which is more typical of clinical samples. In all of these studies, we are able to quickly explore changes in the expression of IFN pathway genes simply by using pre-constructed IFN biosets.

3.8. Global Proteomics

Although DNA microarrays provide a view of the transcriptional changes that occur in response to IFN treatment or virus infection, a more complete picture of the response requires also looking at how the protein content of the cell is affected. We are therefore using quantitative proteomic technologies to evaluate changes in the level of individual proteins in response to IFN treatment and targeted proteomics to identify cellular or viral proteins that interact with specific viral gene products. Although a description of proteomic methods is well beyond the scope of this chapter, it is important to note that proteomics is an important component of a functional genomics approach, and its focus on proteins provides data that are complementary to data obtained from gene expression measurements (reviewed in **ref. 26**).

To quantitatively measure protein levels, we use isotope-coded affinity tag (ICAT) labeling and tandem mass spectrometry *(27)*. The ICAT reagent consists of an affinity tag, a linker that can incorporate stable isotopes (e.g., deuterium), and a reactive group to selectively tag classes of proteins containing a specific functional group. Proteins isolated from two different cell states (e.g., with or without IFN treatment) are denatured, reduced, and labeled with the heavy or light ICAT reagent. The samples are then combined and proteolyzed, and ICAT-labeled peptides are isolated by affinity chromatography and analyzed by microcapillary liquid chromatography and tandem mass spectrometry. The ratio of the ion intensities for an ICAT-labeled pair quantifies the relative abundance of the corresponding proteins, and a tandem mass spectrum reveals the sequence of the peptides providing accurate protein identification. We have recently used this approach to profile the changes in protein levels that occur in Huh7 cells in response to IFN treatment. These studies identified approxy 1200 proteins, including more than 50 proteins that were more abundant in IFN-treated cells *(27a)*. Most of these proteins were the products of known IFN-induced genes, suggesting a good correlation between changes in gene expression and protein abundance and the degree to which changes in gene expression translate into increases in protein level.

3.9. Targeted Proteomics

We also are using a targeted proteomics approach to identify cellular or viral proteins that interact with specific viral gene products. In particular, we are interested in identifying the protein interaction partners of viral proteins that act as IFN antagonists, such as the influenza virus NS1 *(19,21)*, Ebola virus VP35 *(28,29)*, or HCV NS5A proteins *(13,30)*. Because proteins typically interact with one another to perform a particular task, identifying the interaction partners of these proteins can be an important means to discovering their biological function or the molecular mechanism by which a function is carried out. For these studies, we use a tandem affinity purification (TAP) system coupled with mass spectrometry to identify protein interaction partners (reviewed in **ref.** *31*). Viral genes are cloned into a pcDNA3-based TAP-tag expression vector to engineer a C- or N-terminal extension containing the TAP tag, which consists of a calmodulin-binding domain, a tobacco etch virus protease cleavage site, and a protein-A IgG-binding domain. Tagged proteins are then expressed by transient transfection and their biological activity verified prior to further analysis. Once the activity of the tagged protein is verified, protein complexes are purified by affinity purification and individual proteins are identified by mass spectrometry. Our long-term goals are to use this approach to construct a detailed model of the protein–protein interaction networks associated with the IFN response and the mechanisms used by viruses to integrate themselves into this response and evade cellular defense mechanisms.

Ultimately, we are working to integrate data obtained from gene expression profiling and proteomics to gain a comprehensive picture of the IFN response and the various strategies used by viruses to counteract or evade this cellular defense mechanism. We believe this knowledge will contribute greatly to our understanding of virus–host interactions and will eventually lead to improved and rational-designed antiviral therapies.

Acknowledgments

We thank our many collaborators and laboratory colleagues who contributed to the studies described in this chapter. Funding for this work is provided by Public Health Service grants R01AI22646, R01AI47304, R21AI53765, P01AI52106, U19AI48214, P30DA15625, R24RR16354, and P51RR00166 from the National Institutes of Health and by Illumigen Biosciences Inc., Seattle, WA.

References

1. Certa, U., Seiler, M., Padovan, E., and Spagnoli, G. C. (2001) High density oligonucleotide array analysis of interferon-alpha2a sensitivity and transcriptional response in melanoma cells. *Br. J. Cancer* **85,** 107–114.
2. Der, S. D., Zhou, A., Williams, B. R. G., and Silverman, R. H. (1998) Identification of genes differentially regulated by interferon α, β, or γ using oligonucleotide arrays. *Proc. Natl. Acad. Sci. USA* **95,** 15623–15628.
3. de Veer, M. J., Holko, M., Frevel, M., Walker, E., Der, S., Paranjape, J. M., et al. (2001) Functional classification of interferon-stimulated genes identified using microarrays. *J. Leukoc. Biol.* **69,** 912–920.
4. Radaeva, S., Jaruga, B., Hong, F., Kim, W. H., Fan, S., Cai, H., et al. (2002) Interferon-alpha activates multiple STAT signals and down-regulates c-Met in primary human hepatocytes. *Gastroenterology* **122,** 1020–1034.
5. Satoh, J. and Kuroda, Y. (2001) Differing effects of IFNβ vs IFNγ in MS: gene expression in cultured astrocytes. *Neurology* **57,** 681–685.
6. Zimmer, R. and Thomas, P. (2002) Expression profiling and interferon-beta regulation of liver metastases in colorectal cancer cells. *Clin. Exp. Metastasis* **19,** 541–550.
7. García-Sastre, A. (2002) Mechanisms of inhibition of the host interferon α/β-mediated antiviral responses by viruses. *Microbes Infect.* **4,** 647–655.
8. Grandvaux, N., tenOever, B. R., Servant, M. J., and Hiscott, J. (2002) The interferon antiviral response: from viral invasion to evasion. *Curr. Opin. Infect. Dis.* **15,** 259–267.
9. Katze, M. G., He, Y., and Gale, M. Jr. (2002) Viruses and interferon: a fight for supremacy. *Nat. Rev. Immunol.* **2,** 675–687.
10. Brazma, A., Hingamp, P., Quackenbush, J., Sherlock, G., Spellman, P., Stoeckert, C., et al. (2001) Minimum information about a microarray experiment (MIAME) toward standards for microarray data. *Nat. Genet.* **29,** 365–371.
11. Quackenbush, J. (2001) Computational analysis of microarray data. *Nat. Rev. Genet.* **2,** 418–427.
12. Valafar, F. (2002) Pattern recognition techniques in microarray data analysis: a survey. *Ann. NY Acad. Sci.* **980,** 41–64.
13. Geiss, G. K., Carter, V. S., He, Y., Kwieciszewski, B. K., Holzman, T., Korth, M. J., et al. (2003) Gene expression profiling of the cellular transcriptional network regulated by alpha/beta interferon and its partial attenuation by the hepatitis C virus nonstructural 5A protein. *J. Virol.* **77,** 6367–6375.
14. Basler, C. F. and García-Sastre, A. (2002) Viruses and the type I interferon antiviral system: induction and evasion. *Int. Rev. Immunol.* **21,** 305–337.
15. Frese, M., Pietschmann, T., Moradpour, D., Haller, O., and Bartenschlager, R. (2001) Interferon-α inhibits hepatitis C virus subgenomic RNA replication by an MxA-independent pathway. *J. Gen. Virol.* **82,** 723–733.
16. Guo, J. T., Bichko, V. V., and Seeger, C. (2001) Effect of alpha interferon on the hepatitis C virus replicon. *J. Virol.* **75,** 8516–8523.

17. Geiss, G. K., An, M. C., Bumgarner, R. E., Hammersmark, E., Cunningham, D., and Katze, M. G. (2001) Global impact of influenza virus on cellular pathways is mediated by both replication-dependent and -independent events. *J. Virol.* **75**, 4321–4331.
18. Geiss, G. K., Salvatore, M., Tumpey, T. M., Carter, V. S., Wang, X., Basler, C. F., et al. (2002) Cellular transcriptional profiling in influenza A virus-infected lung epithelial cells: the role of the nonstructural NS1 protein in the evasion of the host innate defense and its potential contribution to pandemic influenza. *Proc. Natl. Acad. Sci. USA* **99**, 10736–10741.
19. García-Sastre, A., Egorov, A., Matassov, D., Brandt, S., Levy, D. E., Durbin, J. E., et al. (1998) Influenza A virus lacking the NS1 gene replicates in interferon-deficient systems. *Virology* **252**, 324–330.
20. Wang, X., Li, M., Zheng, H., Muster, T., Palese, P., Beg, A. A., and Garcia-Sastre, A. (2000) Influenza A virus NS1 protein prevents activation of NF-kappaB and induction of alpha/beta interferon. *J. Virol.* **74**, 11566–11573.
21. Talon, J., Horvath, C. M., Polley, R., Basler, C. F., Muster, T., Palese, P., and García-Sastre, A. (2000) Activation of interferon regulatory factor 3 is inhibited by the influenza A virus NS1 protein. *J. Virol.* **74**, 7989–7996.
22. Kash, J. C., Basler, C. F., García-Sastre, A., Carter, V., Billharz, R., Swayne, D. E., et al. (2004) Global host immune response: pathogenesis and transcriptional profiling of type A influenza viruses expressing the hemagglutinin and neuraminidase genes from the 1918 pandemic virus. *J. Virol.* **78**, 9499–9511.
23. Baskin, C. R., García-Sastre, A., Tumpey, T. M., Bielefeldt-Ohmann, H., Carter, V. S., Nistal-Villán, E., et al. (2004) Integration of clinical data, pathology, and cDNA microarrays in influenza virus-infected pigtailed macaques (*Macaca nemestrina*). *J. Virol.* **78**, 10420–10432.
24. Smith, M. W., Yue, Z. N., Geiss, G. K., Sadovnikova, N. Y., Carter, V. S., Boix, L., et al. (2003) Identification of novel tumor markers in hepatitis C virus-associated hepatocellular carcinoma. *Cancer Res.* **63**, 859–864.
25. Smith, M. W., Yue, Z. N., Korth, M. J., Do, H. A., Boix, L., Fausto, N., et al. (2003) Hepatitis C virus and liver disease: global transcriptional profiling and identification of potential markers. *Hepatology* **38**, 1458–1467.
26. Aebersold, R. and Mann, M. (2003) Mass spectrometry-based proteomics. *Nature* **422**, 198–207.
27. Gygi, S. P., Rist, B., Gerber, S. A., Turecek, F., Gelb, M. H., and Aebersold, R. (1999) Quantitative analysis of complex protein mixtures using isotope-coded affinity tags. *Nature Biotechnol.* **17**, 994–999.
27a. Yan, W., Lee, H., Yi, E. C., et al. (2004) System proteomic analysis of the interferon response in human liver cells. *Genome Biol.* **5**, R54.
28. Basler, C. F., Wang, X., Mühlberger, E., Volchkov, V., Paragas, J., Klenk, H. D., et al. (2000) The Ebola virus VP35 protein functions as a type I IFN antagonist. *Proc. Natl. Acad. Sci. USA* **97**, 12289–12294.
29. Basler, C. F., Mikulasova, A., Martinez-Sobrido, L., Paragas, J., Muhlberger, E., Bray, M., et al. (2003) The Ebola virus VP35 protein inhibits activation of interferon regulatory factor 3. *J. Virol.* **77**, 7945–7956.

30. Gale, M., Jr., Korth, M. J., Tang, N. M., Tan, S.-L., Hopkins, D. A., Dever, T. E., et al. (1997) Evidence that hepatitis C virus resistance to interferon is mediated through repression of the PKR protein kinase by the nonstructural 5A protein. *Virology* **230,** 217–227.
31. Puig, O., Caspary, F., Rigaut, G., Rutz, B., Bouveret, E., Bragado-Nilsson, E., et al. (2001) The tandem affinity purification (TAP) method: a general procedure of protein complex purification. *Methods* **24,** 218–229.

4

Genomic DNA Affinity Chromatography

A Technique to Isolate Interferon-Inducible DNA Binding Factors

Jyothi Kumaran and Eleanor N. Fish

Summary

Cytokines elicit responses in target cells by inducing changes in gene expression. For interferons (IFNs), this involves receptor-mediated activation of specific transcription factors, which then translocate into the nucleus to bind to cognate gene elements in the promoters of IFN-inducible genes. The prototypic IFN-inducible transcription factors are the signal transducer and activator of transcription (STAT) proteins. IFN-receptor interactions invoke Janus kinase activation via phosphorylation events, which in turn leads to the recruitment and phosphorylation of STAT proteins on tyrosine residues. Activated STATs then dimerize to form STAT complexes. IFNs-α/β will activate STAT-1, STAT-2, STAT-3, and STAT-5, whereas IFN-γ will predominantly activate STAT-1. In this chapter, we describe a procedure to identify IFN-inducible deoxyribonucleic acid (DNA) binding factors independently of any knowledge of their target DNA sequences. This procedure permits the identification of IFN-inducible STAT complexes as well as any other IFN-inducible DNA binding factors. This biochemical technique uses genomic DNA affinity chromatography to isolate DNA binding factors from IFN-inducible cytoplasmic or nuclear extracts.

Key Words: IFN-inducible; nuclear protein; cytoplasmic protein; STAT; GDAC; binding reaction; protein–DNA interactions.

1. Introduction

Until recently, the procedure to identify interferon (IFN)-induced signal transducer and activator of transcription (STAT) complexes was dependent on the previous identification of the target deoxyribonucleic acid (DNA) elements involved. The STAT complex designated ISGF3, comprised of STAT-2, STAT-1 and the DNA binding adapter protein IRF-9, transcriptionally activates a subset of IFN-inducible genes containing an IFN-stimulated response element (ISRE), with a consensus sequence AGTTTCNNTTTCNC/T *(1)*. Homodimers and heterodimers of STAT-1 and STAT-3 recognize an element designated the palindromic IFN response element, with a consensus sequence TTC/ANNNG/TAA, regulating expression of a distinct set of IFN-inducible genes *(1)*.

A number of experimental techniques have been used to assay transcription factor-DNA element interactions. One routinely used assay, the electrophoretic mobility shift assay, is sensitive and easy to perform *(2,3)*. In this assay, the mobility of a DNA element of known sequence is monitored under electrophoretic conditions. When complexed with protein, the mobility of the DNA element is retarded in the gel. The DNA element must be visualized, either by incorporating a radiolabel into the element or by tagging the element with peroxidase, biotin, or fluorescent tags *(4–6)*. Notably, electrophoretic mobility shift assays are difficult to quantify. Chromatin immunoprecipitation (ChIP) assays permit the detection of DNA binding factors in the context of genomic DNA *(7)*. In this instance, previous knowledge of both the activated transcription factors and the target elements are required. Although this method is considered more physiologically relevant, functional immunoprecipitation antibodies are required for the protocol. This may limit the types of complexes and DNA elements that can be isolated, based on accessibility of the molecular epitope; an antibody that recognizes a particular epitope on a transcription factor may not necessarily recognize the transcription factor when bound to DNA. Moreover, there have been reports of antibody cross-reactivities confounding ChIP results *(8–10)*. Less widely available are the newer sophisticated technologies that incorporate laser-induced detection *(11)* and computer-based genomic approaches with ChIP, for the detection of protein–DNA complexes *(12–14)*. The newly emergent technique of ChIP–chip assays, combining ChIP with gene microarray analysis, holds promise, yet outstanding unresolved issues relating to annotation of all gene sequences, which types of internal controls must be included and the preferred number of replicates that should be performed for accuracy, have also precluded this approach from being widely accepted to date *(15)*.

In recent years, to address the need for an accurate and reliable assay for the detection of IFN-inducible DNA binding factors, we have developed a technique based on genomic DNA affinity chromatography (GDAC). Using this approach we have identified previously uncharacterized IFN-inducible ISGF-3-independent STAT-2-containing complexes *(16,17)* and STAT5-CrkL complexes *(18–20)*. Briefly, this procedure permits the identification of IFN-inducible DNA binding factors from relatively crude cytoplasmic or nuclear extracts, without any prior knowledge of target DNA elements. IFN-inducible cell extracts are mixed with genomic DNA–cellulose in the presence of excess nonspecific poly(dI-dC). DNA-binding proteins are eluted from the DNA–cellulose in high salt buffer, resolved by sodium dodecyl sulfate polyacrylamide gel electrophoresis (SDS-PAGE) and analyzed by Western immunoblots.

2. Materials
2.1. IFN Treatment and Protein Extraction
2.1.1. IFN Treatment of Suspension/Adherent Cells
1. Phosphate-buffered saline.

2.1.2 Nuclear Protein Extraction
1. Hypotonic buffer (HB): 12 mM HEPES, pH 7.9, 4 mM Tris-HCl, pH 7.9, 10 mM potassium chloride (KCl), 250 µM ethylene diamine tetraacetic acid (EDTA), 5 mM magnesium chloride (MgCl$_2$), 1 mM sodium orthovanadate (Na$_3$VO$_4$), 1.05 mM sodium fluoride (NaF), 1 mM sodium pyrophosphate (NaP$_2$O$_7$), 600 µM dithiothreitol (DTT), 500 µM PMSF, 10 µg/mL aprotinin, 20 µg/mL leupeptin, 2 µg/mL pepstatin. Make just prior to use and keep on ice.
2. High salt buffer minus KCl: HB without KCl, 12% v/v glycerol. Make just prior to use and keep on ice.
3. 2 M KCl. Store at 4°C for up to 6 mo.
4. 1-mL syringes and 25-gage, 1.5-in needles.

2.1.3. Cytoplasmic Protein Extraction
1. Hypotonic buffer (*see* **Subheading 2.1.2.** for recipe).
2. 1 M NaF. Store at 4°C for up to 6 mo.
3. 2M KCl. Store at 4°C for up to 6 mo.
4. 10% v/v Triton X-100.
5. Glycerol.
6. 1-mL syringes and 25-gage, 1.5-in needles.

2.1.4. GDAC
1. Tris EDTA buffer (TE buffer/DNA–cellulose buffer): 10 mM Tris-HCl, pH 7.9, 1 mM EDTA, pH 8.0, and 60 mM KCl. May be stored at 4°C for up to 1 yr.
2. 2X WBEBS buffer with KCl: 24 mM HEPES, pH 7.9, 16 mM Tris-HCl, pH 7.9, 1.2 mM EDTA, pH 8.0, 10 mM MgCl$_2$, 24% v/v glycerol, 0.1% v/v TX-100, and 120 mM KCl. May be stored at 4°C for up to 3 mo.
3. 2X WBEBS buffer without KCl: prepare as in **item 2** in **Subheading 2.1.4.** without KCl (*see* **Note 1**).
4. Washing buffer: 1X WBEBS with KCl, 2 mM Na$_4$P$_2$O$_7$, 2 mM Na$_3$VO$_4$, 2 mM sodium NaF, 250 µg/mL bovine serum albumin, 1.2 mM DTT, 1 mM phenylmethyl sulfonyl fluoride (PMSF; *see* **Note 2**). Prepare fresh and keep on ice.
5. Binding buffer: 1X WBEBS with KCl, 2 mM Na$_4$P$_2$O$_7$, 2 mM sodium Na$_3$VO$_4$, 2 mM NaF, 250 µg/mL bovine serum albumin, 1.2 mM DTT, 1 mM PMSF, 10 µg/mL aprotinin, 2 µg/mL leupeptin, and 2 µg/mL pepstatin (*see* **Note 2**). Prepare fresh and keep on ice.
6. Elution buffer: 1X WBEBS without KCl, 2 mM Na$_4$P$_2$O$_7$, 2 mM Na$_3$VO$_4$, 2 mM NaF, 600 mM KCl, 12 mM DTT, 1 mM PMSF, 20 µg/mL aprotinin, 4 µg/mL leupeptin, and 4 µg/mL pepstatin (*see* **Note 2**). Prepare fresh and keep on ice.

7. 200 µg of cytoplasmic extract and/or 100 µg of nuclear extract.
8. 5X sample reducing buffer (5X SRB): 4% w/v SDS, 20% glycerol, 200 mM Tris-HCl, pH 6.8, 8% v/v β-mercaptoethanol, and bromphenol blue powder. Aliquot and store at –20°C indefinitely, or store at room temperature for up to 1 mo.
9. Poly (dIdC) from Amersham, cat. no. 27-7880-01. Store at 4°C.
10. DNA–cellulose (5 g) from Sigma, cat. no. D8515. Store in dessicant at –20°C.
11. MICROCON YM30 mircroconcentrators from Millipore, cat. no. 424.

3. Methods

Refer to **Fig. 1** for a schematic flowchart of the GDAC protocol.

3.1. IFN Treatment and Protein Extraction

All steps, unless otherwise indicated, are to be conducted at 4°C/on ice. Use 30 million cells for each treatment condition. Cells should be actively growing on the day of IFN treatment.

3.1.1. IFN Treatment of Suspension Cells

1. For cytoplasmic protein extraction, pretreat the cells with complete medium containing 10 mM NaF for 1 h at 37°C (*see* **Note 3**). Pellet the cells at 380g (1500 rpm) for 5 min at room temperature. Discard the medium and wash the cells twice with 10 mL of fresh medium without NaF, pelleting the cells between washes.
2. Treat cells for 15 min at 37°C with 1×10^4 U/mL or 5 ng/mL IFN in the same growth medium used for cell culture (*see* **Note 4**).
3. Add 20 mL of cold phosphate-buffered saline (PBS) to the cells and pellet the cells at 380g for 5 min. Remove the supernatant, resuspend the cell pellet in 10 mL of cold PBS, and pellet the cells once more.
4. Remove the supernatant and collect the cells in 1.5-mL Eppendorf tubes in 1 mL of PBS. Pellet the cells at ≥10,000g for 30 s. Remove the supernatant. Keep the cell pellets on ice for all subsequent steps (*see* **Note 5**).

3.1.2. IFN Treatment of Adherent Cells

1. For cytoplasmic protein extraction, pretreat the cells for 1 h at 37°C in complete medium containing 10 mM NaF. Discard the medium and wash the cells twice with 10 mL of fresh medium without NaF.
2. Treat the cells for 15 min at 37°C with 1×10^4 U/mL or 5 ng/mL IFN in the same growth medium used for cell culture.
3. Discard the medium at the end of the treatment time and wash the cells twice with 10 mL of cold PBS.
4. Add 10 mL of cold PBS to the cells, scrape the cells from the culture dish and collect the cells in 50-mL tubes. Pellet cells by centrifuging at 380g for 5 min.
5. Remove the supernatant, wash the cells once with 10 mL of cold PBS and pellet the cells again. Collect the cells in 1.5-mL Eppendorf tubes in 1 mL of PBS and pellet the cells at ≥10,000g for 30 s. Remove the supernatant. Keep the cell pellets on ice for all subsequent steps (*see* **Note 5**).

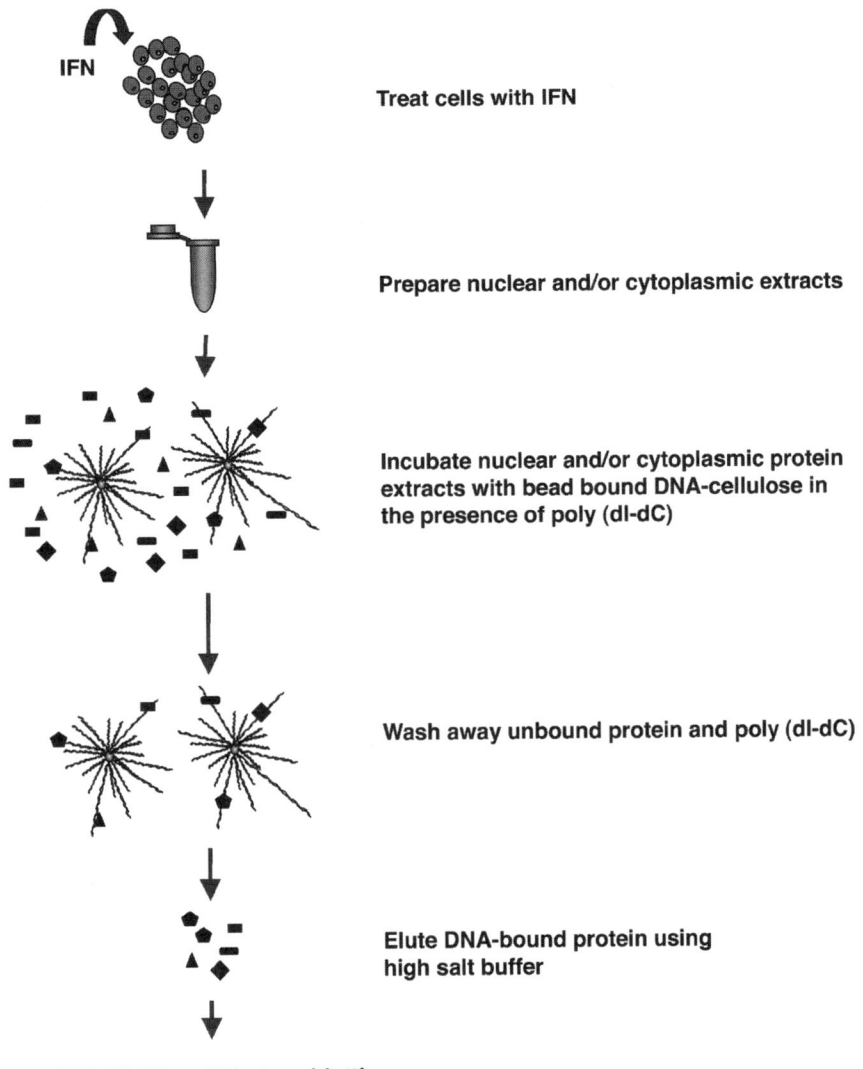

Fig. 1. Flowchart outlining the GDAC protocol.

3.1.3. Nuclear Protein Extraction

1. Resuspend the cell pellets in 700 µL of HB buffer. Shear the cells with a syringe fitted with a 25-gage, 1.5-in needle. The cells must be kept on ice and passed gently through the syringe 20 times. Use minimal force to pass the cells through the syringe to avoid frothing, as this may lead to protein denaturation.
2. Centrifuge the cell lysate at ≥10,000g for 40 s and discard the supernatant.

3. Resuspend the nuclear pellets to homogeneity in 102 μL of HSB minus KCl. Add 18 μL of 2 M KCl and mix (see **Note 6**).
4. Leave the samples on ice for a minimum of 30 min. Vortex occasionally. A longer incubation on ice (e.g., 2 h) may improve protein yields.
5. Centrifuge the tubes at $\geq 10,000g$ for 20 min at 4°C. Collect the supernatants and determine the protein concentrations using conventional protein quantifying methods.
6. The protein extracts may be stored frozen at –80°C until required for GDAC.

3.1.4. Cytoplasmic Protein Extraction (see Note 7)

1. Resuspend cell pellets in 1 mL of HB. Centrifuge the cells at $\geq 10,000g$ for 5min. Discard the supernatant.
2. Add 250 μL of HB to each cell pellet. Shear cells with a syringe fitted with a 25-gage, 1.5-in needle. The cells must be kept on ice and passed gently through the syringe 20 times. Use minimal force to pass the cells through the syringe to avoid frothing as this may lead to protein denaturation.
3. Centrifuge the lysates at $\geq 10,000g$ for 30 s and collect the supernatants in 1.5-mL Eppendorf tubes.
4. Add 6.42 μL of 2 M KCl to each supernatant to bring the salt concentration to 60 mM. Mix and centrifuge at $\geq 10,000g$ for 30 min.
5. Collect 240 μL of each supernatant in 1.5-mL Eppendorf tubes and add 32.73 μL of glycerol and 1.37 μL of 10% v/v Triton X-100. The extracts will now contain 12% v/v glycerol and 0.05% v/v Triton X-100.
6. Vortex briefly to mix the protein extract. The extracts may be stored at –80°C until required for GDAC.

3.2. GDAC

All steps, unless otherwise indicated, are to be carried out at 4°C/on ice.

1. Warm the DNA–cellulose to room temperature.
2. Use 100 μL of hydrated, packed DNA–cellulose per protein extract sample. To prepare hydrated DNA–cellulose, use 29 mg of DNA–cellulose per sample. Suspend the weighed DNA–cellulose in 10 mL of ice-cold TE buffer in a 15-mL tube (see **Note 8**) and keep the DNA–cellulose on ice for a few min.
3. Centrifuge the DNA–cellulose at 112g (1000 rpm) for 3 min. Discard the supernatant.
4. Resuspend the DNA–cellulose in 10 mL of washing buffer. Centrifuge again and discard the supernatant.
5. Add 5 mL of binding buffer containing 60 mM salt to the DNA–cellulose. Centrifuge and discard the supernatant.
6. Resuspend the DNA–cellulose in binding buffer containing KCl such that the DNA–cellulose is diluted in four times the volume needed for each sample, that is, 4 × 100 μL × Number of samples (see **Note 9**).

Genomic DNA Affinity Chromatography

7. Add 400 µL of the hydrated DNA–cellulose into 1.5-mL Eppendorf tubes. Centrifuge the tubes at 112g for 1 min. Remove 300 µL of supernatant to obtain 100 µL of hydrated, packed DNA–cellulose. Keep the DNA–cellulose on ice.
8. For nuclear protein extracts, add binding buffer containing KCl to 100 µg of protein (see **Note 10**). Add 25 µg of poly (dI-dC) to the protein extract and use the binding buffer without KCl to bring the total volume to 200 µL. Add the 200 µL of protein and poly (dI-dC) mixture to the 100 µL of hydrated, packed DNA–cellulose. Mix and incubate on ice for 20 min.
9. For cytoplasmic protein extracts, the salt concentration of the samples is already at 60 mM and does not need to be adjusted. Add 25 µg of poly (dI-dC) to 200 µg of protein extract and make up the total volume to 200 µL using the binding buffer containing KCl. Add the 200 µL of protein and poly (dI-dC) mixture to the 100 µL of hydrated, packed DNA–cellulose. Mix and incubate on ice for 20 min.
10. Leave the samples gently mixing for 2 h at 4°C.
11. Centrifuge the DNA–cellulose at 112g, remove the supernatant, and transfer the DNA–cellulose to 15-mL tubes.
12. Wash the DNA–cellulose 3 times with 3 mL of washing buffer, centrifuging at 112g, for 3 min, discarding the supernatant from each wash.
13. Resuspend the DNA–cellulose in 1 mL of washing buffer and transfer to 1.5-mL Eppendorf tubes. Centrifuge the tubes at 112g for 3 min and remove as much of the supernatant as possible without disturbing the DNA–cellulose.
14. Resuspend the DNA–cellulose in 200 µL of elution buffer and leave the mixture on ice for 30 min.
15. Resuspend the mixture and centrifuge the tubes at 112g to pellet the DNA–cellulose.
16. Transfer 200 µL of supernatant from each sample into 1.5-mL Eppendorf tubes. Centrifuge the tubes at $\geq$10,000g for 2 min.
17. Transfer 180 µL of supernatant from each sample into MICROCON YM30 tubes. Centrifuge the tubes at approx 15,000g for 30 min at 4°C.
18. Add 30 µL of room temperature 5X SRB to the top of each membrane. Invert the membrane chambers into 1.5-mL Eppendorf tubes and centrifuge the tubes at $\geq$10,000g for 30 s at room temperature to collect the concentrated protein.
19. Boil the samples at 100°C for 5 min. Store the samples at –80°C if they are not being used immediately in an SDS-PAGE/Western blotting protocol.
20. Resolve 15 µL of each sample by 10% SDS-PAGE and transfer the proteins to nitrocellulose. Western blot with appropriate anti-STAT, anti-phospho-STAT, anti-CrkL, or anti-IRF9 antibodies. Refer to **Fig. 2** for a representative GDAC result. In this experiment, nuclear extracts from 2fTGH fibrosarcoma cells treated with IFN-α were subjected to GDAC, then the DNA-bound fraction was resolved by SDS-PAGE and immunoblotted for STAT-2. STAT-2 bound DNA in an IFN-dependent manner.

4. Notes

1. Binding buffers with and without salt must be prepared to achieve the appropriate salt concentration (60 mM) for STAT binding.

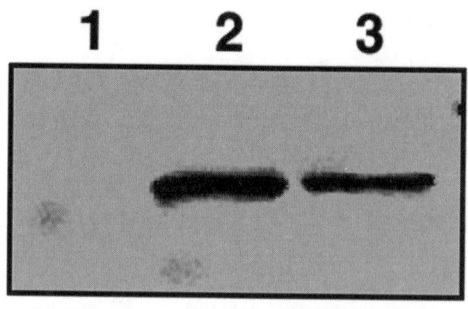

blot: anti-STAT2

Fig. 2. Identification of IFN-inducible STAT-2 by GDAC. Actively growing 2fTGH human fibrosarcoma cells were either left untreated or were treated with 5 ng/mL of IFN-α for 15 min at 37°C. Nuclear extracts were prepared and analyzed for IFN-inducible DNA-binding STAT-2 using GDAC. Eluates from genomic DNA were resolved by SDS-PAGE and analyzed by Western blotting. The blot was probed with an anti-STAT-2 antibody. Lane 1, lysate from untreated cells; Lane 2, lysate from IFN-treated cells; Lane 3, lysate from IFN-treated cells incubated with ISRE. An ISRE element from the promotor region of the human 2'-5' oligoadenylate synthetase gene was added during GDAC to compete for ISGF-3 complex binding to DNA (*see* **Note 11**).

2. Volumes required for each buffer: 10 mL of washing buffer per sample, 10 mL of washing buffer for DNA–cellulose, 1.2 mL of binding buffer per sample and 250 μL of elution buffer per sample.
3. Pretreatment with NaF is required to stop the translocation of STAT containing complexes into the nucleus and concentrate them in the cytoplasm *(21)*.
4. To ensure maximum STAT activation, an IFN dose range of 5×10^3 to 1×10^4 U/mL or 1 to 5 ng/mL IFN is used. Published reports provide evidence for maximal IFN-α/β-induced STAT activation at 15 min *(16,17,22–24)*. Mix suspension cells occasionally during the treatment time to ensure that they are evenly distributed in the IFN conditioned medium.
5. Cell pellets may be stored at –80°C and the protocol can be completed at a later time. Thaw the cell pellets on ice before proceeding with protein extraction.
6. The salt concentration in nuclear extracts is 300 m*M* and must be adjusted to 60 m*M*. We have empirically determined that STATs optimally bind DNA in vitro at a salt concentration of 60 m*M* *(16,17)*. This condition may not be optimal for other DNA binding proteins and so, it is advisable to determine optimal salt concentrations for binding prior to carrying out a GDAC protocol. In addition, if the nuclear pellet is judged to be relatively small, the final elution volume for nuclear protein extraction should be kept to a minimum to maximize the final protein concentration of the extracts.
7. The cytoplasmic fraction contains relatively few other DNA-binding proteins *(16)*.

8. Hydrated DNA–cellulose expands four times in size and this has already been taken into account in our calculations.
9. The equation 4 × 100 µL × number of samples was arrived at by taking into account that the final volume of DNA–cellulose required in the protocol would be 100 µL and that DNA–cellulose quadruples in volume once hydrated. In effect, 400 µL of hydrated DNA–cellulose is required per sample so that, once centrifuged prior to adding protein, 300 µL of supernatant can be removed to obtain 100 µL hydrated, packed DNA–cellulose.
10. Nuclear protein extracts are in 300 mM KCl. The 100-µg aliquot of protein extract will only introduce part of the salt necessary to bring the final salt concentration to 60 mM in 200 µL. The remaining required salt must be calculated and added using the binding buffer containing KCl. Use the binding buffer without KCl to bring the total volume of the protein and poly (dI-dC) mix to 200 µL. This volume is then added to the DNA–cellulose, which has been previously washed with 60 mM KCl binding buffer.
11. Within the context of the ISGF3 complex, STAT-2 contributes its potent transcriptional activation domain whereas Stat-1 and IRF-9 mediate DNA binding *(25)*. Only ISGF-3 complex binding to DNA will be competed upon addition of ISRE. Other STAT-2-containing complexes, for example, STAT-2:STAT-1 heterodimers, will be free to interact with the bead-bound DNA–cellulose. In this example, 100 ng of ISRE was used in the competition experiment. It is advisable to carry out a dose response experiment to determine the ideal amount of DNA element needed to observe competition. STAT-2 antibody was obtained from Santa Cruz Biotechnology, cat. no. sc-476

Acknowledgments

The authors acknowledge Dr. Julien Ghislain, who developed, tested, and established the GDAC protocol in this laboratory. He is currently based at the Ecole Normale Supérieure, Département de Biologie, Paris, France. We would like to thank M. Brierley for contributing the GDAC experiment data shown in Fig. 2. The authors also thank B. Majchrzak-Kita and R. Deonarain for providing technical advice and for critical reading of this manuscript.

References

1. Li, X., Leung, S., Burns, C., and Stark, G. R. (1998) Cooperative binding of Stat1-2 heterodimers and ISGF3 to tandem DNA elements. *Biochimie* **80,** 703–710.
2. Kerr, L. D. (1995) Electrophoretic mobility shift assay. *Methods Enzymol.* **254,** 619–632.
3. Laniel, M. A., Beliveau, A., and Guerin, S. L. (2001) Electrophoretic mobility shift assays for the analysis of DNA-protein interactions. *Methods Mol. Biol.* **148,** 13–30.
4. Gubler, M. L., and Abarzua, P. (1995) Nonradioactive assay for sequence-specific DNA binding proteins. *Biotechniques* **18,** 1008, 1011–1004.

5. Jagelska, E., Brazda, V., Pospisilova, S., Vojtesek, B., and Palecek, E. (2002) New ELISA technique for analysis of p53 protein/DNA binding properties. *J. Immunol. Methods* **267,** 227–235.
6. Zhang, N., Xu, Y., Zhang, Z., and Xiong, W. (2003) A nonradioactive method for detecting DNA-binding activity of nuclear transcription factors. *J. Huazhong. Univ. Sci. Technol. Med. Sci.* **23,** 227–229.
7. Solomon, M. J., and Varshavsky, A. (1985) Formaldehyde-mediated DNA-protein crosslinking: a probe for in vivo chromatin structures. *Proc. Natl. Acad. Sci. USA* **82,** 6470–6474.
8. Weitzmann, M. N., and Savage, N. (1994) Cloning of an antibody binding DNA sequence: pitfalls of DNA/protein immunoprecipitation reactions. *J. Immunol. Methods* **173,** 7–10.
9. Johnson, T. A., Wilson, H. L., and Roesler, W. J. (2001) Improvement of the chromatin immunoprecipitation (ChIP) assay by DNA fragment size fractionation. *Biotechniques* **31,** 740, 742.
10. Kang, S. H., Vieira, K., and Bungert, J. (2002) Combining chromatin immunoprecipitation and DNA footprinting: a novel method to analyze protein-DNA interactions in vivo. *Nucleic Acids Res.* **30,** e44.
11. Phillips, T. M., and Smith, P. (2003) Analysis of intracellular regulatory proteins by immunoaffinity capillary electrophoresis coupled with laser-induced fluorescence detection. *Biomed. Chromatogr.* **17,** 182–187.
12. Shannon, M. F., and Rao, S. (2002) Transcription. Of chips and ChIPs. *Science* **296,** 666–669.
13. Haverty, P. M., Hansen, U., and Weng, Z. (2004) Computational inference of transcriptional regulatory networks from expression profiling and transcription factor binding site identification. *Nucleic Acids Res.* **32,** 179–188.
14. Taverner, N. V., Smith, J. C., and Wardle, F. C. (2004) Identifying transcriptional targets. *Genome Biol.* **5,** 210.
15. Buck, M. J., and Lieb, J. D. (2004) ChIP-chip: considerations for the design, analysis, and application of genome-wide chromatin immunoprecipitation experiments. *Genomics* **83,** 349–360.
16. Ghislain, J. J., and Fish, E. N. (1996) Application of genomic DNA affinity chromatography identifies multiple interferon-alpha-regulated Stat2 complexes. *J. Biol. Chem.* **271,** 12408–12413.
17. Ghislain, J. J., Wong, T., Nguyen, M., and Fish, E. N. (2001) The interferon-inducible Stat2:Stat1 heterodimer preferentially binds in vitro to a consensus element found in the promoters of a subset of interferon-stimulated genes. *J. Interferon Cytokine Res.* **21,** 379–388.
18. Grumbach, I. M., Mayer, I. A., Uddin, S., Lekmine, F., Majchrzak, B., Yamauchi, H., Fujita, S., Druker, B., Fish, E. N., and Platanias, L. C. (2001) Engagement of the CrkL adaptor in interferon alpha signalling in BCR-ABL-expressing cells. *Br. J. Haematol.* **112,** 327–336.
19. Lekmine, F., Sassano, A., Uddin, S., Majchrzak, B., Miura, O., Druker, B. J., Fish, E. N., Imamoto, A., and Platanias, L. C. (2002) The CrkL adapter protein is

required for type I interferon-dependent gene transcription and activation of the small G-protein Rap1. *Biochem. Biophys. Res. Commun.* **291,** 744–750.
20. Uddin, S., Lekmine, F., Sassano, A., Rui, H., Fish, E. N., and Platanias, L. C. (2003) Role of Stat5 in type I interferon-signaling and transcriptional regulation. *Biochem. Biophys. Res. Commun.* **308,** 325–330.
21. Levy, D. E., Kessler, D. S., Pine, R., and Darnell, J. E., Jr. (1989) Cytoplasmic activation of ISGF3, the positive regulator of interferon-alpha-stimulated transcription, reconstituted in vitro. *Genes Dev.* **3,** 1362–1371.
22. Li, X., Leung, S., Qureshi, S., Darnell, J. E., Jr., and Stark, G. R. (1996) Formation of STAT1-STAT2 heterodimers and their role in the activation of IRF-1 gene transcription by interferon-alpha. *J. Biol. Chem.* **271,** 5790–5794.
23. Li, X., Leung, S., Kerr, I. M., and Stark, G. R. (1997) Functional subdomains of STAT2 required for preassociation with the alpha interferon receptor and for signaling. *Mol. Cell. Biol.* **17,** 2048–2056.
24. Wagner, T. C., Velichko, S., Vogel, D., Rani, M. R., Leung, S., Ransohoff, R. M., Stark, G. R., Perez, H. D., and Croze, E. (2002) Interferon signaling is dependent on specific tyrosines located within the intracellular domain of IFNAR2c. Expression of IFNAR2c tyrosine mutants in U5A cells. *J. Biol. Chem.* **277,** 1493–1499.
25. Bluyssen, H. A. and Levy, D. E. (1997) Stat2 is a transcriptional activator that requires sequence-specific contacts provided by stat1 and p48 for stable interaction with DNA. *J. Biol. Chem.* **272,** 4699–4605.

5

Protein Engineering of Interferon Alphas

Renqiu Hu, Ke-jian Lei, Joseph Bekisz, and Kathryn C. Zoon

Summary

Interferon (IFN)-αs constitute a family of proteins exhibiting high degree of homology in primary, secondary, and tertiary structure and display a high level of species specificity in their biological properties. However, small structural differences in these proteins may be responsible for a significant variety of biological actions. Understanding the structure and function of human IFN-α is very important. Recombinant techniques are important tools for the production and modification of IFN proteins. The first IFN hybrid, IFN-α1/α2 was constructed using recombinant technology in 1981. Subsequently, a number of IFN hybrids and mutants have been constructed, expressed and characterized. These hybrids and mutants have resulted in novel IFNs that either combine different biological properties from the parental proteins or have significantly different biological activity. Therefore, IFN hybrids and mutants have provided a powerful tool for studying the structure and function of these molecules. Also, these engineered IFNs may have important new therapeutic applications and may provide greater sights into understanding of the clinical activities of these molecules.

Key Words: Interferon (IFN)-α; structure–function relationship; recombinant techniques; site-directed mutagenesis; cassette mutagenesis; hybrid IFNs; mutant IFNs; polymerase chain reaction (PCR); gene expression.

1. Introduction

Protein engineering can be defined as the use of genetic and chemical techniques to change the structure and function of a protein, thus producing a novel product with specific properties. Site-directed mutagenesis (SDM) is an important method of protein engineering. SDM is the ability to change one amino acid into another by changing the gene sequence for the protein *(1)*. Cassette mutagenesis (CM) is an efficient method for the insertion of oligodeoxynucleotide cassettes, which allows saturation of a target amino acid codon with multiple mutations *(2,3)*. It is one approach for determining the contributions of individual base pairs and their resulting amino acids to the structure and function of the protein.

Using recombinant deoxyribonucleic acid (DNA) technology, it has been possible to create new hybrids that provide novel combinations of the amino acid regions from the parental protein sequences *(4)*. They can be used to study structure–function relationships and to create analogs with novel properties for potential therapeutic applications. Our research goal is to understand how the structure of each of the human interferon (IFN)-α family members correlate with its biological functions. Human IFN-α21a demonstrates a 10-fold increase in antiproliferative activity compared to IFN-α2c *(5)*. Based on these data, studies were continued to further elucidate the role of the different regions of the IFNs in the antiproliferative activity of these molecules. Five human IFN-α hybrids (HY-1 to HY-5) from IFN-α2c and IFN-α21a were constructed and amplified using polymerase chain reaction (PCR), and six human IFN-α mutants (SDM-1, SDM-2 and CM-1, CM-2, CM-3, and CM-4) were obtained by SDM and CM *(6,7)*. The construction scheme of the human IFN-α hybrids and mutants are shown in **Fig. 1**. The amino acid sequences of the constructs are shown in **Fig. 2**. All hybrids and mutants were cloned into a pQE-30 expression vector. The recombinant proteins were expressed in *Escherichia coli* and their biological activities were compared. From these studies, we found that the amino acid region between residues 81 and 95 and, in particular, amino acid residues at positions 86 and 90, were very important for the antiproliferative activity of these molecules *(6,7)*.

2. Materials

2.1. PCR Primers

All oligonucleotide primers were synthesized based on the complementary DNA coding region for the parental IFN proteins (*see* **Fig. 3**). The sequences of inside (within the coding region) primers for SDM and CM should contain the mutant nucleotide sequence for the mutant amino acid residue. For cloning purposes, adaptors of *Bam*H1(5' primer) and *Sph*1(3' primer) were included in all outside (outside the coding region) primers separately.

2.2. PCR Templates

Plasmid DNAs Bluescript/A2 and pQE30/A21 were used as PCR templates for HY-2. Plasmid DNA pQE30/HY-4 is used as template for SDM-2 and plasmid DNA pQE30/SDM-1 is used as template for all cassette mutagenesis.

2.3. Restriction Enzymes

The restriction enzymes *Bam*H1 and *Sph*1 were purchased from Invitrogen (San Diego, CA), and stored at –20°C (not frost-free).

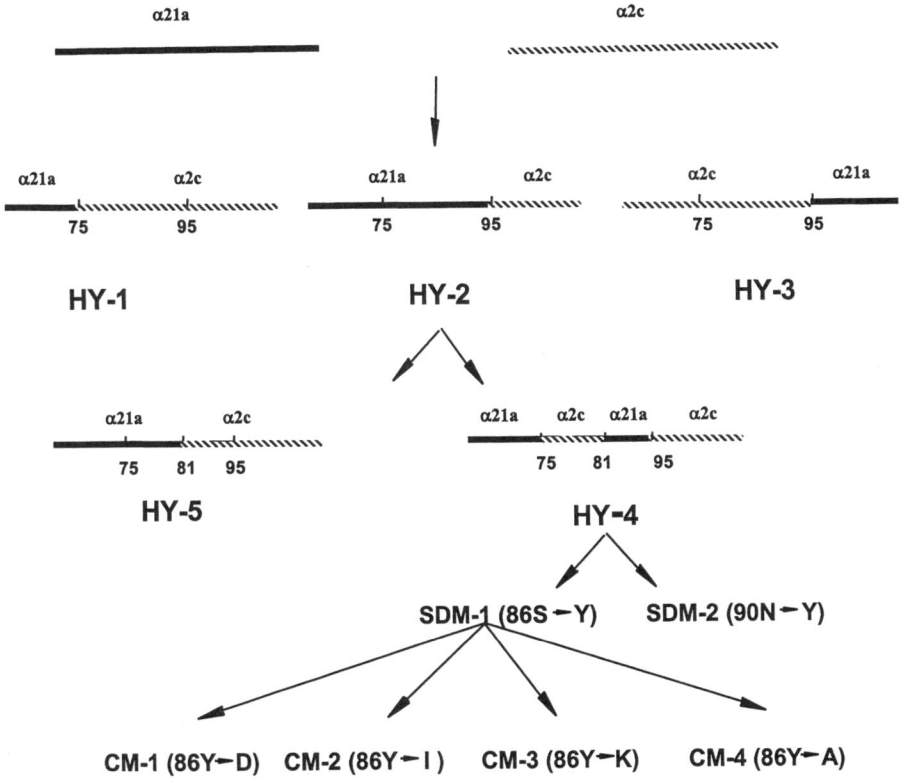

Fig. 1. Construction scheme of human IFN-α hybrid and mutants.

2.4. QIA Expression Kit

The kit was purchased from Qiagen (Valencia, CA) and contains the pQE vector, *E. coli* host strain M15[pREP4], and SG13009 [pREP4], Ni–NTA (nickel–nitrilotriacetic acid) agarose, sodium phosphate stock solution, 1 M imidazole, isopropyl-1-thio-β-D-galactopyranoside (IPTG), and control expression plasmid DNA. The Ni-NTA matrices, *E. coli* host strain, buffers, and imidazole stock solution should be stored at 2 to 8°C. The *E. coli* host strain can be stored under these conditions for up to 3 mo. Cultures should be prepared and stored as soon as possible after receipt of the kit. All other kit components can be stored under these conditions (2–8°C) for up to 1 yr. Lyophilized pQE-30 vector should be resuspended in TE buffer (10 mM Tris, 1 mM ethylene diamine tetraacetic acid, pH 7.4) and stored at −20°C.

Fig. 2. Amino acid sequences of IFN-α2c, IFN-α21a, and IFN-α hybrids and mutants.

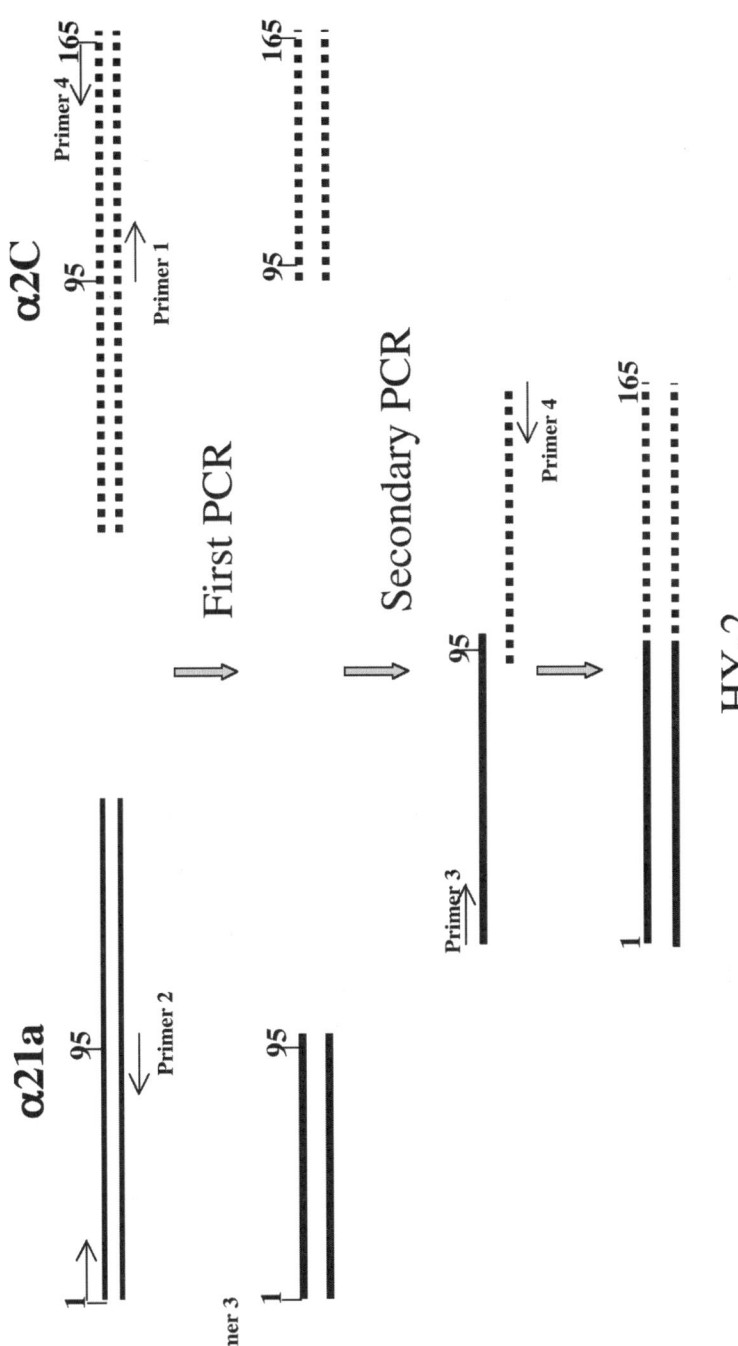

Fig. 3. HY-2 gene construction by PCR technique.

2.5. Culture Medium and Antibiotics

Ampicillin and kanamycin were purchased from Sigma (St. Louis, MO). LB broth was purchased from Biofluids (Camarillo, CA). The stock solutions of 100 mg/mL ampicillin and 25 mg/mL kanamycin should be stored at –20°C.

2.6. Ligation Kit

The Ligation Kit was purchased from Invitrogen (San Diego, CA). The kit contains T4 DNA ligation Buffer (2X conc.), DNA dilution buffer (5X conc.), and T4 DNA ligase (5 U/μL). The kit should be stored at –20°C.

2.7. Purification Components

MinElute PCR Purification Kit was purchased from Qiagen (Valencia, CA). The kit contains MinElute spin columns, binding buffer, wash buffer, elution buffer, and collection tubes. The kit can be stored at room temperature. Wizard PCR Preps DNA Purification System was purchased from Promega (Medison, MI). This purification system contains Wizard PCR Preps DNA Purification Resin, Wizard PCR Preps Direct Purification Buffer (50 mM KCl, 10 mM Tris-HCl pH 8.8, 1.5 mM MgCl$_2$, 0.1% TritonX-100) and Wizard Minicolumns. It can be stored at room temperature. The resin should be protected from exposure to direct sunlight. NK2 Monoclonal antibody affinity columns were prepared as described by our laboratory *(8)* and stored at 4°C (*see* **Note 1**).

2.8. TFB2 Buffer

Mix 10 mM MOPS, 10 mM RbCl, 75 mM CaCl$_2$, and 15% glycerol. Adjust to pH 6.8 with KOH).

2.9. Purification Buffers

Lysis buffer (50 mM NaH$_2$PO$_4$, 300 mM NaCl, 10 mM imidazole, adjusted to pH 8.0 using NaOH); wash buffer, (50 mM NaH$_2$PO$_4$, 300 mM NaCl, 20 mM imidazole, pH 8.0); elution buffer (50 mM NaH$_2$PO$_4$, 300 mM NaCl, 250 mM imidazole, pH 8.0).

2.10. Antibody Affinity Chromatography Buffers

Pre-wash buffer, 0.067 M citric acid and 0.2 M NaCl, pH 2.0; wash buffer 1: 0.5 M NaCl, 0.025 M Tris, pH 7.5; 0.2% Triton X-100; 15 mL of 0.15 M NaCl, 0.1% Triton X-100. Wash buffer 2: 0.018 M citric acid, 0.064 M Na$_2$HPO$_4$, pH 6.0. Wash buffer 3, 0.024 M citric acid, 0.051 M Na$_2$HPO$_4$, pH 5.0. Elution buffer, 67 mM citric acid, 0.2 M NaCl, pH 2.0.

3. Methods

The production of HY-2 [IFN-α21a(1-95)/IFN-α2c(96-165)] and SDM-2 [HY-4(90N→Y)] are used as examples to describe the methods for the preparation of an IFN-α hybrid and a site-directed mutagenesis variant.

3.1. Construction of IFN-α Hybrid and Mutants

The recombinant PCR method is based on two PCR products that overlap in their sequences. Both products contain the same mutation introduced as part of the PCR primer (for mutants) or overlapped parental sequence by using the inside and outside primers separately (for hybrids). These overlapping, primary products can be denatured and allowed to reanneal resulting in two possible heteroduplex products. The heteroduplexes that have recessed 3' end can be extended by DNA polymerase to produce a fragment that is the sum of two overlapping products. A subsequent reamplification of this fragment with only the outside primers results in the enrichment of the full-length, secondary product *(9)*.

3.1.1. IFN-α Hybrid 2 (HY-2)

The construction scheme of IFN-α hybrid 2 (HY-2) is shown in **Fig. 3**. The PCR primers and template for HY-2 are primer 1, 5'-CTG AAT GAC CTC GAG GCC TGC GTG-3' (sense) containing nucleotides 848–871 of IFN-α2c coding region; primer 2, 5'-CAC GCA GGC CTC GAG GTC ATT CAG-3' (antisense) containing nucleotides 399–413 of IFN-α21a coding region are used as inside primers for the PCR reaction, primer 3, 5'-TCC **GGA TCC** TGT GAT CTG CCT CAG ACC-' (sense) containing nucleotides 118-135 of IFN-α21a coding region and BamH1 adaptor (bold bases); and primer 4, 5'-GAG CTC **GCA TGC** TCA TCA TTC CTT CCT CCT TAA TCT-3' (antisense) containing nucleotides 1057–1074 of IFN-α2c coding region. The Sph1 adaptor (bold bases) are used as outside primers for the secondary PCR. The BamH1 restriction site is on the 5' outside primer (primer 3 bold bases), and the Sph1 restriction site is on the 3' outside primer (primer 4 bold bases). Both plasmid DNAs, Bluescript/A2 and pQE30/A21, were used as the templates.

1. The first PCR yields two separate PCR products from IFN-α2c and IFN-α21a.
2. A secondary PCR combines two fragments with an overlapping sequence into one longer product.
3. The PCRs are performed in a 50-μL reaction containing 20 mM Tris-HCl (pH 8.3), 50 mM KCl, 1.5 mM MgCl$_2$, 200 mM dNTP, 1.25 μM each primer, and 10 ng of template DNA. Two drops of mineral oil are added to each reaction tube.
4. The PCRs are run at 94°C for 3 min (predenaturation), followed by 94°C for 30 s (denaturation) then 54°C for 30 s (primer annealing) and, subsequently, 72°C for 30 s (primer extension).

5. Thirty cycles are performed and then the final extension follows at 72°C for 10 min. The reaction is terminated by chilling to 4°C.
6. The PCR products are purified by agarose gel electrophoresis and the bands of purified DNA fragments are excised.
7. The DNA is extracted from the gel by using the Wizard PCR Preps DNA Purification System.
8. The two extracted DNA fragments are then mixed and used as templates.
9. Primers 3 and 4 were used as outside primers for the secondary PCR. The secondary PCR is conducted for 30 cycles using same conditions as the first PCR.
10. Final PCR products are purified using MinElute PCR Purification Kit (*see* **Note 2**).

3.2. Site Directed Mutagenesis (SDM)

3.2.1. SDM-2

Mutagenesis of PCR fragments can be made by chemical synthesis of mismatched primer sequences. These mutations can be made anywhere on the target gene *(2)*.

1. SDM-2 was constructed from HY-4 [IFN-α21a(1-75)/α2c (76-81)/α21a(82-95)/α2c(96-166)] by site-directed mutagenesis. Asparagine (N) at position 90 of HY-4 was replaced with tyrosine (Y).
2. Primer 5, 5'-ACT GAA CTT TAC CAG CAG CTG-3' (sense) containing nucleotides 377–397 of IFN-α21a coding region and mutant residue N(AAC) to Y(TAC) and primer 6, 5'-CAG CTG CTG GTA AAG TTC AGT-3' (antisense) containing nucleotides 377 to 397 of IFN-α21a coding region and mutant residue are used as inside primers (the underlined bases are modified) for PCR.
3. Primers 3 and 4 (*see* **Subheading 3.1.1.**) are used as outside primers. Plasmid DNA pQE30/HY-4 is used as the template for mutant SDM-2 construction.
4. The PCR is performed as described previously (**Subheading 3.1.**; *see* **Note 3**).

3.3. Cassette Mutagenesis (CM)

CM is used to generate multiple mutations of codons at amino acid position 86 in the SDM-1 [HY-4(86S → Y)] to construct CM-1 [SDM-1(86Y→D)], CM-2 [SDM-1(86Y→I)], CM-3 [SDM-1(86Y→K)], and CM-4 [SDM-1(86Y→A)] *(7)*. The two degenerate inside primers for CM-1 (86Y→D), CM-2(86Y→I), CM-3(86Y→K), CM-4(86Y→A) mutants are primers 7, 5'-GAA AAA TTT (A/G/T) (C/T/A)(T/A) ACT GAA CTT AAC-3' (sense), and primer 8, 5'-GTT AAG TTC AGT (T/A) (A/G/T) (C/T/A) AAA TTT TTC-3' (antisense). Primers 3 and 4 are used as outside primer and plasmid DNA pQE30/SDM-1 is used as template. PCRs were performed using standard protocol described previously.

3.4. Ligation of the PCR Fragments With pQE-30 Expression Vector

The pQE-30 vector with a 6 histidine affinity tag is used as expression vector. The His tag is small and uncharged. Therefore, it does not generally interfere with the structure or function of the expressed protein.

3.4.1. Preparation of Vector and Insert DNA for Ligation

1. The insert DNA and pQE-30 vector are digested separately with restriction enzymes *Bam*H1 and *Sph*1.
2. The digested vector is extracted with phenol:chloroform:isoamyl alcohol (25:24:1), and the aqueous phase is removed and extracted with chloroform again.
3. The phases are separated and 1/10 volume of 3 M sodium acetate is added into the water phase and left on dry ice for 30 min.
4. The mixture is centrifuged at 12,000g for 20 min at 0 to 4°C to pellet the DNA.
5. The DNA pellet is resuspended with TE buffer to a final concentration of 0.1 µg/µL.
6. The insert fragments are purified by Wizard PCR Prep DNA Purification System. The Wizard PCR preps DNA Purification System provides a reliable and inexpensive way to purify double-stranded PCR product.
7. The separated PCR product is excised from agarose gel and suspended into 1 mL of purification resin.
8. The DNA is eluted from the resin in water or TE buffer.
9. The ligation of the insert with the prepared vector is carried out using T4 DNA ligase. The efficiency of the subcloning should be monitored by the transformation of non-ligated and self-ligated vector controls.

3.4.2. Ligation

1. A 20-µL ligation reaction mixture containing 50 ng of pQE-30 vector, 70 ng of insert DNA (10-fold molar excess over vector DNA), 1X ligation buffer, and 0.5 µL of T4 ligase is incubated at room temperatures for 5 min (*see* **Note 4**).
2. The ligated insert DNA and vector are ready for transformation (*see* **Note 5**).
3. Confirmatory DNA sequencing was performed on the final constructs (*see* **Note 6**).

3.5. Transformation of Competent SG13009 Cells

3.5.1. Preparation of Competent E. coli

1. A trace of SG13009 [pREP4] cells is removed from the vial with an inoculating needle and streaked onto a LB agar plate containing 25 µg/mL kanamycin.
2. The plate is then incubated at 37°C overnight.
3. A single colony is picked and inoculated into 10 mL of Luria-Bertani (LB)-kanamycin (25 µg/mL) and grown overnight at 37°C.
4. One milliliter of overnight culture was added to 100 mL of prewarmed LB medium containing 25 µg/mL kanamycin in a 250-mL flask and shaken at 37°C until an OD_{600} 0.5 is reached.

5. The culture is cooled on ice for 5 min, and the cells are collected by centrifugation at 4000g at 4°C for 5 min.
6. The supernatant was discarded and the cells are resuspended in sterile cold TFB1 buffer (100 mM RbCl, 50 mM MnCl$_2$, 30 mM potassium acetate, 10 mM CaCl$_2$, 15% glycerol, pH 5.8).
7. The suspension is maintained on ice for an additional 90 min and the cells are harvested by centrifugation at 4000g at 4°C for 5 min. The supernatant was discarded and the cells were resuspended in 4 mL of ice-cold sterile TFB2 buffer. The competent cells are stored at –70°C.

3.5.2. Transformation of Competent SG13009 Cells

1. Competent SG13009 cells (100 µL) are added to a tube with the 10 µL of ligated DNA mix.
2. They are incubated on ice for 20 min and then transferred to a 42°C water bath for 90 s.
3. LB broth (500 µL) is added to the cells and they are shaken at 250 rpm for 90 min at 37°C.
4. Next 50-, 100-, and 200-µL aliquots are dispensed on LB-agar plates containing 25 µg/mL kanamycin and 100 µg/mL ampicillin, and the plates were incubated at 37°C overnight.

3.6. Expression and Purification

3.6.1. Expression

The pQE-30 vector has a 6 Histidine (6X His) tag so that the IFN constructs are expressed as fusion proteins with 6xHis affinity tag on the N-termini *(10)*.

1. Bacteria are grown in 20 mL of LB broth containing 100 µg/mL ampicillin and 25 µg/mL kanamycin at 37°C overnight with shaking.
2. The cultures were diluted 1:50 in LB broth containing the appropriate antibiotics and incubated at 37°C with shaking to an A_{600} of 0.8 to 0.9.
3. Protein expression is induced by addition of 1 mM of IPTG.
4. The bacteria are then incubated at 37°C for 4 to 5 h and harvested by centrifugation at 4000g for 20 min at 4°C. The cell pellets are stored at –20°C.

3.6.2. Purification

In most cases recombinant DNA techniques permit the construction of fusion proteins in which specific affinity tags (e.g., 6X His tag) are added to expressed protein (*see* **Note 7**). The use of these affinity tags simplifies the purification of the recombinant fusion protein by using affinity chromatography methods (*see* **Note 8**). The QIA expression kit uses the nickel-nitrilotriacetic acid (Ni-NTA) affinity chromatography matrix for biomolecules that have been tagged with 6 histidine residues (*see* **Note 9** *[10]*). The expression vector from QIAGEN has the DNA sequence of 6 histidines that can be used for expression of 6X His-tagged recombinant protein in bacteria. The purification of the IFN, HY-2 is accomplished using Ni- NTA affinity column *(10)* followed by NK2 monoclonal antibody affinity chromatography *(8)*.

1. The cell pellet was thawed on ice and the cells were resuspended in lysis buffer.
2. Lysozyme is added to 1 mg/mL, incubated on ice for 30 min, and sonicated on ice (10-s bursts at 200–300W with a 10-s cooling period between each burst).
3. The lysate is centrifuged at 10,000*g* for 30 min at 4°C.
4. 50% Ni-NTA slurry is added to the supernatant by shaking at 4°C for 60 min.
5. The mixture is loaded into a column.
6. The column is washed twice with wash buffer and the protein is eluted with elution buffer *(10)*.
7. NK2 monoclonal antibody affinity chromatography is used as a second step of the purification.
8. The NK2 monoclonal antibody column is pre-washed with 20 mL of phosphate-buffered saline(PBS; pH 7.4) followed by 10 mL of citrate buffer pH 2.0 and finally 20 mL of PBS.
9. The sample is applied to the column and the pass through was re-run on the column.
10. The column is washed sequentially with 50 mL of PBS, 30 mL of wash buffer 1, 20 mL of wash buffer 2, and 20 mL of wash buffer 3 followed by the elution buffer (*see* **Subheading 2.10.**).
11. The eluate is neutralized to pH 7.0 with 2 *N* NaOH.
12. The protein concentration is determined using the Coomassie Plus protein assay, and the purity of HY-2 is assessed by reducing SDS-PAGE and the specific antiviral activity (*see* **Note 10 *[6]***).

4. Notes

1. All buffers and solutions were stored at 4°C.
2. A critical factor in the PCR primer design is the primer length. In general, oligonucleotides between 18 and 24 bases are appropriate *(9)*.
3. The best way to do site directed mutagenesis is placing the mutated base pair in the middle of the primer and there should not be more than three mutated base pairs in a 23-base pair long primer *(9)*.
4. For insertion of DNA into plasmid vectors, especially using only one restriction site for ligation, the vector DNA should be dephosphorylated with alkaline phosphatase *(10)*.
5. Insert to vector ratio is important for ligation reaction. Use 5- to 10-fold molar excess of insert DNA over vector DNA for ligation reaction *(10)*.
6. Check DNA sequence after ligation to make sure that coding sequence is ligated into the correct reading frame, otherwise protein will not be expressed *(10)*.
7. Some proteins expressed intracellularly in *E. coli* are frequently sequestered into insoluble inclusion bodies. This protein can sometimes be solubilized with 6 *M* guanidine-HCl or 8 *M* urea and be purified under denaturing conditions and then refolded *(10)*.

8. Some expressed proteins are not stable in *E. coli* and may be degraded rapidly by proteases. This may be overcome by reducing the growth temperature to 30°C, inducing with IPTG for a shorter period of time, adding glycerol into the purification buffers and/or trying a different host strain *(10)*.
9. If expressed protein does not bind to the Ni-NTA resin, there may be several problems. One should check the sequence of the ligation junctions to ensure that the reading frame is correct, examine whether the 6X His tag is associated with a portion of the protein that is processed, and/or check the binding conditions, the pH and composition of all buffers. The pH of the solution should be checked immediately prior to use and verify the concentration of imidazole is not too high *(10)*.
10. If expressed protein elutes in the wash buffer, the wash stringency may be too high or the buffer condition incorrect. This can be overcome by lowering the concentration of imidazole in the wash buffer and lowering the pH *(10)*.

Acknowledgments

We thank Drs. Dominic Esposito and Nga Y. Nguyen for review of the manuscript.

References

1. Ishii, T. M., Zerr, P., Xia, M. X., Bond, T. C., Maylie, J., and Adelman, P. J. (1998). site-directed mutagenesis. *Methods Enzymol.* **293,** 53.
2. Wells, J.A., Vasser, M., and Powers, D. B. (1985). Cassette mutagenesis: an efficient method for generation of multiple mutations at defined sites. *Gene* **34,** 315–323.
3. Lei, K. J., Pan, J. C., Liu, J. L., Shelly, L. L., and Chou, J. Y. (1995). Structure-function analysis of human glucose-6-phosphatase, the enzyme deficient in glycogen storage disease type 1a. *J. Biol. Chem.* **270,** 11882–11886.
4. Horisberger, M. A. and DiMarco, S. (1995) Interferon-a hybrids. *Phamacol. Ther.* **66,** 507–534.
5. Hu, R., Gan, Y., Liu, J., Miller, and Zoon, C. K. (1993). Evidence for multiple binding sites for several components of human lymphoblastoid interferon-α. *J. Biol. Chem.* **268,** 12591–12595.
6. Hu, R., Bekisz, J., Hayes, M., Audet, S., Beeler, J., Petricoin, E., and Zoon, K. (1999) Divergence of binding, signaling and biological responses to recombinant human hybrid IFNs. *J. Immunol.* **163,** 854–860.
7. Hu, R., Bekisz, J., Schmeisser, H., McPhie, P., and Zoon, K. (2001) Human IFN-α protein engineering: The amino acid residues at positions 86 and 90 are important for antiproliferative activity. *J. Immunol.* **167,** 1482–1489.
8. Zoon, K. C., Miller, D., Bekisz, J., ZurNeddn, D., Enterline, C. J., Nguyen, N., and Hu, R. (1992) Purification and characterization of multiple components of human lymphoblastoid interferon-α. *J. Biol. Chem.* **267,** 15210–15219
9. Innis, M. A., Gelfand, D. H., Sninsky, J. J., and White, T. J. (eds) (1990) *PCR Protocols: A Guide to Methods and Applications.* Academic Press Inc. San Diego, .
10. Qiagen. 2003. *The QIA expressionist: A Handbook for High-Level Expression and Purification of 6xFis-Tagged Proteins.* Qiagen, Santa Clara, CA.

6

Assays for the Interferon-Induced Enzyme 2',5' Oligoadenylate Synthetases

Saumendra N. Sarkar, Mitali Pandey, and Ganes C. Sen

Summary

Inhibition of protein synthesis by interferon treatment is mediated by two major pathways: the 2'-5'-linked oligoadenylates [2-5 (A)] synthetase-RNase L pathway and the double-stranded ribonucleic acid-dependent protein kinase-mediated pathway. 2-5 (A) synthetases are unique interferon-inducible enzymes that, upon activation by double-stranded RNA, polymerize adenosine triphosphate (ATP) to 2-5 (A) synthases. These 2-5 (A) synthetases bind and activate the latent RNase L, causing RNA degradation. In addition to the three major size classes of enzymatically active oligoadenylate synthetase proteins, at least one inactive oligoadenylate synthetase is known in human and mouse. Structure–function studies and recent crystal structure determination have identified several distinct sites in these proteins responsible for different biochemical functions. RNase L is the only known protein that binds to 2-5 (A) synthetases with very high affinity. Gene knockout studies of RNase L have identified its role in antiviral actions of interferon and in apoptosis. Recently, it has also been implicated in prostate cancer metastasis. In this chapter we describe several methodologies for studying biochemical and physiological properties of the 2-5 (A) synthetase-RNase L pathway.

Key Words: 2'-5' Oligoadenylate synthetase; RNase L; interferon; virus.

1. Introduction

The 2'-5' Oligoadenylate synthetases (OAS) were among the first characterized interferon (IFN)-induced antiviral proteins *(1,2)*. IFN treatment induces several isozymes of this family as latent enzymes. They are activated by binding to the cofactor double-stranded ribonucleic acid (dsRNA *[3]*). The active enzyme converts ATP to PPi and 2'-5' linked oligoadenylates] 2-5 (A)] ranging from dimers up to 30 mers *(4,5)*. The only known function of 2-5 (A) is to bind and activate the latent ribonuclease RNase L through its dimerization *(6)*. The activated RNase L degrades all cellular and viral RNA to inhibit viral replication (**Fig. 1**). Hence, the 2-5 (A) system constitutes a regulated RNA decay

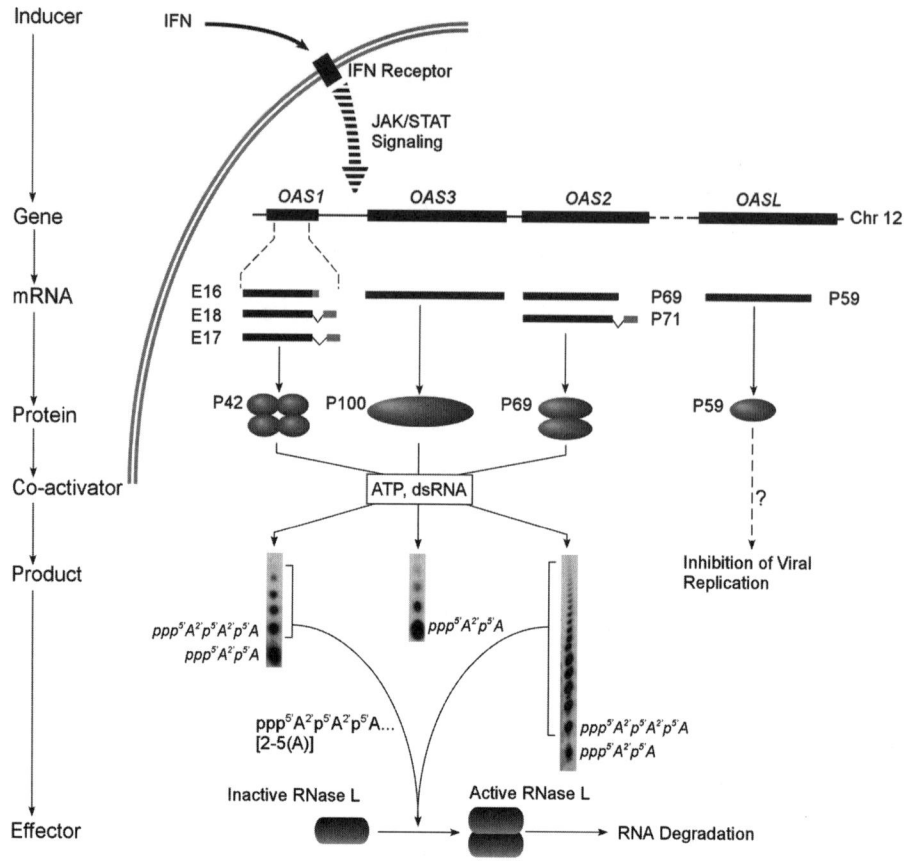

Fig. 1. The 2-5 (A) System. Type I Interferons through IFN receptors and Janus kinase–signal transducer and activator of transcription (JAK/STAT) signaling molecules induce messenger RNA (mRNA) for all four OAS isozymes. The mRNAs for two of these isozymes, OAS1 and OAS2, undergo alternative splicing to generate further variants. Proteins encoded by these mRNAs (except P59) catalyze the polymerization of ATP to 2-5 (A) in the presence of dsRNA. 2-5 (A), in turn, binds to latent RNase L, activates it to an active ribonuclease, which degrades RNA.

pathway, which is activated in response to viral infection, diminishing the production of viral proteins (for reviews, *see* **refs.** *7–12*).

OAS proteins are highly conserved and bear no significant overall sequence homology to other known proteins. There are four OAS genes present in human: *OAS1*, *OAS2*, *OAS3*, and *OASL* (**Fig. 1** *[13]*). On the other hand, mouse has a more complicated OAS locus, which consists of 8 *OAS1* genes, single *OAS2* and *OAS3* genes, and two copies of *OASL* *(14)*. All members of the *OAS* gene family share the same general organization consisting of a basic exon/intron unit of five translated exons: exons A to E. This unit is found once in the *OAS1* and *OASL* genes, is repeated twice in the *OAS2* gene and three times in the *OAS3* gene. A molecular evolutionary analysis of *OAS* sequences suggests that the vertebrate genes are members of a multigene family and underwent successive gene duplication resulting in three size classes of active enzymes *(15)*. There are three major forms of OAS proteins in human cells: 40- to 46-kDa small isoforms (OAS1), 69- to 71-kDa medium isoforms (OAS2), and 100-kDa large isoform (OAS3). Beside these three enzymatically active OAS, there are several OAS-like proteins (OASL) found in humans that are not enzymatically active *(16,17)*. Within the three major classes of enzymes, alternative splicing produces multiple isozymes with different carboxyl terminal regions (**Fig. 1**). The small isozymes function as tetramers, the medium isozymes as dimers, and the large isozyme as monomer. The different isozymes are located in different cellular compartments because of the intrinsic properties of the proteins or because of their differential post-translational modifications that include additions of both lipids and sugars *(4,18)*. There are differences between the enzymatic properties of the three forms of OAS. Most notable is the length of 2-5 (A) oligomers synthesized. The OAS1 isozymes, synthesize up to hexamers of 2-5 (A), and tend to be processive. The OAS2, P69 isozyme, synthesizes longer, up to 30 mers of 2-5 (A), and the reaction is nonprocessive *(4)*. OAS3 makes mostly dimers of 2-5 (A) (**Fig. 1** *[19]*). Because dimeric 2-5 (A) is incapable of activating RNase L, the contribution of OAS3 in the 2-5 (A)-RNase L system remains elusive.

The biological significance of OAS function in the inhibition of viral replication was shown in case of picornavirus *(20,21)*. Recently, the nonenzymatic functions of OAS family of proteins have become apparent from several studies. Resistance to West Nile virus infection was mapped to one of the enzymatically inactive OAS family member *(22,23)*. One of the alternatively spliced OAS1 isozyme has been shown to cause apoptosis through its C-terminal BH3 domain *(24)*. This activity is independent of its enzymatic activity and RNase L. The inactive OAS like protein, P59 OAS L, also has been shown to confer antiviral activity against EMCV when expressed stably in cell line *(25)*. This activity was attributed to the C-terminal ubiquitin-like domain.

The structure function studies using numerous biochemical techniques on recombinant OAS1 and OAS2 have identified several functional domains important for 2-5 (A) synthesis, such as the acceptor, donor, and catalytic sites *(26–28)*. The recently described crystal structure of OAS1 has shown its similarity with other nucleotidyl polymerases *(29)*. However, the structural basis of the unique 2'-5' nucleotidyl transferase activity and the dsRNA-mediated activation are yet to be understood. Major obstacles for working with these proteins are their low affinities for substrate and co-factor. In this chapter we will present methodologies developed in our laboratory to overexpress, purify, and enzymatically characterize several OAS isozymes. We also discuss novel methodologies developed for testing the dsRNA binding and substrate binding properties using crosslinking.

2. Materials

1. Tissue culture cells and appropriate media (serum free as well as complete media supplemented with required antibiotics).
2. Tissue culture dishes (60-mm, 100-mm and 150-mm dishes; 150-mm flasks).
3. Baculovirus shuttle vector, pFastBac1 (Invitrogen, Carlsbad, CA).
4. Isopropyl β-D-thiogalactopyranoside (IPTG; Fisher Scientific, Fair Lawn, NJ).
5. *Escherichia coli* DH10BAC cells (Invitrogen).
6. S-Gal LB agar (Sigma, St. Louis, MO).
7. Antibiotics: ampicillin (Fisher), kanamycin (Fisher), gentamicin (Invitrogen), and tetracycline (Fisher).
8. CELLFECTIN (Invitrogen).
9. Neutral red.
10. Ice-cold 1X phophate-buffered saline (PBS).
11. Complete ethylene diamine tetraacetic acid-free protease inhibitor tablets (Roche Molecular Biochemicals, Indianapolis, IN).
12. 1X FLAG lysis buffer: 300 mM NaCl, 20 mM Tris-HCl, pH 7.5, 10% glycerol, 0.2%Triton X-100, 5 mM β-mercaptoethanol, 1X protease inhibitor.
13. FLAG wash buffer: 300 mM NaCl, 20 mM Tris-Cl, pH 7.5, 10% glycerol, 5 mM β-mercaptoethanol.
14. FLAG elution buffer: 300 mM NaCl, 20 mM Tris-HCl, pH 7.5, 10% glycerol, 5 mM β-mercaptoethanol, 20 μg/mL FLAG peptide.
15. Anti-FLAG M2 monoclonal antibody (Sigma).
16. Anti-FLAG M2 agarose (Sigma).
17. FLAG peptide (Sigma).
18. 1X His binding/lysis buffer: 400 mM NaCl, 20 mM HEPES, pH 7.0, 0.25% Nonidet-P40 (NP-40), 10% glycerol, 3 mM imidazole, 5 mM β-mercaptoethanol, 1X protease inhibitor.
19. His wash buffer: 400 mM NaCl, 20 mM HEPES, pH 7.0, 0.25% NP-40, 10% glycerol, 20 mM imidazole, 5 mM β-mercaptoethanol.
20. His elution buffer: 400 mM NaCl, 20 mM HEPES, pH 7.0, 0.25% NP-40, 10% glycerol, 500 mM imidazole, 5 mM β-mercaptoethanol.
21. His dialysis buffer: 20 mM HEPES, pH 7.0, 200 mM NaCl, 10% glycerol.
22. Enzyme incubation buffer: 20 mM Tris-HCl, pH 7.4, 20 mM magnesium acetate, 2.5 mM dithiothreitol (DTT), 5 mM ATP, 5 μCi of [α-^{32}P] ATP (specific activity, 800 Ci/mmol), and 50 μg/mL poly(I):poly(C).
23. Ni-NTA agarose (Qiagen, Valencia, CA).
24. PEG-8000 (Sigma).

25. Anti-His, H-15 polyclonal antibody (Santa Cruz Biotechnology, Santa Cruz, CA).
26. Coomassie Brilliant Blue R-250 (Bio-Rad, Hercules, CA).
27. 10X Synthetase Assay Buffer: 200 mM Tris-HCl, pH 7.4, 200 mM magnesium acetate, 25 mM DTT, and 50 mM ATP. Dilute to 1X, add 5 µCi of [α-^{32}P] ATP (specific activity, 800 Ci/mmol), and 50 µg/mL poly(I):poly(C) for the assay.
28. Calf Intestinal Alkaline phosphatase (Roche).
29. Polyethylenimine cellulose TLC plates (EM Scientific, Carson City, NV).
30. TLC running Buffer: 0.75 M K$_2$HPO$_4$, pH 3.5.
31. 40% Acrylamide/Bis (29:1; Bio-Rad).
32. 2-5 (A) sample loading buffer: 25% formamide, 0.5% bromophenol blue, 0.5% xylene cyanol.
33. P^1, P^3 -di(adenosine-5')triphosphate (ApppA; Sigma).
34. Methylene blue.
35. Megashortscript transcription kit (Ambion, Austin, TX).
36. Sephadex 25 Quick Spin column (Roche).
37. Polynucleotide kinase (New England Biolabs, Beverly, MA).
38. RNA Annealing Buffer: 50 mM potassium acetate; 10 mM HEPES, pH 7.5, 0.1 mM MgCl$_2$.
39. RNA/OAS1 binding buffer: 200 mM NaCl, 25 mM HEPES, pH 6.8, 0.5 mM ethylene diamine tetraacetic acid, 0.5 mM DTT, and 5% glycerol.
40. poly(A) (Amersham Pharmacia, Upsala, Sweden).
41. P69 labeling buffer: 5 mM 8-Azido ATP; 5 mM dATP; 50 µg/mL poly(I):poly(C); and 200 µCi α–^{32}P dATP (3000 Ci/mmol, 4 mCi/mL).
42. Coupled Transcription and Translation (TNT) rabbit reticulocyte lysate system (Promega, Madison, WI).
43. High-performance liquid chromatography (HPLC) Solvent A: 20 mM N-hydroxy-ethylpiperazine-N'-2-ethanesulfonate (HEPES), pH 8.0.
44. HPLC Solvent B: The same as Solvent A HEPES buffer but also containing 800 mM NaCl.
45. poly(I):poly(C) (Pharmacia).
46. 8-Azido ATP (ICN, Costa Mesa, CA).

3. Methods

3.1. Production of OAS1 and OAS2 From Insect Cell Using Baculovirus Expression System

High-level protein expression using recombinant baculovirus expression vectors to express heterologous genes in cultured insect cells has become a commonly used method to express eukaryotic proteins *(30,31)*. The posttranslationally modified, overexpressed proteins that get targeted to the subcellular locations similar to their authentic counterparts in mammalian cells are generally soluble and can be easily recovered. Previous experience in our laboratory revealed that overexpression of OAS proteins in *E. coli* resulted in either low yield or low specific activity. In some cases, mutants that were inactive in *E. coli* were active when expressed in insect cells *(32)*. Hence, insect cells are the most convenient source of large quantities of recombinant OAS proteins. We have used the Bac-to-Bac Baculovirus expression system from Invitrogen (Carlsbad, CA) to express the E17 (previously called 9–2) and the E16 isozymes of OAS1 and the P69 isozyme of OAS2 in insect cells. In brief, there is site-specific transposition of an expression cassette containing an appropriately opitope tagged with FLAG (Sigma) and/or hexahistidine OAS complementary DNA into a baculovirus shuttle vector (bacmid) propagated in *E. coli*. Recombinant bacmid is selected in the presence of a chromogenic substrate and IPTG and used to transfect insect cells. Viruses harvested from transfected cells are used to generate expanded viral stocks and to infect insect cells to generate protein for purification and analysis (**Fig. 2A**).

1. Subclone OAS1 or its mutants containing a C-terminal His and/or FLAG tag and OAS2 and its mutants containing either a N-terminal His tag or/and a C-terminal FLAG tag into the donor vector pFastBac (*see* **Note 1**).
2. Transform the recombinant plasmids into *E. coli* DH10Bac cells by the $CaCl_2$ method as described in the Bac-to-Bac manual. Select transformants on S-Gal LB agar, supplemented with 50 µg/mL kanamycin, 7 µg/mL gentamicin, and 10 µg/mL tetracycline (*see* **Note 2**).
3. Select three colonies per plate and isolate bacmid DNA from a 3-mL culture using the standard alkali-lysis method described in Bac-to-Bac user manual. The bacmid DNA can be visualized by the overnight electrophoresis of the DNA in 0.5% agarose gel stained with ethidium bromide.
4. Transfect High Five cells with recombinant bacmid DNA using Cellfectin reagent without any further purification as described below.
    a. Insect High Five (H5) cells are grown in Grace Supplemented Insect Cell medium (Invitrogen) with 10% fetal bovine serum at 27°C. 0.5×10^6 cells are seeded in 3 mL of complete media in 60-mm dishes and grown overnight.
    b. The next day, mix 6 µL of the bacmid DNA with 100 µL of serum-free media (approx 2 µg of total DNA) while in another tube, mix 6 µL of - Cellfectin reagent with 100 µL of serum-free medium. Allow both tubes to stand for 5 min, after which add the DNA-media mix to the tube containing the Cellfectin reagent and allow to stand for 20 min at room temperature.
    c. Meanwhile, wash the H5 cells twice with 3 mL of serum-free media. Dilute the transfection mixture with 0.8 mL of serum-free media and add drop wise to the cells.
    d. Incubate cells with the transfection mixture for 5 h at 27°C, after which aspirate the transfection media and grow the cells in 3 mL of complete media for at least 72 h or till all the cells on the plate are floating.
5. Scrape the cells and centrifuge at 300*g* for 5 min at 4°C and collect the supernatant as the initial virus stock (P1).

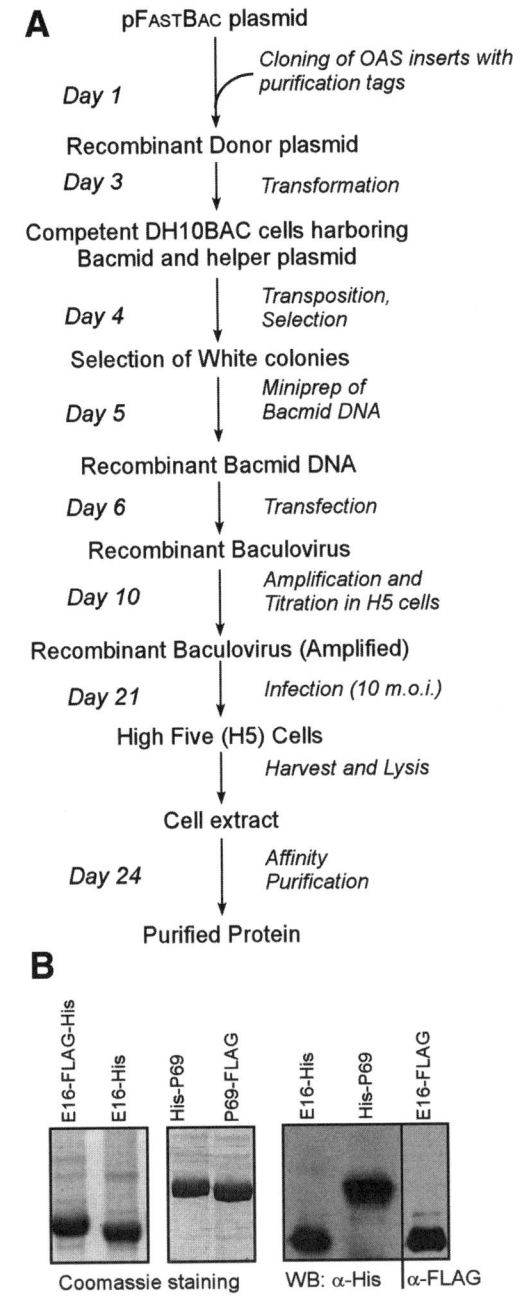

Fig. 2. Expression and purification of OAS proteins using insect cell-baculovirus expression system. (**A**) Flowchart and the time line for the OAS expression procedure from baculovirus expression system. (**B**) Purified human OAS1 P42 and OAS2 P69 isozymes and their detection by western blotting with anti-His (α-His) and anti-FLAG (α-FLAG) antibody.

6. Use the P1 viral stock to infect High Five cells (described below) and analyze protein production by western blotting to check for the highest expression. The viral stock with the highest-level of protein expression should be further amplified and used for large-scale protein production using High Five cells.
   a. To amplify the virus seed 0.75×10^7 cells in a 150-mm dish and allow to grow overnight.
   b. The next day cover the cells with 3 mL of complete media containing the P1 virus at an approximate multiplicity of infection (m.o.i.) of 0.1 (*see* **Note 3**). Rock the plates at room temperature for 45 min to allow the virus to adhere to the cells.
   c. Cover the cells with an additional 17 mL of complete media and allow it to amplify at 27°C for 72 h.
   d. Collect cells and media, centrifuge at 300g for 5 min at 4°C, collect supernatant in tubes, wrap in aluminum foil, and store at 4°C.

Typically each stock needs to go through three rounds of amplification to get a titer of 10^8 to 10^9 PFU/mL. Viral titer of each stock is determined by plaque assay. To produce large-scale protein, insect High Five cells were infected in the same way as described previously; however, an m.o.i. of 20 was used.

3.2. Purification of Tagged Proteins

We have regularly used FLAG or hexahistidine tags for purifying OAS isozymes. Both tagged proteins are purified in one-step by affinity chromatography using either anti-FLAG M2-agarose or Ni-NTA-agarose.

3.2.1. Purification of FLAG-Tagged Protein

1. Infect high five cells with recombinant baculovirus for 40 to 42 h at 20 m.o.i.
2. Collect cells on ice and centrifuge at 5200 rpm for 15 min at 4°C.
3. Wash the cells twice in ice-cold 1X PBS.
4. Resuspend the cell pellet (for each 150-mm plate of cells, use 1 mL of lysis buffer) in FLAG lysis buffer and freeze thaw on dry ice three times.
5. In the meantime equilibrate the anti-FLAG M2-agarose beads with 20 bead volume of FLAG lysis buffer.
6. Sonicate the lysate at 4 to 5 amp for 14 s on ice and centrifuge at 13,000g for 30 min at 4°C.
7. Add the cell lysate to equilibrated anti-FLAG M2-agarose beads (80 µL of beads per 1 mL of cell lysate) and allow it to bind for 4 h with gentle rocking on a rotary shaker.
8. Wash the beads with FLAG wash buffer five times for 15 min each.
9. Elute the protein with FLAG peptide present in the FLAG elution buffer in a volume of 0.5 mL per 1 mL of cell lysate.

3.2.2 Purification of the His-Tagged Protein

1. Initial infection and collection of the cells are done the same way as above.
2. After washing with PBS, resuspend the cells in His binding/lysis buffer and prepare clarified cell lysate as described previously. Mix the clarified cell lysate with Ni-NTA beads that had been equilibrated with the His binding/lysis buffer and let the suspension rock for 4 h on a rotary shaker.
3. Wash the protein-bound beads, 15 min each, for five times with His-wash buffer.
4. lute the protein for 1 h in His elution buffer.

Both the FLAG and the His-tagged protein should be dialyzed against His dialysis buffer for 6 h before it can be used for activity assay. The purified protein can also be concentrated after dialysis, using PEG-8000 till a volume of 100 µL/mL of cell lysate is obtained (*see* **Note 4**). Protein can be stored in aliquots at −80°C. The purified protein is homogenous (**Fig. 2B**) and can be used for further experiments.

3.3. Enzyme Assays

Synthesis of 2'-5' oligoadenylates can be monitored in several different ways. The most common method is by incubating enzymes (1 µg/mL purified protein) with enzyme incubation buffer in a 10-µL volume at 30°C for at least 3 h. The reaction is stopped by heating for 5 min at 95°C. The 2-5(A) products are analyzed by two methods.

3.3.1. Thin-Layer Chromatography (TLC)

After stopping the 2-5 (A) synthesis reaction, centrifuge the samples at 12,000 rpm for 5 min, and transfer 7 µL (for a 10-µL enzyme reaction) clear supernatant in a fresh tube containing 3 µL of alkaline phosphatase (1 U/µL).

1. Allow the phosphatase reaction to go on for at least 4 h, but can be extended overnight.
2. Heat the reaction mixture for 5 min at 95°C to inactivate the phosphatase, centrifuge for 30 s, and spot (2 mL of each sample) on polyethylenimine cellulose TLC plates.
3. Develop the TLC plate in 0.75 M K_2HPO_4, pH 3.5, air-dry, and expose to a phosphorimager screen or autoradiograph.

In this assay, the dephosphorylated 2-5(A) core products of varying lengths $A(^{2'}p^{5'}A)_n$ migrate more slowly than the free phosphate (top of the TLC plate; **Fig. 3A**). This is a simple and convenient method for obtaining rough estimates of relative activities between different samples in one experiment. There are other methods for separating 2-5 (A) products by TLC, which separates 2-5 (A) dimmers from trimers. *(33,34).*

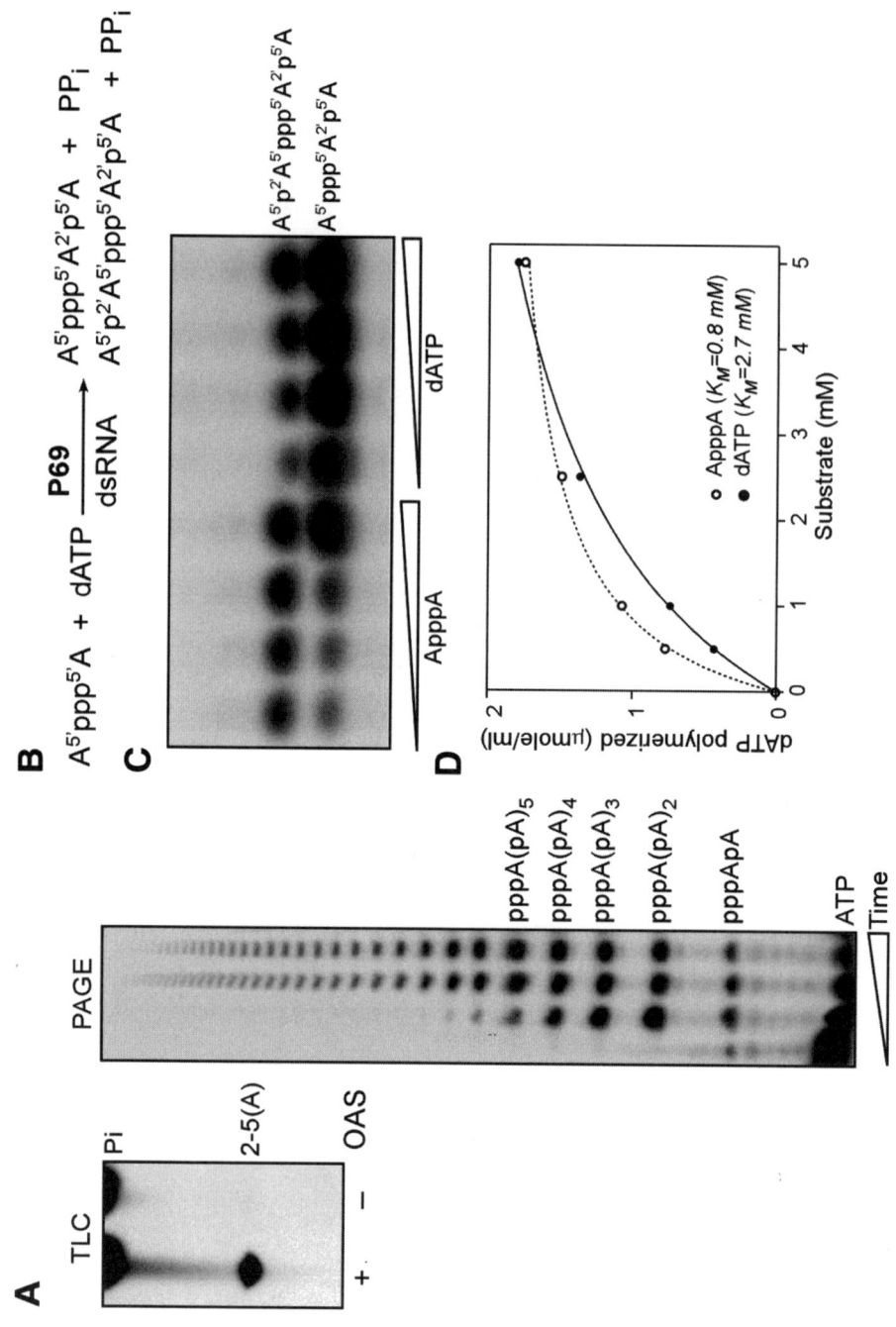

3.3.2. Polyacrylamide Gel Electrophoresis (PAGE)

A more sensitive and complete analysis of all 2-5 (A) products is obtained by separating the heat inactivated reaction mixture in 20% polyacrylamide–urea (7 *M*) gel *(35)*. We use 0.8-mm thick gels that are cast and run in a standard DNA sequencing gel apparatus in 1X TBE buffer.

1. Set the gel cassette with clean, silica gel coated glass plates and appropriate spacers (*see* **Note 5**).
2. Mix 33.65 g of urea, 40 mL 40% acrylamide/Bis solution (Bio-Rad), and 8 mL of 10X TBE. Make up the volume to 80 mL with water. Filter and degass the mixture (*see* **Note 6**).
3. Aliquot out 5 mL of the above mixture, add 12.5 µL of 10% ammonium persulfate and 5 µL of TEMED, mix well, and pour in the gel cassette to seal the bottom of the cassette.
4. After the bottom seal has been set, add 200 µL of 10% ammonium persulfate and 30 µl TEMED to the rest of the gel mixture, and carefully fill the gel cassette, avoiding bubbles, with the content.
5. Set a square toothcomb on the top to make wells and let the gel solidify overnight (*see* **Note 7**).
6. Next morning, clean the gel cassette off unnecessary dried urea, carefully remove the comb and pre-run the gel for 2 h at 1400V.
7. One microliter from a 10-µL heat-inactivated reaction mixture (without phosphatase treatment) is diluted in 4 µL of gel loading buffer, from which 2 µL of each sample is loaded in alternate lanes and electrophoresed for 4 to 5 h at 1600V until the bromophenol blue of the loading dye runs halfway through the gel, which ensures the retention of unused ATP (*see* **Note 8**).
8. At the end of the electrophoresis, transfer the gel on a X-ray film support, cover with plastic wrap, and directly expose to the phosphorimager screen (**Fig. 3A**).

3.3.3. Determination of Kinetic Parameters

The amount of ATP polymerized by the enzyme for each reaction can be determined by quantifying the PAGE autoradiogram as follows. Each experiment includes a blank sample without the enzyme that is processed in the same

---

Fig. 3. *(opposite page)* OAS activity assays. (**A**) Analysis of 2-5(A) products generated by purified recombinant OAS using two different methods: TLC and PAGE. (**B**) Schematic representation of the reaction catalyzed by OAS using ApppA as acceptor and dATP as donor substrates. (**C**) Product analysis by PAGE using above two substrates. In the first four lanes, dATP was kept constant at 4 m*M*, with increasing ApppA concentrations (0.5, 1, 2.5, and 5 m*M*), whereas in next four lanes dATP was increased same way in presence of constant ApppA (4 m*M*). (**D**) Determination of acceptor (○)- and donor (●)-specific kinetic parameters of P69 using ApppA and dATP.

way as the experimental samples. After analyzing the products by gel electrophoresis, the total radioactivity in each lane is quantified and normalized with respect to the blank sample lane to normalize for loading variations. The PhosphorImager count obtained in the blank sample lane is equivalent to 50 nmol of ATP present in a 10 µL of reaction mixture. The nanomoles of ATP polymerized in each reaction is then determined by comparing the total counts from 2-5(A) products with the blank lane. Appropriate normalization against reaction time, gives the reaction velocity that when plotted against substrate concentration and fitted with Michaelis-Menten equation gives the kinetic parameters for ATP.

In addition to ATP or 2-5 (A), OAS2 or OAS1 can use several other nucleic acids containing a penultimate adenine, such as P^1,P^3-di(adenosine-$5'$)triphosphate (ApppA) as acceptor substrate to elongate the chain with ATP or dATP *(27,36)*. If the reaction is conducted using only ApppA and dATP, each of the substrate can exclusively act as acceptor or donor molecule, respectively, because ApppA does not have free 5' phosphates and dATP lacks the 2'OH group (**Fig. 3B**). Under these circumstances, keeping the concentration of one substrate high, the concentration of the other substrate is changed and the rates of the enzyme reactions can be measured (**Fig. 3C,D**). This method can very effectively be used for determining separate K_M for acceptor and donor substrates that can be used as an indirect measure of affinities of the two substrate binding sites *(27)*.

An indirect nonradioactive assay for OAS enzymes that measures the inorganic pyrophosphate produced during oligoadenylate synthesis has been described *(37,38)*. In this assay, a coupled enzymatic reaction results in a mole-to-mole formation of NADPH from the inorganic pyrophosphate through the use of the three enzymes UDP-Glc pyrophosphorylase, phosphoglucomutase and glucose-6-phosphate dehydrogenase. The strong fluorescence of resulting NADPH is spectrophotometrically measured in a multi-well format. Thus, this method can provide a high throughput for measuring OAS activity.

3.4. RNA Binding Assays

Unlike PKR family of dsRNA binding proteins, OAS proteins do not have any defined dsRNA-binding motif. The low affinity of OAS enzymes for the coactivator dsRNA has always been the major technical problem in characterizing dsRNA binding properties of these enzymes. To overcome this problem, we have recently used a crosslinking method to stabilize the protein–dsRNA complex *(29)*.

3.4.1. dsRNA Crosslinking

Unlike conventional ultraviolet (UV)-mediated RNA protein crosslinking, which is more efficient for ssRNA–protein crosslinking, methylene blue can be used for efficient crosslinking of protein and double-stranded nucleic acid in presence of visible light *(39,40)*. We have used a 34-bp synthetic dsRNA, which is long enough for the activation of OAS1 or OAS2 *(4,37)*.

1. Transcribe each strand of the dsRNA from synthetic DNA template with Megashortscript transcription kit according to the manufacturer's instruction (*see* Note 9 for the template description).
2. Dephosphorylate the templates by treating with 20 U of calf intestinal phosphatase for 1 h at 37°C, phenol extract and precipitate with ethanol (5 vol), and sodium acetate (0.3 *M*, pH 5.2).
3. Redissolve the pellet in water and purify the transcripts from free NTPs by passing through a Sephadex 25 Quick Spin column.
4. End label equimolar amounts of 34-bp sense and antisense RNA using γ-^{32}P ATP and polynucleotide kinase and anneal in RNA annealing buffer by heating to 85°C for 2 min followed by slow cooling to room temperature.
5. Mix 0.6 µg of protein-purified OAS1 (P40) protein with 0.6 µg of labeled dsRNA from above on ice in a 9-µL volume of RNA/OAS1 binding buffer.
6. To reduce nonspecific cross-linking, 0.25 µg of poly(A) can be included in the reaction.
7. Immediately transfer the mixture to single wells of a microwell plate containing 1 µL of methylene blue (100 µg/mL).
8. Irradiate the mixture with visible light for 30 min on ice by placing the plates 4 cm under a 60-W fluorescent tube light.
9. Boil the mixture in 1X sodium dodecyl sulfate (SDS)-PAGE loading buffer and analyze by SDS-PAGE (**Fig. 4**).

3.5. 2-5 (A) Binding and Crosslinking

It has been shown previously that the acceptor substrates have higher affinity for OAS enzymes than donor substrates *(26)*. Thus, to characterize the substrate binding sites we prefer to use crosslinkable 2-5 (A) molecules rather than ATP. We have used purified P69 to prepare radiolabeled azido 2-5 (A) dimer using 8-azido ATP and radioactive dATP (**Fig. 5A**). Because dATP does not have an acceptor 2' OH group, the desired dimer is the exclusive radiolabeled product. Conditions have been developed using a high enzyme concentration and a short incubation time to ensure that almost all input substrates had been converted to dimers containing both ppp-azidoA-p-azidoA and ppp-azidoA-p*-dA molecules. The dimers is purified by HPLC and used as the ligand in subsequent experiments.

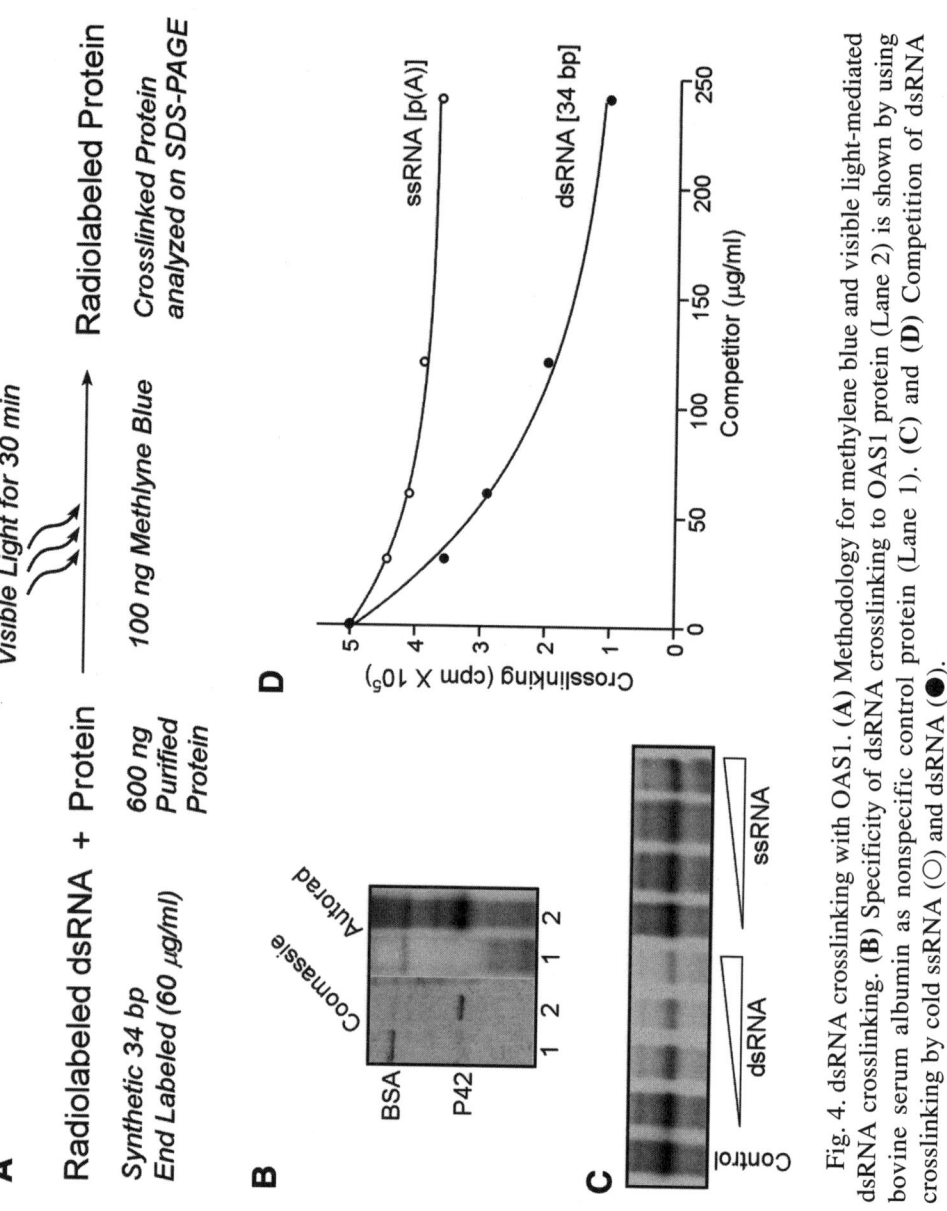

Fig. 4. dsRNA crosslinking with OAS1. (**A**) Methodology for methylene blue and visible light-mediated dsRNA crosslinking. (**B**) Specificity of dsRNA crosslinking to OAS1 protein (Lane 2) is shown by using bovine serum albumin as nonspecific control protein (Lane 1). (**C**) and (**D**) Competition of dsRNA crosslinking by cold ssRNA (○) and dsRNA (●).

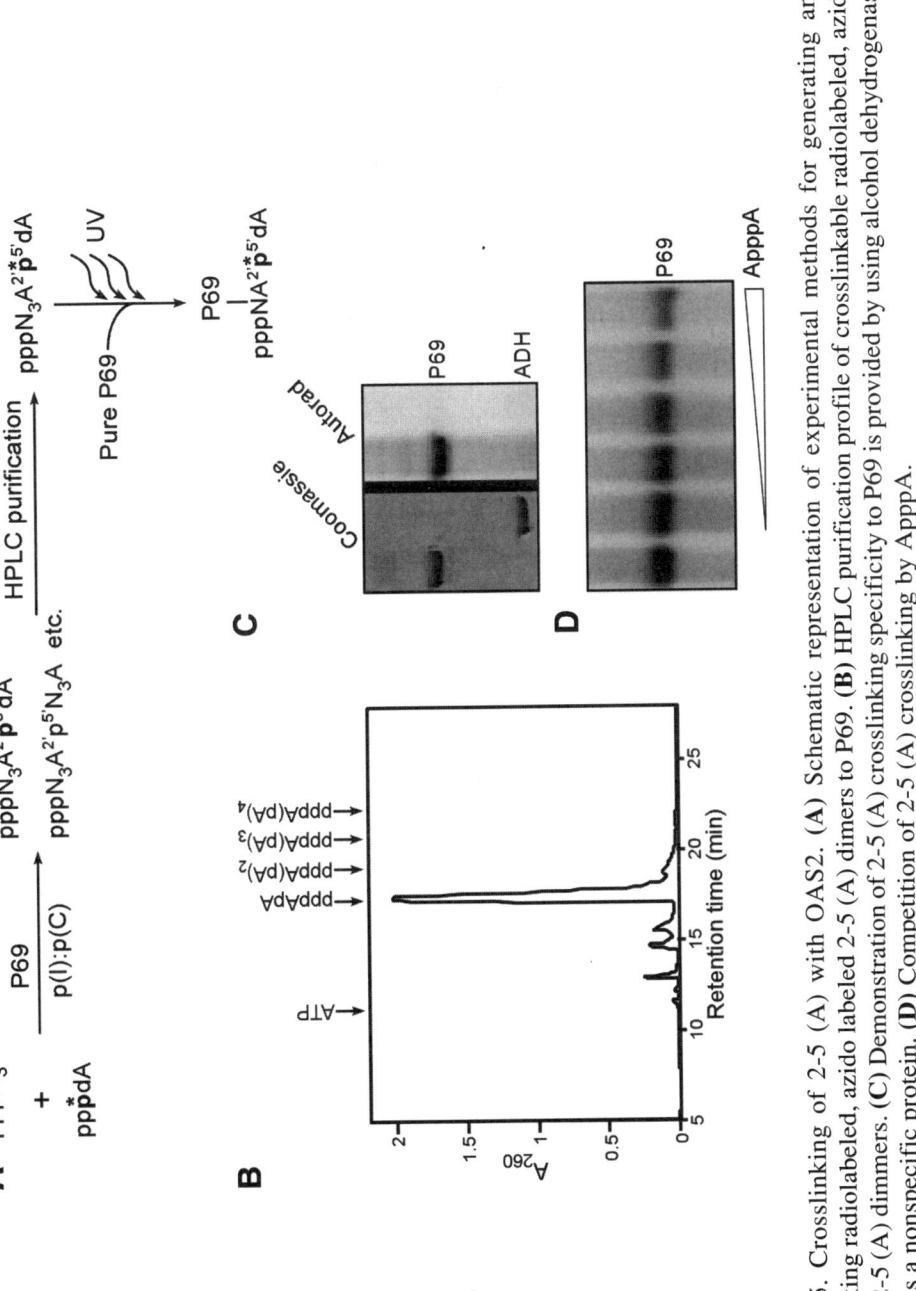

Fig. 5. Crosslinking of 2-5 (A) with OAS2. (**A**) Schematic representation of experimental methods for generating and crosslinking radiolabeled, azido labeled 2-5 (A) dimers to P69. (**B**) HPLC purification profile of crosslinkable radiolabeled, azido labeled 2-5 (A) dimmers. (**C**) Demonstration of 2-5 (A) crosslinking specificity to P69 is provided by using alcohol dehydrogenase (ADH) as a nonspecific protein. (**D**) Competition of 2-5 (A) crosslinking by ApppA.

3.5.1. Preparation of Radiolabeled Azido-2-5 (A) Dimers

Incubate 0.3 mg/mL P69 in 50-μL aliquots of P69 labeling buffer for 3 h at 30°C. After 3 h, heat the reaction mixture for 90 s, centrifuge, and collect the supernatant.

3.5.2. HPLC Purification of 2-5 (A)

2-5 (A) generated by OAS reactions can be separated by HPLC using an anion exchange column (Rainin Pure-Gel SAX Column: 7 mm particle size, 500 Å pore size, 10 mm × 10 cm) run at a flow rate of 1 mL/min. We use the following gradient: $t = 2$ min, Solvent B = 0%, $t = 2.2$ min, Solvent B = 10%, $t = 30$ min, Solvent B = 40%, $t = 32$ min, Solvent B = 100%. Collect 2-5 (A) dimer peaks from several HPLC runs (**Fig. 5B**). Turn off the UV lamp during peak elution to avoid photo activation of azido group. Dialyze pooled fractions against 20 mM HEPES (pH 8.0) using Spectrapor CE Float-A-Lyzer, (500 Da MWCO) overnight at 4°C. Concentrate the dialyzed sample in a speedvac followed by another round of dialysis for 4 h. Determine the concentration of radiolabeled azido 2-5 (A) by measuring OD260 (*see* **Note 10**).

3.5.3. Radiolabeled Azido 2-5 (A) Dimer Crosslinking to P69

1. Mix 0.83 mM radiolabeled azido 2-5 (A) dimer, 0.1 mg/mL P69 in 20 mM Tris-Cl (pH 7.5), and 20 mM Mg–acetate (pH 7.5).
2. Incubate the reaction mixture on ice for 30 min and aliquot in a 25-μL volume on a Nunc 96-well mini tray.
3. Place the tray on ice and photolyze the samples for 2 min with 254 nm radiation from a hand-held UV mineralight lamp at a distance of 4 cm.
4. Boil the samples for 1 min in SDS-PAGE sample loading buffer and electrophorese.
5. Visualize the protein bands by Coomassie blue staining.

For analytical experiments, the extent of cross-linking can be determined by exposing dried gels to Phosphorimager screen followed by scanning and quantification. In the ApppA competition experiment (**Fig. 5D**), increasing concentrations of ApppA was present in the reaction mixture during the incubation before crosslinking.

4. Concluding Remarks

Despite the long history of the OAS enzymes, several biologically relevant questions about these enzymes remain unanswered, partly because of the technical difficulties of working with these proteins. The lack of good recombinant expression methodology and partly insoluble nature of these proteins has always been a major hurdle for biochemical characterization. The baculovirus-insect cell expression system described here thus far has worked satisfactorily for several structure–function studies. Recently, the crystal structure of porcine OAS1 has shown that these enzymes have very similar structural features as other nucleotidyl transferases such as Poly A polymerase *(29)*. However, in the absence of a crystal structure of the enzyme with bound substrate, the mechanism of the unique 2'-5' phosphodiester bond formation remains elusive. Similarly, the exact mechanism of dsRNA-mediated activation is not known yet.

The physiological aspects of these enzymes are not completely explored. The presence of different isozymes with apparently similar functions is intriguing. Though there have been hints of non-enzymatic anti-viral role of some isozymes, other physiological roles of these enzymes are not clear. Presence of several isozymes and multiple genes for the same isozyme (8 genes for mouse OAS1), have made it very difficult choice for gene knock-out studies. Mouse overexpression studies with OAS1 isozyme have shown that in vitro apoptosis-causing isozyme 9-2 does not cause apoptosis when expressed in vivo *(41)*. Recently developed siRNA technology may be useful in addressing some of these questions in the future.

5. Notes

1. Unlike purification of the P69 isozyme of OAS2 by using a N-terminal His-tag *(4,5)*, all tags (either FLAG or His or both) used to purify OAS1 isozymes have to be at the C-terminal region because the N-terminal region in OAS1 is believed to be inaccessible *(29)*. For OAS2 both N-terminal and C-terminal can be used.
2. This gives white colonies on a background of brown/black colonies overnight thereby eliminating the need to incubate the plates at 4°C to develop the blue tetramer in conventional X-gal/IPTG containing plates as described in the BAC-TO-BAC user manual.
3. Plaque assay for Baculovirus
   a. Plate 1×10^6 High Five cells in 6-well dishes (each dilution is checked in triplicates) for overnight.
   b. Make an eight log serial dilution (starting from 10^{-3}) of the harvested virus by sequentially diluting 0.5mL of the previous dilution in 4.5 mL of serum-free Grace insect cell media.
   c. Aspirate all media from the cells and add 1 mL of viral inoculum from each dilution.
   d. Shake for 1 to 4 h at room temperature on a rocker platform.
   e. While the virus is getting adsorbed on the cell surface, prepare the Grace's plaquing overlay. In a 50-mL tube, combine 25 mL of Grace Insect cell media (2X) supplemented with 20% fetal bovine serum and 2X antimycotic-antibiotic + 12.5 mL sterile H_2O + 12.4 mL of 4% low-melt agarose (in water) and keep at 40°C for 3 to 4 h.
   f. After the incubation, sequentially remove the viral inoculum from the wells (move from high to low dilution) and replace with 3 mL of the agarose over-

lay prepared earlier. Working very quickly, remove all traces of the viral inoculum and do not let the cells dry.

g. Allow the agarose to dry in the hood for 10 min and place plates in the incubator for 4 d and visualize plaques by putting 2 mL of neutral red containing agarose overlay.

h. Prepare the neutral red containing agarose overlay by making the agarose overlay as described before except add 1/100th vol of 1% neutral red solution.

i. Leave plates overnight in the incubator before counting. An optimum range of count is 3 to 20 plaques per well. Calculate the viral titer by the formula:

$$PFU/mL = \frac{1}{Dilution\ Factor} \times No.\ of\ plaques \times \frac{1}{mL\ inoculum\ per\ plate}$$

4. All the human OAS isozymes have solubility problems. It is very difficult to obtain highly concentrated protein preparation in a low salt buffer. Thus we have always maintained at least 200 mM NaCl in all buffers and the eluted protein is dialyzed against dialysis buffer containing 200 mM NaCl.

5. It is absolutely essential to completely clean the glass plates with soap and dry before using to avoid air bubbles in the gel. We use Sigmacoat (Sigma) to coat the gel side of each glass plate and dry under fume-hood before setting the gel cassette.

6. To dissolve urea in the 40% Acrylamide/Bis and TBE solution, the mixture needs to be warmed up in a 42°C water bath. The volume of the gel mix after dissolving urea becomes close to 80 mL, very little water is needed to make up the volume. Thus, do not add water to the mix before everything is dissolved.

7. While pouring the gel, it is recommended to over fill the gel cassette with the gel mix, and then set the comb for creating wells. After setting the comb, we wrap the gel top with plastic wrap, to prevent evaporation and let it solidify overnight.

8. After the pre-run, the wells should be carefully cleaned before loading samples, by passing running buffer through them with a syringe. We always use a flat tipped gel-loading tip for sample loading.

9. We use partially single-stranded DNA templates containing T7 promoter for transcribing two strands of 34-bp dsRNA. The templates are created by annealing T (top) and two B (bottom) oligos as shown below.

5' AATTTAATACGACTCACTATAG

3' TTAAATTATGCTGAGTGATATCCCTCTGGCCGTCTAGACTATA GTAACTCTAGGG

5' AATTTAATACGACTCACTATAG

3' TTAAATTATGCTGAGTGATATCCCTAGAGTTACTATAGTCTAG ACGGCCAGAGGG

10. For measuring the 2-5 (A) concentration, we assumed the extinction coefficient of 2-5 (A) dimer is the same as that of ApppA.

Acknowledgments

Relevant research in the authors' laboratory was supported by the grant CA-68782 from the National Institutes of Health.

References

1. Roberts, W. K., Hovanessian, A., Brown, R. E., Clemens, M. J., and Kerr, I. M. (1976) Interferon-mediated protein kinase and low-molecular-weight inhibitor of protein synthesis. *Nature* **264,** 477–480.
2. Hovanessian, A. G., Brown, R. E., and Kerr, I. M. (1977) Synthesis of low molecular weight inhibitor of protein synthesis with enzyme from interferon-treated cells. *Nature* **268,** 537–540.
3. Lengyel, P., Samanta, H., Pichon, J., Dougherty, J., Slattery, E., and Farrell, P. (1980) Double-stranded RNA and the enzymology of interferon action. *Ann. N. Y. Acad. Sci.* **350,** 441–447.
4. Sarkar, S. N., Bandyopadhyay, S., Ghosh, A., and Sen, G. C. (1999) Enzymatic characteristics of recombinant medium isozyme of 2'-5' oligoadenylate synthetase. *J. Biol. Chem.* **274,** 1848–1855.
5. Sarkar, S. N., and Sen, G. C. (1998) Production, purification, and characterization of recombinant 2', 5'- oligoadenylate synthetases. *Methods* **15,** 233–242.
6. Dong, B. and Silverman, R. H. (1995) 2-5A-dependent RNase molecules dimerize during activation by 2-5A. *J. Biol. Chem.* **270,** 4133–4137.
7. Kerr, I. M. (1987) The 2-5A system: a personal view. *J. Interferon. Res.* **7,** 505–510.
8. Lengyel, P. (1987) Double-stranded RNA and interferon action. *J. Interferon. Res.* **7,** 511–519.
9. Hovanessian, A. G. (1991) Interferon-induced and double-stranded RNA-activated enzymes: a specific protein kinase and 2',5'-oligoadenylate synthetases. *J. Interferon. Res.* **11,** 199–205.
10. Rebouillat, D. and Hovanessian, A. G. (1999) The human 2',5'-oligoadenylate synthetase family: interferon-induced proteins with unique enzymatic properties. *J. Interferon Cytokine Res.* **19,** 295–308.
11. Samuel, C. E. (2001) Antiviral actions of interferons. *Clin. Microbiol. Rev.* **14,** 778–809.
12. Sen, G. (2001) Viruses and Interferons. *Annu. Rev. Microbiol.* **55,** 255–281.
13. Justesen, J., Hartmann, R., and Kjeldgaard, N. O. (2000) Gene structure and function of the 2'-5'-oligoadenylate synthetase family. *Cell Mol. Life Sci.* **57,** 1593–1612.
14. Eskildsen, S., Hartmann, R., Kjeldgaard, N. O., and Justesen, J. (2002) Gene structure of the murine 2'-5'-oligoadenylate synthetase family. *Cell Mol. Life Sci.* **59,** 1212–1222.
15. Kumar, S., Mitnik, C., Valente, G., and Floyd-Smith, G. (2000) Expansion and molecular evolution of the interferon-induced 2'-5' oligoadenylate synthetase gene family. *Mol. Biol. Evol.* **17,** 738–750.

16. Hartmann, R., Olsen, H. S., Widder, S., Jorgensen, R., and Justesen, J. (1998) p59OASL, a 2'-5' oligoadenylate synthetase like protein: a novel human gene related to the 2'-5' oligoadenylate synthetase family. *Nucleic Acids Res.* **26**, 4121–4128.
17. Rebouillat, D., Marie, I., and Hovanessian, A. G. (1998) Molecular cloning and characterization of two related and interferon- induced 56-kDa and 30-kDa proteins highly similar to 2'-5' oligoadenylate synthetase. *Eur. J. Biochem.* **257**, 319–330.
18. Marie, I., Galabru, J., Svab, J., and Hovanessian, A. G. (1989) Preparation and characterization of polyclonal antibodies specific for the 69 and 100 k-dalton forms of human 2-5A synthetase. *Biochem. Biophys. Res. Commun.* **160**, 580–587.
19. Rebouillat, D., Hovnanian, A., Marie, I., and Hovanessian, A. G. (1999) The 100-kDa 2',5'-oligoadenylate synthetase catalyzing preferentially the synthesis of dimeric pppA2'p5'A molecules is composed of three homologous domains. *J. Biol. Chem.* **274**, 1557–1565.
20. Chebath, J., Benech, P., Revel, M., and Vigneron, M. (1987) Constitutive expression of (2'-5') oligo A synthetase confers resistance to picornavirus infection. *Nature* **330**, 587–588.
21. Ghosh, A., Sarkar, S. N., and Sen, G. C. (2000) Cell growth regulatory and antiviral effects of the P69 isozyme of 2-5 (A) synthetase. *Virology* **266**, 319–328.
22. Mashimo, T., Lucas, M., Simon-Chazottes, D., Frenkiel, M. P., Montagutelli, X., Ceccaldi, P. E., et al. (2002) A nonsense mutation in the gene encoding 2'-5'-oligoadenylate synthetase/L1 isoform is associated with West Nile virus susceptibility in laboratory mice. *Proc. Natl. Acad. Sci. USA* **99**, 11311–11316.
23. Perelygin, A. A., Scherbik, S. V., Zhulin, I. B., Stockman, B. M., Li, Y., and Brinton, M. A. (2002) Positional cloning of the murine flavivirus resistance gene. *Proc. Natl. Acad. Sci. USA* **99**, 9322–9327.
24. Ghosh, A., Sarkar, S. N., Rowe, T. M., and Sen, G. C. (2001) A specific isozyme of 2'-5' oligoadenylate synthetase is a dual function proapoptotic protein of the bcl-2 family. *J. Biol. Chem.* **276**, 25447–25455.
25. Hartmann, R., Rebouillat, D., Justesen, J., Sen, G. C., and Williams, B. R. (2001) The P59 Oligoadenylate Synthetase like Protein (P59OASL) does not display oligoadenylate synthetase activity but posses anti-viral properties conferred by an ubiquitin-like domain. *J. Interferon Cytokine Res.* **21**, S-69.
26. Sarkar, S. N., Ghosh, A., Wang, H. W., Sung, S. S., and Sen, G. C. (1999) The nature of the catalytic domain of 2'-5'-oligoadenylate synthetases. *J. Biol. Chem.* **274**, 25535–25542.
27. Sarkar, S. N., Miyagi, M., Crabb, J. W., and Sen, G. C. (2002) Identification of the substrate-binding sites of 2'-5'-oligoadenylate synthetase. *J. Biol. Chem.* **277**, 24321–24330.
28. Sarkar, S. N., Pal, S., and Sen, G. C. (2002) Crisscross enzymatic reaction between the two molecules in the active dimeric P69 form of the 2'-5' oligodenylate synthetase. *J. Biol. Chem.* **277**, 44760–44764.
29. Hartmann, R., Justesen, J., Sarkar, S. N., Sen, G. C., and Yee, V. C. (2003) Crystal structure of the 2'-specific and double-stranded RNA-activated interferon-induced antiviral protein 2'-5'-oligoadenylate synthetase. *Mol. Cell* **12**, 1173–1185.

30. O'Reilly, D. R., Miller, L. K. A., and Luckow, V. A. (1992) *Baculovirus expression vectors : A Laboratory Manual*, W. H. Freeman & Co., New York
31. Griffiths, C. M. and Page, M. J. (1997) Production of heterologous proteins using the baculovirus/insect expression system. *Methods Mol. Biol.* **75,** 427–440.
32. Bandyopadhyay, S., Ghosh, A., Sarkar, S. N., and Sen, G. C. (1998) Production and Purification of Recombinant 2'-5' oligoadenylate Synthetase and its Mutants using the Baculovirus System. *Biochemistry* **37,** 3824–3830.
33. Dougherty, J. P., Samanta, H., Farrell, P. J., and Lengyel, P. (1980) Interferon, double-stranded RNA, and RNA degradation. Isolation of homogeneous pppA(2'p5'A)n-1 synthetase from Ehrlich ascites tumor cells. *J. Biol. Chem.* **255,** 3813–3816.
34. Justesen, J., Ferbus, D., and Thang, M. N. (1980) Elongation mechanism and substrate specificity of 2',5'-oligoadenylate synthetase. *Proc. Natl. Acad. Sci. USA* **77,** 4618–4622.
35. Miele, M. B., Liu, D. K., and Kan, N. C. (1991) Fractionation and characterization of 2',5'-oligoadenylates by polyacrylamide gel electrophoresis: an alternative method for assaying 2',5'-oligoadenylate synthetase. *J. Interferon. Res.* **11,** 33–40.
36. Turpaev, K., Hartmann, R., Kisselev, L., and Justesen, J. (1997) Ap3A and Ap4A are primers for oligoadenylate synthesis catalyzed by interferon-inducible 2-5A synthetase. *FEBS Lett.* **408,** 177–181.
37. Hartmann, R., Norby, P. L., Martensen, P. M., Jorgensen, P., James, M. C., Jacobsen, C., et al. (1998) Activation of 2'-5' oligoadenylate synthetase by single-stranded and double-stranded RNA aptamers. *J. Biol. Chem.* **273,** 3236–3246.
38. Justesen, J. and Kjeldgaard, N. O. (1992) Spectrophotometric pyrophosphate assay of 2',5'-oligoadenylate synthetase. *Anal. Biochem.* **207,** 90–93.
39. Lalwani, R., Maiti, S., and Mukherji, S. (1995) Involvement of H1 and other chromatin proteins in the formation of DNA-protein cross-links induced by visible light in the presence of methylene blue. *J. Photochem. Photobiol. B* **27,** 117–122.
40. Liu, Z. R., Wilkie, A. M., Clemens, M. J., and Smith, C. W. (1996) Detection of double-stranded RNA-protein interactions by methylene blue-mediated photo-crosslinking. *RNA* **2,** 611–621.
41. Gomos, J. B., Rowe, T. M., Sarkar, S. N., Kessler, S. P., and Sen, G. C. (2002) The proapoptotic 9-2 isozyme of 2-5 (A) synthetase cannot substitute for the sperm functions of the proapoptotic protein, Bax. *J. Interferon Cytokine Res.* **22,** 199–206.

7

A Convenient and Sensitive Fluorescence Resonance Energy Transfer Assay for RNase L and 2',5' Oligoadenylates

Chandar S. Thakur, Zan Xu, Zhengfu Wang, Zachary Novince, and Robert H. Silverman

Summary

Interferon action against viruses is mediated in part through a ribonucleic acid (RNA) decay pathway known as the 2-5A system. Unusual 5'-triphosphorylated, 2',5'-linked oligoadenylates (2-5A) are produced in mammalian cells by interferon-inducible 2-5A synthetases (OAS) in response to viral double-stranded RNA. 2-5A activates a uniquely regulated endoribonuclease, RNase L, resulting in the cleavage of single-stranded viral and cellular RNAs, thus suppressing viral replication. In addition, RNase L was recently identified as a strong candidate for the hereditary prostate cancer 1 susceptibility allele. RNase L is ubiquitously expressed at basal levels in a wide range of mammalian cell types. Conventional RNase L assays, which can be inconvenient and cumbersome, typically involve cleavage of radioactively labeled RNA species or of endogenous ribosomal RNA. Here we describe a convenient, rapid, nonradioactive, and relatively inexpensive fluorescence resonance energy transfer (FRET) that may be used to accurately measure levels of either 2-5A or RNase L activity with a high degree of specificity and sensitivity. The RNA probe used in the FRET assay was designed based on a region of respiratory syncytial genomic RNA. We demonstrate the utility of our FRET assay with several novel biostable analogs of 2-5A.

Key Words: Interferon; RNase L; FRET; 2-5A; 2',5' oligoadenylate; endoribonuclease.

1. Introduction
1.1. Background on the Biological Roles of RNase L and 2-5A

RNase L is an essential enzyme in interferon (IFN) action against viruses *(1)*. Activators of RNase L are produced by IFN-induced enzymes ([2',5'-linked oligoadenylates synthetases] or [OASs]) that require double-stranded ribonucleic acid (dsRNA), often of viral origin, to convert adenosine triphosphate (ATP) to a series of short 2'- to 5'-linked oligoadenylates, collectively referred to as 2-5A [$p_x5'(A2'p5')_nA$, x = 1 to 3, n = 2 to ≥4] *(2)*. The degradation of 2-5A is mediated by a recently cloned 2'-phosphodiesterase (2'-PDE) that hydrolyzes 2-5A into 5'-AMP and ATP *(3)*. RNase L has an interesting arrangement of structural and functional domains. The N-terminal half of RNase L contains eight complete ankyrin-like repeats, encompassing the 2-5A binding domain, whereas the C-terminal half has a protein kinase-like region and the ribonuclease domain *(4)*. Sustained activation of RNase L results in stress-response involving the JNK mitogen-activated protein kinases, culminating in caspase-dependent apoptosis through a mitochondrial pathway *(5)*. Interestingly, the human RNase L gene has been recently identified as a strong candidate for the hereditary prostate cancer 1 (*HPC1*) allele, suggesting a protective role for RNase L in suppressing prostate cancer in most men. In a subset of prostate cancer cases, mutations in *RNASEL/HPC1* allow cancer to progress *(6,7)*.

To date, RNase L is the only well-established biochemical receptor for 2-5A *(1)*. Binding of 2-5A causes inactive RNase L monomers to dimerize to the activated enzyme *(8)*. The activated enzyme contains two molecules of RNase L and two molecules of 2-5A *(9)* and cleaves single-stranded RNA preferentially at UU or UA dinucleotides, leaving 3'-phosphoryl groups *(10,11)*.

1.2. Methods for Monitoring RNase L Activity and Its Activator, 2-5A

Several methods have been previously described for measuring RNase L activity. For instance, cell-based rRNA cleavage assays may be used to determine whether a particular type of virus will lead to RNase L activation during the course of infection. RNase L activation in intact cells frequently results in the appearance of specific cleavage products of rRNAs as observed in denaturing agarose gels or in RNA chips *(12–14)*. In cell-free systems, RNase L activity has been previously measured by cleavage of various radiolabeled RNA substrates, including poly(rU) *(15)* and oligoribonucleotides such as $rC_{11}UUC_7$ *(16)*. The degradation of RNA substrates can be monitored by gel electrophoresis methods. Once RNase L is purified, free from contamination of other ribonucleases, cleavage of the RNA substrate becomes completely dependent on the addition of the 2-5A activator. More recently, different laboratories, including our own, have developed more convenient fluorescence resonance energy transfer (FRET) assays for RNase L (**Fig. 1**. *[5,17,18]*). These different FRET assays for RNase L each utilize a synthetic oligoribonucleotide with a fluorophore and a quencher at opposite termini. When the FRET RNA probe is intact and there is exposure to the excitation wavelength of light, energy transfer occurs from the fluorophore to the quencher owing to their proximity. However, once RNA cleavage occurs, physical separation of the quencher from the fluorophore allows light emission as measured by a spectrofluorometer. For an

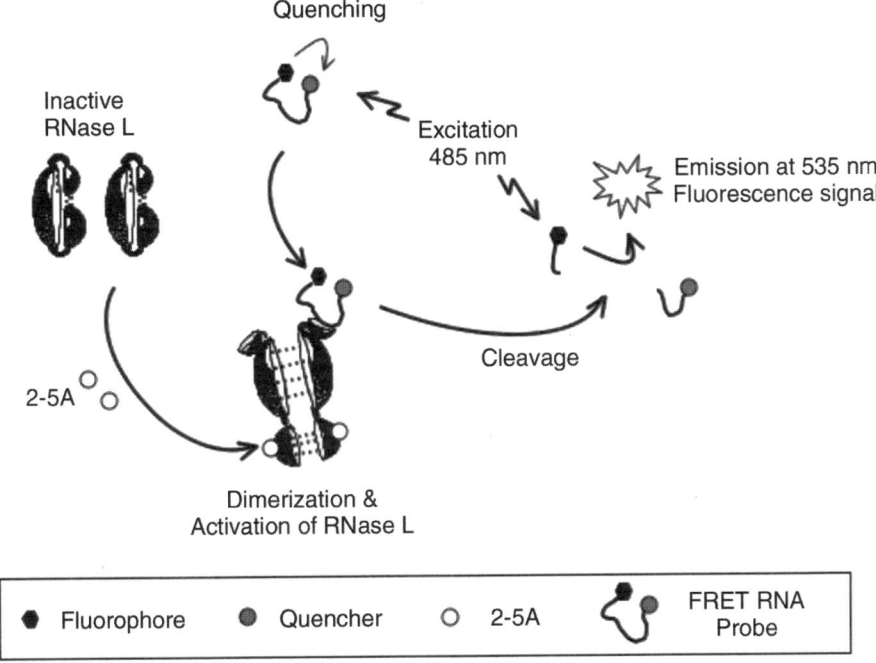

Fig. 1. FRET assay for measuring the activation of RNase L by 2-5A.

excellent discussion of theoretical considerations in the design, interpretation and analysis of FRET assays (*see* ref. *17*).

The assay we describe here differs from previous FRET assays that rely on cleavage of the substrate $rC_{11}U_2C_7$ (*17,18*). Instead, we use an RNA sequence derived from the intergenic region of respiratory syncytial virus genomic RNA that is highly susceptible to cleavage by RNase L owing to a multiplicity of cleavage sites (UU and UA). Our assay may be used to quantitate RNase L activity or to compare the ability of different 2-5A molecules and analogs to activate RNase L (**Figs. 2–4**). For example, the assay may be used to screen or evaluate candidate RNase L activators for the potential to be developed as therapeutic agents for viral infections and cancer. We demonstrate the utility of this method by evaluating the activity of several novel chemical analogs of 2-5A (**Fig. 4** and **Table 1**). Among the advantages of the FRET assay over conventional methods are 1) the assays are non-radioactive; 2) the FRET RNA probe can be stored at –70°C for extended periods (whereas radioactive probes are often subject to rapid decay); 3) the assay allows real-time monitoring of ribonuclease activity; and 4) the assays are performed in microtiter plates allowing large numbers of reactions to proceed simultaneously.

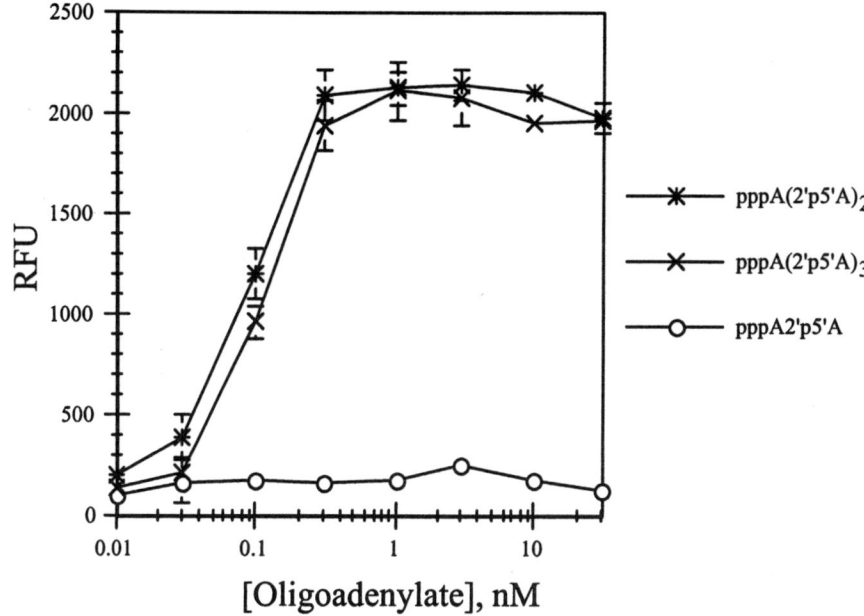

Fig. 2. Dose–response curves with natural activators of RNase L in FRET assays. Reactions were performed for 120 min at 21°C. RFU, relative fluorescence unit.

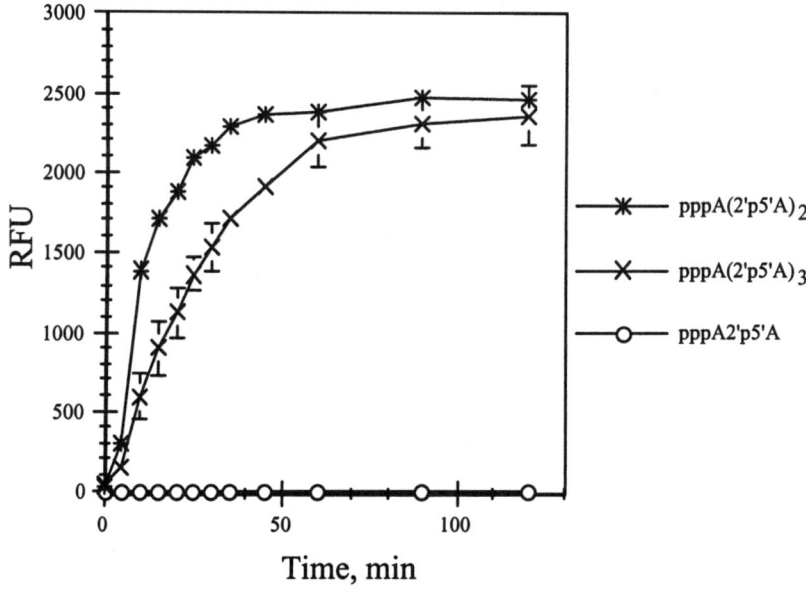

Fig. 3. Kinetics of RNase L activity in response to natural 2-5A activators at 3 nM as determined in FRET assays. Background fluorescence (<200 RFU), which was determined by incubating FRET probe in buffer, was subtracted before plotting data.

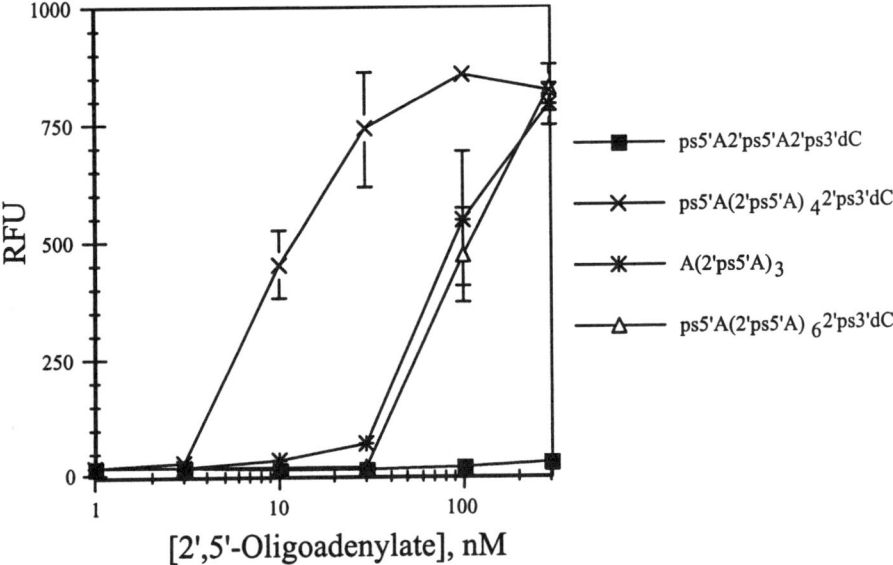

Fig. 4. Dose response curves of novel 2-5A analogs in RNase L FRET assays. Reactions were for 120 min at 21°C. Background fluorescence was subtracted.

Table 1
Relative Activities of 2',5'-Linked Oligoadenylates in RNase L FRET Assay

2-5A or analogs	Number of 2',5'-linked adenylyl residues	Phosphodiester (PO) or phosphorothioate (PS)	EC_{50}
pppA2'p5'A	2	PO	NA
pppA(2'p5'A)$_2$	3	PO	0.1 nM
pppA(2'p5'A)$_3$	4	PO	0.1 nM
A(2'ps5'A)$_3$	4	PS	100 nM
ps5'A(2'ps5'A)$_4$2'ps3'dC	5	PS	10 nM
ps5'A(2'ps5'A)$_6$2'ps3'dC	7	PS	100 nM

EC_{50}, concentration required to produce 50% of the maximal effect; NA, no activity.

1.3. Example 1: RNase L Activation by Natural 2',5'-Phosphodiester-Linked Oligoadenylates (2-5A)

RNase L activation was observed with concentrations of p$_3$A(2'p5'A)$_2$ or p$_3$A(2'p5'A)$_3$ as low as 0.1 nM, with maximal activity in the range of 0.3 to 1.0 nM, under standard conditions (120 min at 21°C; **Fig. 2**). The trimer and tetramer 2-5A species produce similar activation profiles, whereas as the dimer species, pppA2'p5'A, fails to activate RNase L (**Figs. 2** and **3** *[15]*). Results, such as those with trimer 2-5A, may be used as a standard curve to measure or confirm 2-5A levels in an unknown solution, such as from an extract of virus infected cells. The kinetics of RNase L reactions at 21°C shows slightly faster kinetics when the enzyme is activated by the trimer species of 2-5A, compared with tetramer 2-5A (**Fig. 3**; *see* **Note 1**). This could possibly reflect the enhanced ability of RNase L to dimerize into its activated state by trimer 2-5A as compared with tetramer 2-5A *(8)*. The reaction products were first detected after 5 min and reach a plateau at about 1 h at 21°C. The FRET probe was completely stable in control reactions containing pppA2'p5'A and RNase L (**Fig. 3**).

1.4. Example 2: Determining the Abilities of Novel 2-5A Analogs to Activate RNase L

The activities of novel biostable 2-5A analogs with phosphorothioate (PS) internucleotide linkages were analyzed in FRET assays (**Fig. 4** and **Table 1**). There was no activity with the compound ps5'A2'ps5'Aps3'dC, which has only two 2',5'-linked adenylyl residues. The compound, ps5'A(2'ps5'A)$_4$ 2'ps3'dC, was the most active, with an EC_{50} (effective dose 50, required to achieve 50% RNA cleavage) of about 10 nM (approx 1% of the activity of authentic natural 2-5A (**Fig. 2**). The phosphorothioate tetramer core compound, A(2'ps5'A)$_3$ and ps5'A(2'ps5'A)$_6$2'ps3'dC, with seven 2',5'-adenylyl residues, were both approx 10-fold less active, with EC_{50}'s of about 100 nM. These reduced activities are likely owing to absence of 5'-phosphoryl in the former compound and the extended length of the latter compound. Our findings demonstrate the utility of the FRET assay to compare different novel 2-5A analogs and natural 2-5A for their abilities to active RNase L (**Table 1**).

2. Materials

2.1. FRET Assay for RNase L

1. Recombinant purified human RNase L, 2–3 mg/mL, stored as aliquots at –70°C (*see* **Subheading 3**).
2. Cleavage buffer (10X): 250 mM Tris-HCl, pH 7.4, 1 M KCl, 0.1 M MgCl$_2$, 0.5 mM ATP, pH 7.4, and 70 mM β-mercaptoethanol.
3. Diethylpyrocarbonate (DEPC)-treated water (Invitrogen, cat. no. 750024).
4. FRET probe, 6-FAM-UUA UCA AAU UCU UAU UUG CCC CAU UUU UUU GGU UUA-BHQ-1 (custom synthesized by Proligo, Boulder, CO; or Integrated DNA Technologies, Inc., Coralville, IA). The FRET probe (200 µM) in DEPC water is stored in 15-µL aliquots at –70°C. Dilute in DEPC-water to 1 µM on day of use.
5. Black 96-well microtiter round bottom plates (Costar; cat. no. 064432; *see* **Note 2**).
6. Purified 2-5A oligomers: p$_3$A2'p5'A, p$_3$A(2'p5'A)$_2$, and p$_3$A(2'p5'A)$_3$ or 2-5A analogs.

7. Equilibration buffer for Blue Sepharose CL-6B affinity resin (buffer A): 20 mM HEPES, pH 7.4, 5 mM MgCl$_2$, 50 mM KCl, 1 mM ethylene diamine tetraacetic acid, 10% glycerol, 7 mM β-mercaptoethanol, 100 μM ATP, 2 μg/mL leupeptin, 2 μg/mL pepstatin, and 50 μM phenylmethanesulfonyl fluoride.
8. Elution buffer for Blue Sepharose CL-6B affinity resin (buffer B): buffer A supplemented with 1.0 M KCl.
9. Dialysis membrane: Fisher, cat. no. 21-152-15, 12,000–14,000 MW cutoff.

2.2. Equipment

Plate reader: Wallac Victor^2 1420 fluorometer multilabel counter (Perkin-Elmer).

3. Methods

3.1. RNase L Expression and Purification

Baculovirus expression of full-length human recombinant RNase L, without tag, is typically used. Expression and purification of RNase L has been described in detail elsewhere *(19)*. In that protocol, we purified the RNase L to homogeneity through three successive steps involving separation in FPLC columns. However, we have observed that only one column is necessary to obtain optimum preparations of RNase L suitable for this FRET assay. Briefly, the following steps are taken:

1. RNase L is produced in the *Spodoptera frugiperda*-derived cell line Sf-21 or Sf-9.
2. Two liters of Sf-21 suspension culture, maintained at 27°C, are infected at a density of 2.5 × 10^6 cells/mL with RNase L-expressing baculovirus *(15)* at a multiplicity of infection of 5.
3. Seventy-two hours after infection, cells are lysed mechanically with a French Press to harvest the intracellularly produced RNase L monomer. All subsequent steps are carried out at 4°C.
4. The cell lysate, centrifuged twice for 45 min at 40,000g to completely remove debris, is applied to a freshly packed fast protein liquid chromatography (FPLC) column (HR16/10) containing Blue Sepharose CL-6B affinity resin (Amersham Biosciences) equilibrated with buffer A.
5. The bound protein is eluted by a linear gradient of 100% buffer A to 100% buffer B in 60 min, followed by buffer B for an additional 50 min.
6. Fractions containing RNase L, as determined by absorbance are pooled and dialyzed against buffer A.
7. Total protein concentration (RNase L is typically about 80% of the total protein) is about 3 mg per ml, about 50 mg per preparation.
8. Protein is stored in 100-μL aliquots at –70°C in buffer A (*see* **Note 3**).

Alternative modes of RNase L expression and purification have been described, although these methods have not been specifically tested in our laboratory in this particular FRET assay. Others have used in FRET assays GST-RNase L produced in *Escherichia coli* and purified by glutathione-Sepharose 4B affinity chromatography followed by Sephacryl S200HR gel filtration *(18)*. In principal, any RNase L preparation that is free of contaminating ribonucleases should be suitable.

3.2. 2-5A and Analogs

Natural 2-5A [$p_3(A2'p)_nA$, where $n = 1$ to >3] was prepared enzymatically from ATP using hexahistidine tagged and purified, recombinant porcine 42-kDa 2-5A synthetase (a gift from R. Hartmann, Aarhus, Denmark *[20]*). We have previously published a detailed protocol for 2-5A synthetase reactions *(21)*. That protocol was using 2-5A synthetase isolated from extracts of interferon-α treated human HeLa cells, which may be used in place of recombinant 2-5A synthetase. Poly(I):poly(C)-agarose is used for immobilization, purification and activation of 2-5A synthetase. Separation of 2-5A oligomers is performed by high-performance liquid chromatography on Dionex semi-preparative columns or by FPLC on a mono-Q column. 2-5A analogs are chemically synthesized using an ABI model 380B automated DNA synthesizer (Applied Biosystems) as described previously *(14)*.

3.3. FRET Probe

The cleavable RNA substrate is a 36-nucleotide synthetic oligoribonucleotide, derived from the intergenic sequence of respiratory syncytial virus (RSV) RNA, with a fluorophore (6-FAM or 6-carboxyfluorescein) at the 5'-terminus and a black hole quencher-1 (BHQ1), at the 3'-terminus (Materials). It is stored as 200 µM in DEPC water at –80°C. The FRET probe is diluted in DEPC H_2O to 1 µM on the day of use. Because the reporter dye, 6-FAM, is light sensitive, caution should be taken to avoid exposing to light (*see* **Note 4**).

3.4. RNase L/FRET Probe Mixture (5 mL) for 110 Assays

Pipet listed items in the following order in a 15-mL conical tube in ice (*see* **Note 5**):

1. 3.74 mL of DEPC H_2O (Invitrogen, cat. no. 750024).
2. 500 µL of 10X Cleavage Buffer buffer.
3. 750 µL of FRET probe (1 µM, diluted fresh on day of use; final concentration in assay is 135 nM).
4. 10 µL of 2 µg/µL RNase L preparation (180 ng per well. Replace with 10 µL of H_2O for controls lacking RNase L; final concentration is 43 nM).

3.5. Set-Up Reactions in Black 96-Well Microtiter Plates

1. Pipet 45 µL of RNase L/FRET probe mixture or FRET probe mixture without RNase L (**Subheading 3.4.**) into wells. Assays are performed in triplicate with and without RNase L.

2. Pipet (at desired concentrations): 5 µL of 2-5A compound, test compound (e.g., 2-5A analog), sample with unknown amount of 2-5A (e.g., concentration of 2-5A to be determined), or as control, DEPC H_2O, into wells.
3. Incubate plate at 21°C. For kinetics, incubate for 0, 5, 10, 15, 30, 45, 60, 90, and 120 min. For standard concentration curve, incubate for 120 min.
4. Determine fluorescence in plate reader using fluorescein protocol at 485-nm excitation and 535-nm emission wavelengths for 0.1 s.

3.6. Individual Assays

Pipet listed items in the following order directly into wells of plate on ice:

1. 28 µL of DEPC water.
2. 5 µL of 10X Cleavage Buffer.
3. 5 µL of 2-5A or H_2O (as control; *see* **Note 6**).
4. 5 µL of RNase L at 36 ng per µL (*see* **Note 7**)
5. 7 µL of 1 µ*M* FRET probe (*see* **Note 8**).
6. Perform reactions and determine fluorescence as in **Subheading 3.5**.

4. Notes

1. The reaction rate is temperature dependent and can be performed at higher temperatures to achieve more rapid results (e.g., 30–37°C).
2. The assay can also be performed in other platforms besides 96-well plates (384- or 1536-well plate).
3. Dilute RNase L in 1X Cleavage Buffer on day of use. Repeated cycles of freezing and thawing will lower activity of RNase L. Therefore, prepare many aliquots of RNase L for storage at –70°C.
4. To minimize photobleaching of 6-FAM during storage, the FRET probe should be stored in light protected, amber tubes (Fisher Scientific Co., cat. no. 05-408-125).
5. General precaution: always keep working place clean, use fresh disposable gloves, and change them frequently to avoid nuclease contamination.
6. Chemically modified 2-5A analog may be less potent than natural 2-5A (e.g., **Fig. 4**). Therefore, higher concentrations may be required to activate RNase L.
7. RNase L activity may vary between different preparations. Therefore, an RNase L dose curve should be performed with each preparation to determine optimal amount.
8. FRET RNA probe concentration should be optimized for newly synthesized probe. To optimize, keep concentrations of RNase L and 2-5A constant, and use different concentrations of FRET probe between 50 n*M* and 500 n*M*. Include controls with no RNase L or with RNase L but without 2-5A. Select the concentration producing the highest fluorescence signal after reaction. Excessive probe may result in high background and reduced signal-to-noise ratio. The expected signal-to-noise ratio is about 15:1.

Acknowledgments

This work was supported by US Department of Defense Grant W81XWH-04-1-0055 (to R.H.S).

References

1. Zhou, A., Hassel, B. A., and Silverman, R. H. (1993) Expression cloning of 2-5A-dependent RNAase: a uniquely regulated mediator of interferon action. *Cell* **72**, 753–765.
2. Kerr, I. M. and Brown, R. E. (1978). pppA2'p5'A2'p5'A: an inhibitor of protein synthesis synthesized with an enzyme fraction from interferon-treated cells. *Proc. Natl. Acad. Sci. USA* **75**, 256–260.
3. Kubota, K., Nakahara, K., Ohtsuka, T., Yoshida, S., Kawaguchi, J. Fujita, Y., et al. (2004) Identification of 2'-phosphodiesterase, which plays a role in the 2-5A system regulated by interferon. *J. Biol. Chem.* **279**, 37,832–37,834.
4. Dong, B. and Silverman, R. H. (1997) A bipartite model of 2-5A-dependent RNase L. *J. Biol. Chem.* **272**, 22,236–22,242.
5. Li, G., Xiang, Y., Sabapathy, K., and Silverman, R. H. (2004) An apoptotic signaling pathway in the interferon antiviral response mediated by RNase L and c-Jun NH2-terminal kinase. *J. Biol. Chem.* **279**, 1123–1131.
6. Carpten, J., Nupponen, N., Isaacs, S., Sood, R., Robbins, C., Xu, J. et al. (2002) Germline mutations in the ribonuclease L (RNase L) gene in hereditary prostate cancer 1(HPC1)-linked families. *Nat. Genet.* **30**, 181–184.
7. Silverman, R. H. (2003) Implications for RNase L in prostate cancer biology. *Biochemistry* **42**, 1805–1812.
8. Dong, B. and Silverman, R. H. (1995) 2-5A-dependent RNase molecules dimerize during activation by 2-5A. *J. Biol. Chem.* **270**, 4133–4137.
9. Cole, J. L., Carroll, S. S., and Kuo, L. C. (1996) Stoichiometry of 2',5' oligoadenylate-induced dimerization of ribonuclease L. A sedimentation equilibrium study. *J. Biol. Chem.* **271**, 3979–3981.
10. Wreschner, D. H., McCauley, J. W., Skehel, J. J., and Kerr, I. M. (1981) Interferon action—sequence specificity of the ppp(A2'p)nA-dependent ribonuclease. *Nature* **289**, 414–417.
11. Floyd-Smith, G., Slattery, E., and Lengyel, P. (1981) Interferon action: RNA cleavage pattern of a (2'-5')oligoadenylate—dependent endonuclease. *Science* **212**, 1030–1032.
12. Wreschner, D. H., James, T. C., Silverman, R. H., and Kerr, I. M. (1981) Ribosomal RNA cleavage, nuclease activation and 2-5A(ppp(A2'p)nA) in interferon-treated cells. *Nucleic Acids Res.* **9**, 1571–1581.
13. Silverman, R. H., Skehel, J. J., James, T. C. (1983) Wreschner DH, Kerr IM. (1983) rRNA cleavage as an index of ppp(A2'p)nA activity in interferon-treated encephalomyocarditis virus-infected cells. *J. Virol.* **46**, 1051–1055.
14. Xiang, Y., Wang, Z., Murakami, J., Plummer, S., Klein, E. A., Carpten, J. D., et al. (2003) Effects of RNase L mutations associated with prostate cancer on apoptosis induced by 2',5' oligoadenylates. *Cancer Res.* **63**, 6795–6801.
15. Dong, B., Xu, L., Zhou, A., Hassel, B. A., Lee, X., Torrence, P. F., and Silverman, R. H. (1994) Intrinsic molecular activities of the interferon-induced 2-5A-dependent RNase. *J. Biol. Chem.* **269**, 14,153–14,158.

16. Carroll, S. S., Chen, E., Viscount, T., Geib, J., Sardana, M. K., Gehman, J., and Kuo, L. C. (1996) Cleavage of oligoribonucleotides by the 2',5' oligoadenylate-dependent ribonuclease L. *J. Biol. Chem.* **271**, 4988–4992.
17. Geselowitz, D. A., Cramer, H., Wondrak, E. M., Player, M. R., and Torrence, P. F. (2000) Fluorescence resonance energy transfer analysis of RNase L-catalyzed oligonucleotide cleavage. *Antisense Nucleic Acid Drug Dev.* **10**, 45–51.
18. Nakanishi, M., Yoshimura, A., Ishida, N., Ueno, Y., and Kitade, Y. (2004) Contribution of Tyr712 and Phe716 to the activity of human RNase L. *Eur. J. Biochem.* **271**, 2737–2744.
19. Silverman, R. H., Dong, B., Maitra, R. K., Player, M. R., and Torrence, P. F. (2000) Selective RNA cleavage by isolated RNase L activated with 2-5A antisense chimeric oligonucleotides. *Methods Enzymol.* **313**, 522–533.
20. Hartmann, R., Justesen, J., Sarkar, S. N., Sen, G. C., and Yee, V. C. (2003) Crystal structure of the 2'-specific and double-stranded RNA-activated interferon-induced antiviral protein 2'-5'-oligoadenylate synthetase. *Mol. Cell.* **12**, 1173–1185.
21. Rusch, L., Dong, B., and Silverman, R. H. (2001) Monitoring activation of ribonuclease L by 2',5' oligoadenylates using purified recombinant enzyme and intact malignant glioma cells. *Methods Enzymol.* **342**, 10–20.

8

Regulation of Murine Interferon Regulatory Factor Gene Expression in the Central Nervous System Determined by Multiprobe RNase Protection Assay

Shalina S. Ousman and Iain L. Campbell

Summary

Despite a key role in the regulation of interferon (IFN) gene expression and in mediating many downstream actions of the IFNs, the regulation of IFN regulatory factor (IRF) gene expression in the normal and pathological central nervous system and, indeed, other tissues, is poorly defined. We sought to examine the expression and regulation of the IRF genes in a number of different murine models for immune- or virally induced central nervous system disease. Here, we describe the development of a multiprobe RNase protection assay that permits the simultaneous detection and quantification of IRF ribonucleic acid transcripts for multiple family members in murine cells and tissues.

Key Words: Central nervous system; experimental autoimmune encephalomyelitis; interferon; interferon regulatory factor; lymphocytic choriomeningitis virus; RNase protection assay; transgenic mouse.

1. Introduction

After exposure to potentially harmful infectious agents such as viruses, cells initially respond by producing a spectrum of inflammatory mediators in a coordinated effort to decrease dissemination of the foreign agent(s). Among these mediators are the interferons (IFNs), a group of cytokines that form one of the earliest lines of defense during pathological conditions such as viral infection by promoting an antiviral state in uninfected cells, apoptosis of virally infected cells, and coordinating the innate and adaptive arms of antiviral immune response *(1,2)*. However, increased production of IFNs also is associated with the development and progression of a number of diseases such as multiple sclerosis *(3,4)*, insulin-dependent diabetes mellitus *(5)*, and Aicardi–Goutières syndrome *(6)*. Therefore, it is essential to tightly regulate and limit interferon production to protect against possible detrimental actions of this cytokine.

The regulation of IFN synthesis and many downstream actions of the IFNs are mediated by the IFN regulatory factors (IRFs), a family of transcription factors that are produced by a variety of cells and tissues (for reviews, *see* **refs. 7,8**). There are 10 mammalian IRF family members (IRFs 1–10) along with a number of viral forms *(7–9)*. IRFs normally reside in the cytoplasm and after C-terminal phosphorylation (which, for some IRFs, e.g., IRF-3 *[10,11]* occurs in direct response to viral infection of the cell) translocate to the nucleus, where their N-terminal binds to a specific deoxyribonucleic acid (DNA) sequence, 5'-AANNGAAA-3', called the IFN-stimulatory response element, to induce transcription of a number of genes, including IFN-α and IFN-β *(7,8)*. IRFs enable amplification of the peripheral antiviral response through a positive feedback mechanism that involves not only their regulation of IFNs, but their inducibility by IFNs themselves. More specifically, early during viral invasion certain IRFs such as IRF-3 are activated directly by viruses and induce the expression of a number of IFNs including IFN-β and IFN-α4. These cytokines then induce the transcription and translation of another IRF, IRF-7, which proceeds to promote the transcription of other IFN-α genes *(12,13)*. Despite the essential role of IRFs in regulating IFN expression and mediating certain downstream actions of IFNs during viral infection, the role of IRFs in the normal and pathological central nervous system (CNS) is largely unknown. To begin to address this problem, we set about to examine the expression and regulation of the IRF genes in a number of different animal models for immune- or virally induced CNS diseases. To accomplish this objective, it was necessary first to develop the analytical approaches that would allow the detection of IRF gene expression. For this purpose, we chose the RNase protection assay (RPA) method.

RPA allows for the detection and quantification of multiple RNA transcripts in cells and tissues using custom-made multiprobe RPA sets *(14)*. This approach has a number advantages compared with other RNA detection methods, such as northern blot analysis or reverse transcription-polymerase chain reaction (RT-PCR). These include high sensitivity and specificity, small sample requirement, easy quantification, rapid and simultaneous analysis of multiple target transcripts, high-throughput analysis and construction, and use of custom-made probe sets. In this procedure, target RNA [poly (A)$^+$ or total] is incubated with excess radioisotopic-labeled antisense single-stranded RNA as probe leading to the formation of stable double stranded RNA:RNA hybrids. The excess probe is then removed by digestion with single-strand-specific RNase. RNA probes that formed a duplex with complementary messenger RNA targets are "protected" from digestion. These protected hybrids are subsequently denatured and separated using standard polyacrylamide gel electrophoresis. The separated protected probes can then be visualized using routine autoradiography. The protocols discussed here will encompass 1) the design, and 2) con-

Regulation of IRF Gene Expression in CNS 117

struction of an IRF multiprobe RPA set, and 3) the RPA method for the analysis of IRF expression in the CNS in different viral and immune states.

2. Materials

Listed in this heading are the reagents we routinely use along with their commercial suppliers. These suppliers are not exclusive and reagents can be purchased from many other reputable manufacturers.

1. 100 mM dATP (cat. no. U120A), 100 mM dUTP (cat. no. U123A), 100 mM dCTP (cat. no. U122A), 100 mM dGTP (cat. no. U121A), 10X T4 ligase buffer (cat. no. C126B), T4 polynucleotide kinase, 10 U/µL (cat. no. M410A), T4 Ligase, 3 U/µL (cat. no. M180A), pGEM-4Z (cat. no. P2161), 5X transcription buffer (30 mM MgCl$_2$, 50 mM NaCl, 10 mM spermidine, 200 mM Tris-pH 7.9, cat. no. P118B), 10 mM rATP (cat. no. P113B), 10 mM rUTP (cat. no. P116B), 10 mM rCTP (cat. no. P114B), 10 mM rGTP (cat. no. P115B), T7 RNA polymerase 20 U/µL (cat. no. P207B), RNasin, 40 U/µL (cat. no. N211A), DNase-1, 1 U/µL (cat. no. M610A), and 100 mM dithiothreitol (DTT; cat. no. P117B, Promega, Madison, WI).
2. 10X PCR buffer (cat. no. y02028), Taq polymerase, 5 U/µL (cat. no. 18036-042), 1 kb ladder, 1 µg/µL (cat. no. 10787-018), *Eco*R1, 10 U/µL (cat. no. 15202-021), *Hind*III, 10 U/µL (cat. no. 15207-012), 10X restriction enzyme buffer, 50 mM MgCl$_2$ (cat. no. y02016), SUPERSCRIPT II RNase H reverse transcriptase (cat. no. 18064-014), 5X First Strand Buffer (cat. no. y00146), 0.1 M DTT (cat. no. y00147), Oligo d(T) primer (12–18 mer, no. 40-0012), and competent bacteria (DH5α, cat. no. 18258-012, Invitrogen, Carlsbad, CA)
3. 5'-[α-^{32}P] UTP (3000 Ci/mmol, 10 mCi/mL, cat. no. PB 10203, Amersham Biosciences Corp., Piscataway, NJ).
4. Tris-saturated phenol–chloroform (cat. no. 100997, Roche, Indianapolis, IN).
5. SeaKem ME agarose and SeaPlaque GTG low melt agarose (FMC Bioproducts, Rockland, ME).
6. 6X DNA loading buffer: 0.208% bromphenol blue, 0.208% xylene cyanol FF, and 25% glycerol in water. Aliquot and store at –20°C.
7. 1X TE: 10 mM Tris-HCL, 1 mM ethylene diamine tetraacetic acid (EDTA), pH 8.3.
8. SOC medium: add 31 g of SOC powder (Bio 101, Vista, CA) to 1 L of milliQ (mQ) H$_2$O. Autoclave and store at room temperature.
9. Ampicillin plates: add 36 g of LB Agar and 15 g of agarose to 1 L of mQH$_2$O. Autoclave and cool. Add 2 mL of ampicillin, mix, and quickly pour into Petri dishes. Allow to polymerize, cover plates, wrap in foil, and store at 4°C.
10. RNase A (1 mg/mL, cat. no. 2272, Ambion Inc., Austin, TX).
11. Ribonuclease T1 (1188 U/µL, cat. no. R1003, Sigma, St. Louis, MO).
12. RNase buffer (25 mL): mix 250 µL of 1 M Tris, pH 7.5, 1.5 mL of 5 M NaCl, 250 µL of 0.5 M EDTA, pH 8.0, and 23 mL of double dionized (dd) H2O. Immediately before use, add the following to 5 mL of RNase buffer (for 25 samples): 5 µL of RNase A (1 mg/mL) and 1 µL of RNase T1 (125 U/mL).

13. RNase-free yeast tRNA: Dilute RNase-free yeast tRNA (cat. no. 109525, Roche, Indianapolis, IN) in sterile, Rnase-free TE at a concentration of 2 mg/mL. Store in 1-mL aliquots at −20°C. Yeast tRNA obtained from other sources can be made RNAse free by repeated phenol/chloroform extraction.
14. 10% sodium dodecyl sulfate (SDS): Add 10 g of SDS to 100 mL sterile mQH$_2$O.
15. Proteinase K stock 10 mg/mL: Resuspend proteinase K (cat. no. P6556, Sigma, St. Louis, MO) to a concentration of 10 mg/mL in sterile mQH$_2$O. Store 1-mL aliquots at −20°C, where they are very stable.
16. Proteinase K working solution: Make up fresh, for 20 samples: 235 µL of ddH$_2$O, 155 µL of 10% SDS, 30 µL of 10 mg/mL proteinase K, and 30 µL of 2 mg/mL yeast tRNA.
17. RPA hybridization buffer (HB; 5X stock solution): 200 mM PIPES (disodium salt of piperazine-N,N'-bis(2-ethanesulfonic acid, pH 6.4), 2 M NaCl, and 5 mM EDTA. Working solution: 4 parts formamide, 1 part 5X stock. Aliquot and store at 4°C. Stable for approx 6 mo if kept in the dark.
18. RPA loading buffer: Mix 80% formamide, 10 mM EDTA (disodium salt of ethylene diamine tetraacetic acid; pH 8.0), 1 mg/mL xylene cyanol FF, and 1 mg/mL bromophenol blue. Store in 1-mL aliquots at −20°C.
19. 10X TBE: mix together 1.3 M Trizma-base, pH 8.0; 450 mM boric acid, and 25 mM EDTA. Dilute to 1X TBE using sterile mQH$_2$O.
20. 5% Acrylamide mix (1 L): dissolve 420.4 g of urea (7 M) in 500 mL of H$_2$O and 50 mL 10X TBE on a heat plate. Add 125 mL 40% acrylamidebis (19:1) and adjust volume to 1 L of with mQH$_2$O. Filter (0.45 µm), wrap in foil and store at 4°C. Stable for 2 to 3 mo.
21. 10% ammonium persulfate: Prepare fresh in sterile mQH$_2$O.
22. "Rain X" (Unelko Corp., Scottsdale, AZ) can be obtained from general automobile supply stores. However, other siliconizing products may also be used.
23. Sequencing gel apparatus: Standard sequencing gel apparatus with 0.5-mm spacers can be used as long as the length (recommended minimum 30 cm from bottom well) is adequate for good separation of the protected fragments. It is necessary to use square bottom wells rather than standard nucleotide sequencing combs.

3. Methods

3.1. Design of RPA Probe Sets

Before construction of the RPA probe set can be undertaken, it is first necessary to decide upon which genes are to be analyzed and against which probes will be generated and then subsequently, design the probe set. For each gene selected, the DNA sequence is then obtained from genomic database sources, such as the NCBI Entrez Nucleotide database (http://www.ncbi.nlm.nih.gov/entrez/query.fcgi?db=Nucleotide), and the target sequence is determined for the corresponding probe to be generated. A number of factors need to be considered in this exercise. First, optimal separation of the RNA protected hybrids by polyacrylamide gel electrophoresis (*see* **Subheading 3.3.2.**) is achieved over a probe size range of approx 80 to 400 bp. Second, increasingly wider separation of the protected RNA hybrids within the gel occurs with descending size. Therefore, the difference in size between individual probes needs to be increased with increasing size of the probe. Third, it helps to have some information as to the tissue expression levels of each of the genes to be targeted in the RPA. As a general rule, genes with low expression are assigned a larger size probe than those that are expressed abundantly. It should be noted that in the case of abundant targets, there sometimes can be smaller breakdown products that are generated that can interfere with or obscure other protected fragments for shorter length probes in the set. For quantification and quality control it is necessary to include one probe against a "housekeeping" gene. For this purpose we routinely use a probe to the ribosomal protein gene RPL-32 *(15)*. Because such housekeeping genes are usually expressed at high levels it is advisable to make the length of their probes the shortest in the set.

The probes should be directed against unique sequences in the messenger RNA for the gene of interest, and this should be established by comparing the sequences of gene families and other related molecules. This can be done by using sequence alignment programs available on the internet and from other sources. We routinely use BLAST (http://www.ncbi.nlm.nih.gov/cgi-bin/BLAST/nph-blast), which is an efficient, easy-to-use sequence analyzing program. The specificity of the RPA is absolute and requires 100% sequence identity between the probe and the target RNA. Therefore, problems also can arise if the target gene is part of homologous gene family (e.g., as is the case with IFN-α). In this situation varying degrees of sequence homology between the probe and these additional targets give rise, in addition to the authentic protected fragment, to the generation of multiple smaller RNase protected fragments. In such cases it is advisable to run only a limited probe set containing the probe for the gene of interest and the housekeeping probe. Finally, when designing the individual probes it is critical that the selected target sequence does not contain restriction enzyme sites that will be used in the cloning of the synthesized probe fragments (*see* **Subheading 3.2.6.**). Given all the preceding considerations, a probe set was designed for the murine IRFs as shown in **Table 1**.

3.2. Construction of RPA Probe Set

The initial step involves synthesis of the probe template from RNA using reverse transcriptase-polymerase chain reaction (RT-PCR) or if available, directly from the cloned complementary DNA (cDNA) using PCR (*see* **Notes 1 and 2**).

Table 1
Design Features of the Murine IRF Multiprobe RPA Set

No.	Gene	Size (protected)	Target sequence	Genbank No.
1.	IRF-7	285	481–766	U73037
2.	IRF-6	250	301–551	U73029
3.	IRF-5	225	61–286	AF028725
4.	IRF-3	185	4–568 (exonic)	AF036341
5.	IRF-9/p48	150	481–631	U51992
6.	IRF-2	130	431–561	J03168
7.	IRF-1	115	211–326	M21065
8.	L32	78	61–139	K02061

3.2.1. Preparation of RT: (First-Strand cDNA Synthesis Using SUPERSCRIPT II)

Oligo d(T)$_{12\text{-}18}$ (500 µg/mL)	1 µL
Poly (A)$^+$ or total RNA	1.0 or 5.0 µg
Sterile H$_2$O to 12 µL	10 or 6 µL

Heat mixture to 70°C for 10 min and quick chill on ice. Collect the contents of the tube by brief centrifugation and add:

5X First Strand Buffer	4 µL
0.1 M DTT	2 µL
10 mM dNTP mix	1 µL

Mix gently and incubate at 42°C for 2 min. Add 1 µL of SUPERSCRIPT II and mix by pipetting gently up and down. Incubate at 42°C for 50 min. Terminate the reaction by heating at 70°C for 15 min. The cDNA can now be used as a template for amplification in PCR.

3.2.2. PCR

	µL	[Final]
PCR buffer (10X)	8	0.8 X
MgCl$_2$ (50 mM)	8	4 mM
mQ H$_2$O	53.5	
Taq polymerase (5U/µL)	0.5	0.025 U/µL
Total	70	

Then add:

	µL	[Final]
5′ primer (2 nM)	5	100 pM
3′ primer (2 nM)	5	100 pM
RT reaction product (from above)	20	

or

	µL	[Final]
cDNA template (0.5 ng/µL)	20	0.1 ng/µL

Carefully mix by vortexing. The reaction is performed in a thermocycler machine using the following linked programs: program 1: 94°C, 4 min; program 2: 94°C, 30 s, 55°C, 40 s, 72°C, 1 min for 35 cycles; program 3: 72°C, 5 min; program 4: 4°C, hold.

After PCR, perform a diagnostic agarose gel electrophoresis to confirm for correct fragment size and concentration (*see* **Note 3**). Remove 20 µL of the PCR mix and run on a standard 2 to 3% ME agarose gel containing 0.002% ethidium bromide. Run gel approximately one-third the way and photograph under ultraviolet (UV) light. Select the tube that contains the greatest amount of product of the correct size and proceed as follows.

3.2.3. Chloroform Extraction

1. To the remaining 80 µL of PCR mixture, add 100 µL of H_2O and 20 µL of 3 M sodium acetate.
2. Vortex and then add 180 µL of chloroform.
3. Vortex again to an emulsion, centrifuge for 1 min at maximum speed at room temperature, and carefully remove the aqueous (upper) phase.
4. Add 600 µL of 100% ethanol. Mix by inverting tube and freeze in dry ice for 20 min.
5. Thaw and centrifuge for 30 min at 800g at 4°C.
6. Carefully remove the supernatant with a pipet and air-dry the pellet. Dissolve the pellet thoroughly in 8 µL of H_2O by vortexing.

3.2.4. End-Ligation and EcoR1/HindIII Digestion

1. To facilitate efficient restriction enzyme digestion of the PCR DNA fragments, an end-ligation reaction is performed. Set up the following reaction:

	µL	[Final]
PCR mix	8	
T4 ligase buffer (10X)	1.0	1X
T4 polynucleotide kinase (10 U/µL)	0.5	0.5 U/µL

2. Incubate for 20 min at 37°C, then add:

	µL	[Final]
T4 ligase (3U/µL)	0.5	0.15 U/µL

3. Incubate for 20 min at 37°C and then heat inactivate for 15 min at 72°C. Briefly spin and add the following to the end-ligation reaction mix to perform the restriction enzyme digestion reaction:

	µL	[Final]
(end-ligation mix)	(10)	
Restriction enzyme buffer (10X)	3	1X
EcoR1 (12 U/µL)	1.5	0.6 U/µL
HindIII (10 U/µL)	1.5	0.5 U/µL
H_2O	14	

4. In parallel with this reaction, set up a restriction enzyme digestion of the pGEM-4Z transcription vector as follows:

pGEM-4Z plasmid (1 µg/µL)	10	333 ng/µL
Restriction enzyme buffer (10X)	3	1X
EcoR1 (12 U/µL)	1.5	0.6 U/µL
HindIII (10 U/µL)	1.5	0.5 U/µL
H$_2$O	14	

5. Incubate both reactions for 1 h at 37°C, then add 5 µL of 6X DNA loading buffer.

3.2.5. Gel Purification of EcoR1/HindIII Digested PCR Fragment and pGEM-4Z Vector

1. Prepare a 1% ME agarose gel containing 0.002% ethidium bromide. Load samples and run gel at 100 V until leading dye front has run approximately one-fourth to one-third of the way.
2. Visualize gel under UV illumination and photograph. Carefully cut out a block of gel in front of each fragment band using a clean razor-blade.
3. Place gel in cold room and fill cut out wells with 0.8% low-melt gel. In addition, to sample lanes, a block of gel is also removed and the well refilled with low-melt gel from a non-sample loaded lane which will serve as a control gel fragment.
4. After polymerization, run gel again until DNA fragment has migrated into the middle of the low-melt gel.
5. Visualize under UV-illumination and cut out DNA band as well as control gel, trim the excess gel from band and transfer fragments to labeled 1.5-mL microfuge tubes.

3.2.6. Cloning EcoR1/HindIII Gel Fragments in pGEM-4Z

1. For ligation of the fragments in pGEM-4Z, melt gel fragments for 15 min at 72°C, and set up the following ligation reactions:

(i)	µL	(ii)	µL	(iii)	µL
pGEM-4Z gel	1	pGEM-4Z gel	1	pGEM-4Z gel	1
PCR gel fragment	5	Control gel fragment	5	Control gel fragment	5
5X T4 ligase buffer	6	5X T4 ligase buffer	6	5X T4 ligase buffer	6
T4 ligase	1	T4 ligase	1	T4 ligase	0
H$_2$O	17	H$_2$O	17	H$_2$O	17

2. Vortex mixtures and incubate for 2 h at 37°C. Heat for 10 min at 72°C to melt gel, vortex mix, and remove 2 µL for transformation of 25 µL of competent bacteria (XL-2Blue; Stratagene, San Diego, CA).
3. Thaw and prepare bacteria on ice according to the manufacturer's instructions.
4. Place 25 µL of bacterial suspension into a 15-mL snap-cap polypropylene tube.

5. Pipet 2 µL of DNA gel into bacteria and mix *gently*.
6. Incubate on ice for 30 min and then heat shock in a 42°C water bath for 35 s.
7. Add 1 mL of SOC medium and incubate in a 37°C shaker for 1 h.
8. Spin at 1500 rpm for 10 min and carefully remove the supernatant leaving approx 100 µL behind.
9. Resuspend bacteria by gently pipetting and plate on an ampicillin agar plate (equilibrate plate to room temperature before plating bacteria). Incubate plates upside down at 37°C overnight. This should give the following result:

	(i)	(ii)	(iii)
Number of colonies	+++	+/–	–

10. Pick six colonies from plate (i) and perform DNA minipreps using standard methods to confirm insertion of the PCR fragment using *Eco*R1/*Hind*III digestion of miniprep DNA (*see* **Note 4**). Retain an aliquot of each bacterial suspension and store at 4°C pending DNA maxiprep. After confirmation, select a positive DNA clone containing the *Eco*R1/*Hind*III PCR fragment and grow up the bacteria for a DNA maxiprep. The plasmid DNA is now ready for further manipulation.

3.2.7. Linearization of Cloned pGEM-4 Constructs

Set up two restriction enzyme reactions as follows:

	µL	[Final]
Cloned pGEM-4 plasmid (12 µg)	~12	0.12 µg//µL
Restriction enzyme buffer (10X)	10	1X
*Eco*R1 or *Hind*III	6	~ 0.7 U/µL
H$_2$O to	100 µL	

1. Incubate for a minimum of 2 h at 37°C. Remove 1 µL of reaction mix for gel analysis to confirm linearization. To the remaining digest, add 20 µL of 3 *M* sodium acetate, 80 µL of TE, and mix.
2. Add 200 µL of Tris-saturated phenol–chloroform and vortex to an emulsion.
3. Centrifuge at maximum speed for 10 min and remove the aqueous phase.
4. Re-extract the aqueous phase with 180 µL of chloroform. Transfer the aqueous phase to a sterile tube and add 3 volumes (600 µL) of 100% ethanol.
5. Mix and freeze in dry ice for 20 min.
6. Thaw, centrifuge at 800*g* for 20 min at 4°C, wash pellet in 100 µL of 80% ethanol, and recentrifuge.
7. Dry pellet and solubilize in 20 µL of sterile, RNase-free 1X TE.
8. Determine the concentration of the linearized plasmid by spectrophotometry at 260 nm using a 1:50 dilution of the plasmid in sterile H$_2$O. The concentration should be 0.3 to 0.6 µg/µL. To confirm linearization, run a 0.8% diagnostic ME agarose gel electrophoresis using the 1 µL aliquot that was removed after the enzyme digestion.

3.2.8. Preparation of RPA Probe Set

1. Dilute the purified *Eco*R1 linearized DNA (previously prepared) to give a working solution of 150 ng/μL. To prepare a 150 ng/μL solution, apply the following formula:

    Dil = (linearized DNA μg/μL × 1000)/150.

    The individual linearized plasmids can then be combined to generate the probe set. The linearized plasmids are added to RNase-free TE such that the final dilution for each gives a concentration of 15 ng/μL (*see* **Notes 5** and **6**).
2. After addition of each of the components, mix the probe set and store almost indefinitely at –70°C in a sealed microfuge tube.

3.2.9. Synthesis and Purification of Sense Target RNA

1. Set up the following transcription reaction:

	μL	[Final]
Transcription buffer (5x)	20	1X
DTT (100 mM)	10	10 mM
RNasin (40 U/μL)	1.0	0.4 U/μL
rATP, rCTP, rGTP, UTP (each 2.5 mM)	20	0.5 mM
HindIII linearized DNA template (0.5 μg/μL)	10	0.05 U/μL
SP6 RNA polymerase (20 U/μL)	2.0	0.4 U/μL
H$_2$O	37	

2. Incubate at 37°C for 90 min, then add:

	μL	[Final]
RQ 1 DNase (2 U/μL)	3.0	0.06 U/μL

    Incubate at 37°C for 30 min
3. To purify the sense RNA, add 100 μLl of Tris-saturated phenol:chloroform and extract.
4. Centrifuge for 5 min at 800g and carefully remove the aqueous phase.
5. Re-extract aqueous phase with an equal volume of chloroform and centrifuge as above.
6. Remove aqueous phase into a new tube, add 20 μL of 3 M ammonium acetate and 600 μL of 100% ethanol and freeze in dry ice for 20 min.
7. Centrifuge for 20 min at 800g at 4°C.
8. Wash the pellet with 150 μL of 80% ethanol and centrifuge again for 10 min at 800g at 4°C.
9. Air-dry the pellet and add 50 μL of RNase-free TE.
10. Determine the concentration of the RNA by UV spectroscopy at A260 nm.

3.2.10. Preparation of Sense Target Set

1. The final concentration of each sense target RNA in the set is 2 pg/μL. The dilution to achieve this should be in the order of 1: 250,000 > 500,000.

2. Prepare stock solutions of the sense RNA transcripts to give a concentration of 40 pg/µL and then combine each corresponding sense RNA to give a final concentration of 2 pg/µL for each.
3. Store in small (5-µL) aliquots at –70°C (*see* **Note 6**).

3.3. RNase Protection Assay (RPA)

3.3.1. Radioisotopic Probe Labeling (see **Notes 7 and 8**)

1. Add the following to a 1.5-mL sterile microfuge tube:

[^{32}P]UTP (3000 Ci/mmol; 10 mCi/mL)	10 µL
GACU pool (GAC:2.75 mM each; U:61 µM)	1 µL
DTT (100 mM)	2 µL
5X transcription buffer	4 µL
RPA template set	1 µL
RNasin (40 U/µL)	0.8 µL
T7 Polymerase (20 U/µL)	1 µL

    Mix by gently pipetting or flicking the tube and quick spin in a microfuge tube. Incubate at 37°C for 1 h.
2. Terminate reaction by adding 2 µL of DNase I (~1 U/µL). Mix by gently flicking and quick spin in a microfuge tube. Incubate at 37°C for 30 min.
3. Add in order:

20 mM EDTA, pH 8.0	26 µL
Tris-saturated phenol–chloroform	50 µL
Yeast tRNA (2 µg/µL)	2 µL

    Vortex for 30 s and centrifuge at 800g for 5 min at room temperature.
4. Transfer the aqueous phase (top) to a new tube. Add 50 µL of chloroform, vortex, and centrifuge again at 800g for 5 min at room temperature.
5. Transfer the aqueous phase to a new 1.5-mL microfuge tube and add 50 µL of 4 M ammonium acetate and 250 µL of ice-cold 100% ethanol. Invert several times and incubate for 15 min in dry ice. Microcentrifuge for 15 min at 800g at 4°C.
6. Remove the supernatant carefully and add 100 µL of ice-cold 90% ethanol to the pellet. Microfuge again at 800g for 5 min at 4°C.
7. Carefully remove the entire supernatant and dry the pellet. Add 50 µL of hybridization buffer to the pellet and solubilize by gently vortexing for 20 s and quick microfuge.
8. Quantify 1 µL of the labeled probe and store the rest of the probe at –20°C.

3.3.2. Hybridization

1. Aliquot desired amount of RNA to 1.5-mL sterile tubes. A good starting concentration is 1 µg of poly (A+) RNA or 5 µg of total RNA (*see* **Note 9**). As a positive control an additional tube can be included containing 1 µL of the sense RNA mix. Dry RNA samples in a vacuum evaporator (no heat). As a negative control include an additional tube containing no RNA (*see* **Note 10**).

2. Add in order to the RNA containing and negative control tubes:

Hybridization buffer	8 µL
Diluted labeled probe (250,000 dpm/µL)	2 µL

    Vortex the tubes gently for 1 to 2 min to solubilize RNA. Add one drop of mineral oil and quick centrifuge. Transfer the tubes to a heat block set at 95°C and immediately set the temperature to 56°C and incubate overnight (*see* **Note 11**).
3. RNase treatment: Remove the tubes from the heating block and equilibrate to room temperature. Set the heat block temperature to 95°C. To the tubes, add 100 µL of RNase buffer containing RNase A and RNase T1 to each tube. Mix gently by low-speed vortexing. Briefly centrifuge and incubate for 45 min at 32°C water bath.
4. Proteinase K treatment: After incubation at 32°C, carefully transfer the reaction mix (lower phase) to a new tube containing 18 µL of proteinase K working solution (*see* **Notes 12** and **13**). Mix the RNase and Proteinase K mixture by low speed vortexing, briefly centrifuge and incubate for 15 min in a 37°C water bath.
5. Purification and precipitation: after proteinase K digestion, add 150 µL of 1:1 Tris-saturated phenol:chloroform. Vortex vigorously for 30 s and centrifuge at 800*g* for 5 min at room temperature (*see* **Note 14**). Transfer the aqueous phase to a new tube containing 120 µL of 4 *M* ammonium acetate and 650 µL of 100% ethanol. Invert tubes several times and incubate on dry ice for 20 min. Centrifuge at 800*g* at 4°C for 20 min. Carefully remove and discard the supernatant and wash pellet in 100 µL of ice-cold 80% ethanol. Recentrifuge at 800*g* for 5 min at 4°C. Carefully remove the supernatant and dry pellet completely in a vacuum evaporator (no heat). Add 4 µL of loading buffer to each sample. Include an additional tube and add the probe (6000 dpm). Vortex and briefly centrifuge. Incubate samples for 3 min at 95°C and then store on ice pending electrophoresis.
6. Gel electrophoresis: scrape the gel plates gently with a razor-blade to remove any residual acrylamide. Clean with dH$_2$O and wipe dry. Perform one final clean with 70% ethanol and wipe dry with Kim wipe tissues. Coat the short plate by buffing dry with Rain-X solution. Assemble plates and tape. For the gel mixture combine:

5% acrylamide	100 mL
10% ammonium persulfate	600 µL
TEMED	80 µL

7. Mix by swirling and pour into assembled gel plates being careful to avoid bubble formation. Clamp plates, insert appropriate comb and allow gel to polymerize for approximately 1 h. After polymerization remove the comb, insert gel into vertical electrophoresis apparatus, flush wells with 1X TBE and prerun at 50 Watts constant for at least 40 min. Carefully load the samples into the wells and run until the bromophenol blue dye reaches about 30 cm down from the bottom of the wells (*see* **Notes 15** to **18**). Carefully disassemble the gel plates by lifting up the coated (short) plate leaving the gel on the nontreated plate. Place a presized piece of Whatman filter paper on top of the gel and remove the gel. Place gel on gel drying apparatus, cover with plastic wrap and dry for 1 to 2 h. Once the gel is

Regulation of IRF Gene Expression in CNS

dry, place in an autoradiographic cassette and store at −70°C. Develop film to visualize and quantify the separated radioactive protected fragments (*see* **Note 19**).

4. Results and Conclusions

We used the multiprobe RNase protection assay to identify for IRF expression in the CNS during a variety of different inflammatory conditions (**Figs. 1, 2**) that included: intracranial lymphocytic choriomeningitis virus (LCMV) infection (**Fig. 1.**; *[17]*), experimental autoimmune encephalomyelitis (EAE; **Fig. 2A** *[18]*), and in transgenic mice that produced IFN-α (**Fig. 2B** *[19]*) or IL-12 (**Fig. 2C** *[20]*) constitutively in astrocytes.

In the normal CNS (d 0) several IRF genes, including IRF-2, -3, -5, -7, and -9, were constitutively expressed (**Fig. 1A,B**). However, after intracranial LCMV infection in wild-type (WT) mice, expression of the IRF-7 and IRF-9 genes was significantly upregulated by d 2 and remained elevated at d 6 after infection. At this latter time point a significant increase in IRF-5 RNA was also observed (**Fig. 1A,B**). We proceeded to investigate whether a similar profile in IRF gene expression and upregulation was evident in WT mice with myelin oligodendrocyte glycoprotein (MOG)-induced EAE. Indeed, a significant increase in IRF-5, -7, and -9 gene expression also was observed but only in animals that were symptomatic for EAE. The brains of presymptomatic (d 6 after immunization) and postsymptomatic (28 d after immunization) animals did not display a significant change in the expression of any of the IRF genes (**Fig. 2B**).

We also investigated IRF gene expression by RPA analysis in the brains of transgenic mice with astrocyte-targeted expression of the IFN-α and IL-12 genes. The expression of these two genes was driven by the astrocytic-specific promoter for glial fibrillary acidic protein (GFAP). These animals spontaneously exhibit motor deficits that are accompanied by robust inflammatory responses in their brains *(19,20)*. Interestingly, in two lines of IFN-α transgenic animals (GIFN12 and GIFN39), IRF-7 and IRF-9 genes were significantly increased in the brains of phenotypically normal mice compared with their WT counterparts (**Fig. 2A**). Because IFN-α is an inducer of IRFs, the chronic expression of this cytokine in the CNS of these transgenic animals likely mediated the persistent induction of IRF-7 and IRF-9 genes. In contrast to the IFN-α mice, in the IL-12 transgenic animals upregulation of IRF-5, IRF-7, and IRF-9 gene expression was only observed in IL-12 mice that exhibited neurological impairment and not in phenotypically normal animals (**Fig. 2C**). This indicates that IL-12 alone does not regulate cerebral IRF gene expression. It is likely that later infiltration of IFN-γ-producing immune cells into the CNS *(20)* mediates the upregulation of IRF gene expression observed in symptomic

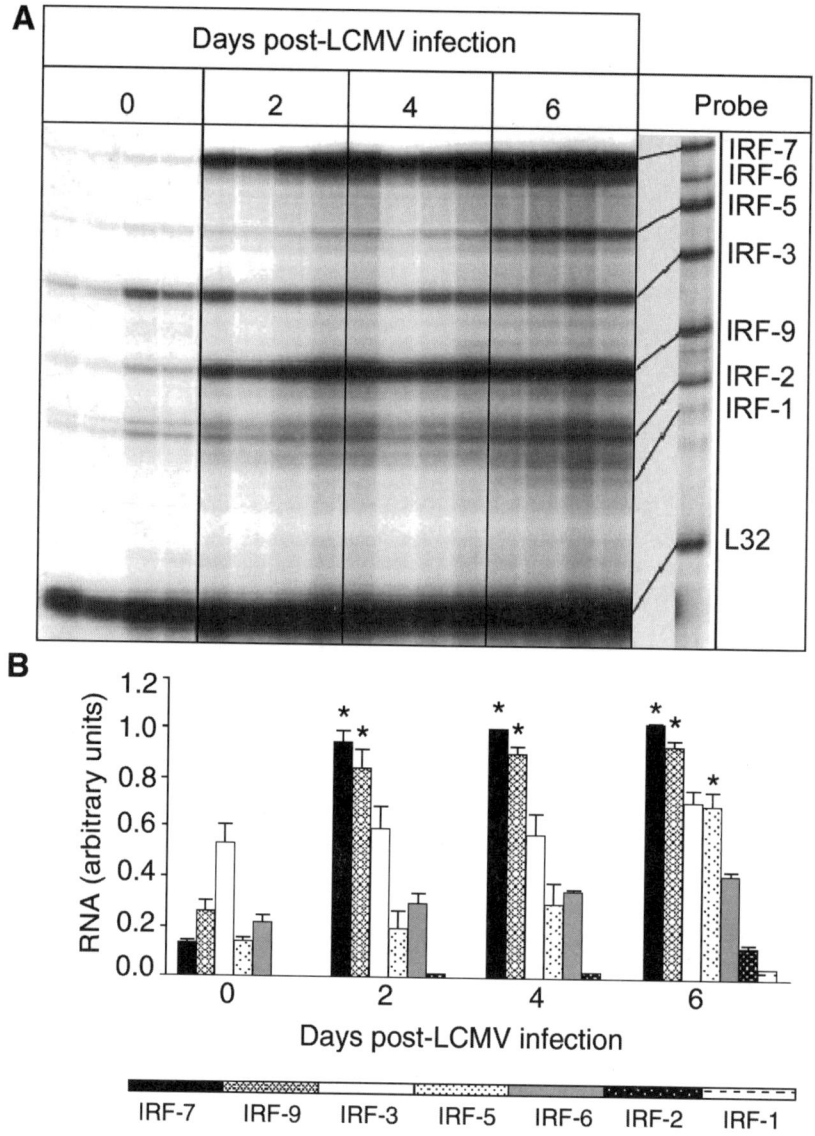

Fig. 1. Multiprobe RPA analysis of IRF gene expression in the brain of mice with LCMV. Adult mice were inoculated intracranially with LCMV-ARM53b as described previously *(17)* and at the times shown mice were euthanized and their brains removed for the isolation of poly (A+) RNA. For the RPA shown, 1 μg of poly (A+) RNA was used. (**A**) represents film autoradiography after a 3-d exposure whereas (**B**) represents densitometric quantification of the individual bands using NIH Image 1.63 software. This was calculated as a ratio of the densitometry of each IRF band relative to its corresponding L32 message. The average of the four samples per time point was then plotted for each IRF.

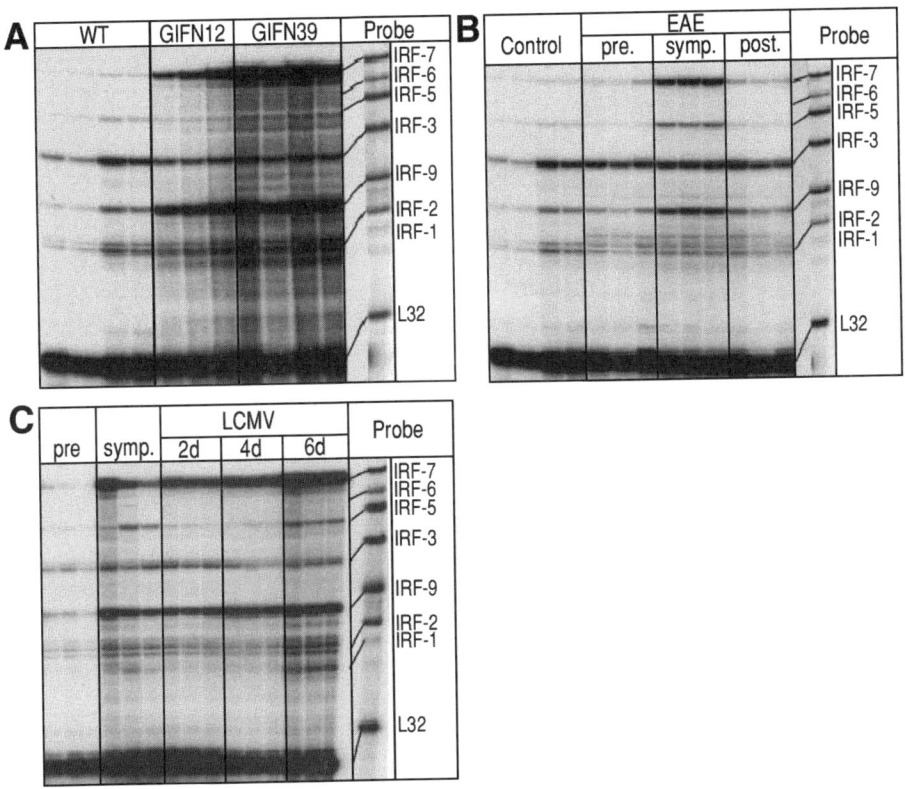

Fig. 2. (**A**) IRF gene expression in the brain of two lines of transgenic mice (GIFN) where the IFN-a gene is placed under control of the GFAP promoter in astrocytes *(19)*. GIFN12 and GIFN39 are low and high expresser lines, respectively. (**B**) IRF gene expression in the brains of mice with EAE. EAE is a mouse model for multiple sclerosis and was induced in C57BL6 mice by active immunization with myelin oligodendrocyte glycoprotein peptide as described previously *(18)*. RNA was isolated from the cerebellum of nonimmunized (Control) or immunized, presymptomatic (pre.; 6 d), symptomatic (symp.; 14 d), and postsymptomatic (post.; 28 d) mice. (**C**) IRF gene expression in the brain of GF-IL12 transgenic mice (GF-IL12 *[20]*) and after intracranial LCMV infection. The GF-IL12 mice chronically produce IL-12 in astrocytes as a result of the IL-12 gene placed under the control of the GFAP promoter. Some of the GF-IL12 mice spontaneously develop a motor deficit including ataxia and tremors. We analyzed for IRF gene expression in the brain of spontaneously sick GF-IL12 transgenic mice as well as presymptomatic GFIL-12 animals infected with LCMV.

IL-12 transgenic mice. When normal IL-12 animals were infected intracranially with LCMV a significant induction of IRF-7 and IRF-9 genes was observed by day 2 and maintained to day 6 post-infection. IRF-5 gene induction was also observed but only at 6d post-infection (**Fig. 2C**).

As illustrated here for the semiquantitative analysis of multiple IRF genes, the multi-probe RPA technique is versatile. It enables the simultaneous identification of multiple genes across a variety of experimental conditions within a single gel. Custom-made RPA probe sets also allow for detection of multiple gene family members within the same batch of RNA. Technically, the RPA method is relatively straightforward, results are obtained rapidly, within 3 d, from the radiolabeling of the probe to development of the autoradiograph. Thus, the RPA technique is a highly sensitive and specific method for multiple gene detection within a variety of tissues and cells.

5. Notes

1. The probe fragments are conveniently synthesized using PCR. After deciding upon the target sequence and length of the probes, upstream and downstream oligonucleotide primers have to be designed that commence with the 5' end of the target region of choice. To facilitate subsequent cloning into the plasmid vector (*see* below) the upstream and downstream primers should also include a 5' sequence extension incorporating a unique restriction enzyme recognition site that will allow directional cloning into the precut transcription vector. In the case of our own studies we routinely use EcoR1 and Hind III for this purpose, respectively. Probe cDNA synthesis can be accomplished by direct PCR using a cDNA clone from the gene of interest. If this is not available RT-PCR synthesis can be used to synthesize cDNA from cellular or tissue total or poly (A)+ RNA that is known to express the gene of interest.
2. To reduce variation in transcriptional efficiency, it is advisable to use the same plasmid vector for the cloning of each of the individual probes in the set. We routinely use the pGEM-4Z plasmid that has a multiple cloning sites containing *Eco*R1 and *Hind*III restriction enzyme recognition sites and allows for T7 and SP6 RNA polymerase-driven transcription. Other plasmid vectors also can be used as long as they contain flanking RNA polymerase promoters to the site of probe fragment insertion.
3. If the ligation reaction worked, a ladder of progressively fainter DNA fragments should be apparent when the gel is visualized under UV. Conversely, there should only be a single band after the *Eco*R1/*Hind*III digestion.
4. Once the probes of desired length have been cloned, they should be sequenced and their identity confirmed again using the BLAST program.
5. For most cases the final concentration of the probe for the labeling reaction should be 15 ng/µL. As an example, to make a probe set of final volume 20 µL, 2 µL of each diluted linearized plasmid (150 ng/µL) would be added. Clearly, only 10 individual probes could be combined in this set. For probe sets containing more than 10 components, the linearized plasmids above should be diluted to 300 ng/µL, thus giving a 1:20 dilution.
6. The diluted sense RNA target sets are not stable to repeated freeze thawing and degrade progressively with each cycle. It is recommended that these be stored in small aliquots at –70°C and used for no more than three to five cycles of freeze

thawing or until the appearance of the sense bands in the autoradiographs begins to deteriorate.

7. Because the RPA method entails the use of RNA, certain standard RNase free precautions should be taken. We recommend separation of all reagents used on the first and second days of the assay. (If care is taken to maintain RNase free technique at all times then separation of reagents is not necessary). All plastic ware (e.g., pipet tips, 1.5-mL Microfuge tubes, etc.) and glassware should also be autoclaved and powder free latex gloves should always be worn. We do not routinely treat solutions with DEPC.

8. Initially, both sensitivity and specificity of the RPA probes should be tested by titration against synthetic sense and target tissue RNA. This step is necessary to determine the sensitivity and specificity of the probe set as well as to determine that the probe is in excess of the target over a range of RNA concentrations. The potential for misidentification of the protected band increases with the number of probes in a given RPA. Therefore the correct identity of each protected band seen with the target RNA sample should be established by comparison with the corresponding protected sense RNA band as well as by incubating each probe individually with target RNA.

9. Either poly (A)+ RNA or total RNA can be used for target RNA. However, poly (A)+ RNA offers greater sensitivity for detection of more rare target RNA and gives a higher signal to background ratio. For poly (A)+ RNA isolation, the protocol of Badley et al. *(16)* is effective whereas for total RNA isolation, commercially available reagents such as TRIZOL (Gibco/BRL, Gaithersburg, MD) work well.

10. As a control for both the DNase and RNase digestion steps, a negative control sample should always be included in the assay. This sample is simply probe (diluted to the same concentration used for the target RNA samples) alone incubated in the hybridization buffer and subsequently processed in parallel with the target RNA containing samples. Following autoradiography the negative control lane should always appear completely clear. However, if bands appear, in our experience, it is most likely that these are attributable to incomplete digestion of the linearized probe DNA template by the DNase 1 resulting in the formation of DNA/RNA hybrids. Thus, these protected RNA probe hybrids will run with the same apparent molecular size as the probe alone. In this event discard the DNase and use a new batch. Additional bands in the negative control lane likely indicate inefficient RNase digestion. In these circumstances check RNase concentrations and incubation conditions and adjust if necessary.

11. Because the labeled probes are single-stranded RNA, they are very susceptible to chemical and physical degradation and deteriorate in quality and specific activity progressively. The probes should therefore be made fresh and used immediately (or within 24 h). The amount of probe to add to the hybridization reaction is calculated on the basis of 500 CPM/µL/UTP residue in the probe set. The number of UTPs per probe present in the RPA set therefore should be determined (for example, a probe with 100 UTP residues would be diluted to 5×10^4 CPM/µL). Before hybridization, count the freshly made probe and dilute accordingly.

12. When taking the aqueous solution from under the oil it is important to completely avoid the mineral oil because it may interfere with the subsequent purification steps. Setting the pipet to approx 105 µL will prevent any uptake of mineral oil.
13. It is convenient to use the time during the incubations to prepare for the following steps: (a) Two sets of marked tubes, one set for the proteinase K digestion and the other for the transfer of the aqueous phase from the phenol:chloroform extraction and precipitation. (b) The polyacrylamide gel.
14. The phenol:chloroform extraction step destroys the RNAse and efficiently purifies the protected fragments. It is therefore very important to vortex for at least 20 s to obtain an emulsion of the phenol:chloroform with the aqueous solution. Make absolutely sure to avoid the protein interface when removing the clarified aqueous phase. Setting the pipette to approx 120 µL will prevent uptake of the organic interface.
15. The polyacrylamide gels used are standard sequencing gels of 0.5-mm thickness. It is necessary to coat one of the glass plates with an agent that prevents sticking of the gel. For this purpose we use "Rain X" solution. After thoroughly cleaning the glass plates with 70% ethanol and drying, the "Rain X" is applied over the entire surface of the glass. In addition, to prevent sticking of the gel to the comb it is also necessary to coat the comb with Rain-X.
16. The width of the gel and the number of wells should be chosen in a way that, at least, the outermost wells on either side are not loaded with sample, since these sometimes run distorted. It is also advisable to always load all wells that are not used with loading buffer to decrease distortion during running.
17. The gels (approx 20 cm width) are initially prerun for 30–45 min at 45–50 watts and after sample loading at the same power. For larger (approx 30 cm width) gels, prerun and run at 55 to 60 watts.
18. To increase the comparability between different RPAs, we advise that each gel electrophoresis be run the same distance. To optimally separate probes between 300 to 87 bp length, we run the Bromophenol Blue dye band a distance of 30 cm from the bottom of the well.
19. Sometimes double or even multiple bands will appear for a specific probe in the RPA. Depending on their size, these may reflect inefficient RNase processing or be due to a sequence mismatch between the probe and the target RNA. In the case of inefficient RNase processing the bands will be close together at the correct protected fragment size and include an additional band with the same size as the sense target RNA. This problem can usually be corrected by adjusting the conditions for the RNase digestion step. When sequence mismatch occurs, the protected bands will usually run at an inappropriately small size. Carefully check the sequence of each synthesized probe to ensure it is identical to the target sequence. If there is no difference, the extra bands may indicate the reported target sequence contains an error or that there are homologous target RNAs. It is advisable to resynthesize the probe to a different region in the target sequence. If multiple bands still occur it may be advisable to remove this particular probe entirely from the RPA set.

Acknowledgments

This study was supported by NIH grants MH62231; MH62261 and NS36979 to I.L.C. S.O. is a postdoctoral fellow of the National Multiple Sclerosis Society (NMSS) and Multiple Sclerosis Society of Canada. This is manuscript number 16320-NP from the Scripps Research Institute.

References

1. Barnes, B., Lubyova, B., and Pitha, P. M. (2002) On the role of IRF in host defense. *J. Interferon Cytokine Res.* **22**, 59–71.
2. Levy, D. E., Marie, I., and Prakash, A. (2003) Ringing the interferon alarm: differential regulation of gene expression at the interface between innate and adaptive immunity. *Curr. Opin. Immunol.* **15**, 52–58.
3. Navikas, V. and Link, H. (1996) Review: Cytokines and the pathogenesis of multiple sclerosis. *J. Nuerosci. Res.* **45**, 322–333.
4. Benveniste, E. N. (1998) Cytokine actions in the central nervous sytem. *Cytokine Growth Factor Rev.* **9**, 259–275.
5. Huang, X., Yuang, J., Goddard, A., Foulis, A., James, R. F., Lernmark, A., et al. (1995) Interferon expression in the pancreases of patients with type I diabetes. *Diabetes* **44**, 658–64.
6. Lebon, P., Badoual, J., Ponsot, G., Goutieres, F., Hemeury-Cukier, F., and Aicardi, J. (1988) Intrathecal synthesis of interferon-alpha in infants with progressive familial encephalopathy. *J. Neurol. Sci.* **84**, 201–208.
7. Taniguchi, T., Ogasawara, K., Takaoka, A., and Tanaka, N. (2001) IRF family of transcription factors as regulators of host defense. *Annu. Rev. Immunol.* **19**, 623–655.
8. Grandvaux, N., tenOever, B., Servant, M. J., and Hiscott, J. (2002) The interferon antiviral response: from viral invasion to evasion. *Curr. Opin. Infect. Dis.* **15**, 259–267.
9. Nehyba, J., Hrdlickova, R., Burnside, J., and Bose, H. R. J. (2002) A novel interferon regulatory facotr (IRF), IRF-10, has a unique role in immune defense and is induced by the v-Rel oncoprotein. *Mol. Cell. Biol.* **22**, 3942–3957.
10. Qin, B. Y., Liu, C., Lam, S. S., Sumpter, R., Jr., Ikeda, M., Lemon, S. M., and Gale, M., Jr. (2003) Crystal structure of IRF-3 reveals mechanism of autoinhibition and virus-induced phosphoactivation. *Nat. Struct. Biol.* **10**, 913–921.
11. Foy, E., Li, K., Wang, C., Sumpter, R., Jr., Ikeda, M., Lemon, S. M., and Gale, M., Jr. (2003) Regulation of interferon regulatory factor-3 by the hepatitis C virus serine protease. *Science* **300**, 1145–1148.
12. Sharma, S., tenOever, B. R., Grandvaux, N., Zhou, G. P., Lin, R., and Hiscott, J. (2003) Triggering the interferon antiviral response through an IKK-related pathway. *Science* **300**, 1148–1151.
13. Levy, D. E., Marie, I., Smith, E., and Prakash, A. (2002) Enhancement and diversification of IFN induction by IRF-7-mediated positive feedback. *J. Interferon Cytokine Res.* **22**, 87–93.
14. Stalder, A., Pagenstecher, A., Kincaid, C., and Campbell, I. L. (1999) Analysis of gene expression by multiprobe RNase protection assay, in *Neurodegeneration*

Methods and Protocols. (Harry, J., and Tilson, H. A., eds.), Humana Press, Totowa, NJ, pp. 53–66.
15. Dudov, K. P. and Perry, R. P. (1984) The gene family encoding the mouse ribosomal protein L32 contains a uniquely expressed intron-containing gene and an unmutated processed gene. *Cell* **37,** 457–468.
16. Badley, J. E., Bishop, G. A., St. John, T., and Frelinger, J. A. (1988) A simple, rapid method for the purification of poly A$^+$ RNA. *Biotechniques.* **6,** 114–116.
17. Campbell, I. L., Hobbs, M. V., Kemper, P., and Oldstone, M. B. A. (1994) Cerebral expression of multiple cytokine genes in mice with lymphocytic choriomeningitis. *J. Immunol.* **152,** 716–723.
18. Lassmann, S., Kincaid, C., Asensio, V. C., and Campbell, I. L. (2001) Induction of type I immune pathology in the brain following immunization without central nervous system autoantigen in transgenic mice with astrocyte-targeted expression of IL-12. *J. Immunol.* **167,** 5485–5493.
19. Akwa, Y., Hassett, D. E., Eloranta, M. L., Sandberg, K., Masliah, E., Powell, H., Whitton, J. L., Bloom, F. E., and Campbell, I. L. (1998) Transgenic expression of IFN-α in the central nervous system of mice protects against lethal neurotropic viral infection but induces inflammation and neurodegeneration. *J. Immunol.* **161,** 5016–5026.
20. Pagenstecher, A., Lassmann, S., Carson, M. J., Kincaid, C. L., Stalder, A. K., and Campbell, I. L. (2000) Astrocyte-targeted expression of IL-12 induces active cellular immune responses in the central nervous system and modulates experimental allergic encephalomyelitis. *J. Immunol.* **164,** 4481–4492.

9

Mitogen-Activated Protein Kinase Pathways in Interferon Signaling

Antonella Sassano, Amit Verma, and Leonidas C. Platanias

Summary

There is recent evidence that in addition to the classic JAK/STAT pathways, mitogen-activated proteins (MAP) kinase pathways play important roles in Type I interferon signaling and the generation of interferon responses. In particular, the p38 MAP kinase cascade exerts positive regulatory roles on transcriptional activation of interferon-sensitive genes (ISGs) and the induction of the antiproliferative and antiviral properties of interferons. In this chapter, methodologies to detect activation of p38 and various upstream and downstream effectors are provided. Also, the methodological approaches used to examine the role of this pathway on the regulation of hematopoiesis are discussed.

Key Words: Interferon; MAP kinase; p38, Rac1; hematopoiesis.

1. Introduction

Several studies *(1,2)* have established that interferons (IFNs) have clinical activity against many cancers and are potent regulators of normal hematopoiesis. The mechanisms by which type I interferons (IFN-α, -β, and -ω) transduce signals have been elucidated to a great extent during the last few years. The binding of IFNs to their receptors results in activation of two tyrosine kinases of the Janus family, Tyk-2 and Jak-1, those are constitutively associated with the different receptor subunits (reviewed in **refs. 3,4**). Activation of these tyrosine kinases results in phosphorylation of several signaling proteins. Such phosphorylations result in the ultimate activation of multiple cellular pathways, including the Stat pathway (reviewed in **refs. 3–8**), the CBL/Crk cascade *(9–11)*, and the IRS-PI 3'-kinase pathway *(12–15)*. There is adequate evidence that has established that the type I IFN-dependent transcription of target genes is mainly regulated by the Jak–Stat pathway *(3–8)*.

Despite the substantial advances in our understanding of these pathways, the molecular mediators of interferon's actions in normal and malignant hematopoiesis had been unknown. Previous work has shown that type I IFNs activate members of the MAP family of kinases (mitogen-activated protein kinase; MAPK), including Erk kinases *(16)* and the p38 MAP kinase *(2,17–20)*. Our work has established that activation of the p38 MAPK is required for transcriptional activation of IFN-sensitive genes, elucidating an important role for p38 activation in interferon signaling. In addition, our studies have demonstrated that such transcriptional regulation of IFN-sensitive genes is unrelated to effects on deoxyribonucleic acid (DNA) binding of Stat complexes or serine phosphorylation of Stats *(18)*, apparently involving a Stat-independent nuclear mechanism. Thus, coordination of the functions of the IFN-activated Stat and p38 pathways is necessary for full transcriptional activation in response to interferons. Most importantly we have been able to show that activation of the p38 MAPK pathway plays a central role in the generation of the inhibitory effects of type I IFNs against leukemic and normal hematopoietic progenitors *(2,19)*.

In the present chapter, we discuss experimental methods used to study the role of MAP kinases in interferon signaling. Because the p38 MAPK appears to be a very important regulator of the biological activities of IFNs, we will restrict this chapter to this particular MAP kinase. For these experiments, we have used specific pharmacological inhibitors of the p38 MAPK, that is, SB203580 and SB202190. These are pyridinyl imidazole compounds that act by binding to the adenosine triphosphate (ATP) site of the p38 molecule and inhibit its kinase activity *(21)*. Both SB203580 and SB202190 appear to exhibit similar specificities and, in addition to inhibiting p38 (also called p38α), they inhibit the p38β2 kinase isoform, but not the p38γ and p38δ isoforms of the same family *(22)*.

2. Materials

The materials listed below outline (1) the immunoblotting assay to detect phosphorylation of p38, (2) the p38 MAP kinase assay, (3) the MAPKAP Kinase-2 and MAPKAP Kinase-3 assays, (4) the Rac1 activation assay, (5) the study of the role of p38 MAP kinase on interferon-regulated gene transcription (luciferase assays), (6) the study of the role of the p38 MAPK in the biological effects of interferons on hematopoiesis (methylcellulose colony-forming assays).

2.1. Immunoblotting to Detect p38 MAP Kinase Phosphorylation

1. Anti-p38 antibody (Santa Cruz, CA).
2. Secondary anti rabbit antibody-HRP (Amersham Biosciences, NJ).
3. Antiphospho-p38 (Thr180/Tyr182) antibody (Cell Signaling, MA).

MAP Kinase Pathways in Interferon Signaling 137

4. Sodium dodecyl sulfate polyacrylamide gel electrophoresis (SDS-PAGE) gel apparatus.
5. 5X SDS gel-loading buffer: 3 mL of 1 M TRIS-HCl, pH 6.8, 25 mL of 50% glycerol, 10 mL of 10% SDS, 2.5 mL of 2-mercaptoethanol, 4.5 mL of distil water, and 5 mL of 1% bromophenol blue.
6. Kodak film.
7. Polyvinylidene difluoride (Immobilon-P Transfer Membrane).
8. Phosphorylation lysis buffer (PLB): 50 mM N-hydroxyethylpiperazine-N'-2-ethanesulfonate (Hepes), pH 7.3, 150 mM NaCl, 1.5 mM MgCl$_2$, 1 mM ethylene diamine tetraacetic acid, pH 8.0; 100 mM NaF, 10 mM sodium pyrophosphate, and 200 µM sodium orthovanadate, at 4°C.
9. Complete lysis buffer: in PLB add 10% glycerol, fresh 0.5% Triton X-100, fresh protein inhibitors, and fresh 20 to 100 µg/mL phenylmethyl sulfonyl fluoride (PMSF).
10. Tris-Buffered saline Tween-20 (TBST): dissolve 8.8 g of NaCl, 0.2 g of KCl, and 3 g of Tris base in distilled H$_2$O, add 500 µL of Tween-20, adjust the pH to 7.4 with HCl, add distilled water to 1 L.
11. Blocking buffer: 5% bovine serum albumin and 0.2% sodium azide in TBST.
12. Erasing buffer: 62.5 mM Tris-HCl, pH 6.8; 0.2% SDS; and 100 mM 2-mercaptoethanol.

2.2. p38 MAP Kinase Assay

1. Refrigerated centrifuge
2. PLB (*see* **Subheading 2.1.**, **item 8**).
3. Complete lysis buffer (*see* **Subheading 2.1.**, **item 9**).
4. TBST (*see* **Subheading 2.1.**, **item 10**).
5. Blocking buffer (*see* **Subheading 2.1.**, **item 11**).
6. Washing buffer: PLB and fresh 0.1% Triton X-100.
7. Kinase buffer: 25 mM Hepes, pH 7.3, 25 mM MgCl$_2$, 25 mM β-glycerophosphate, 2 mM dithiothreitol, 0.1 mM sodium orthovanadate, 20 µM ATP (*see* **Note 1**).
8. 1.5-mL screw cap tubes.
9. Protein G-Sepharose (Amersham Pharmacia Biotech, NJ).
10. Control nonimmune Rabbit IgG (Sigma, MO).
11. Anti p38 Antibody (Santa Cruz, CA).
12. Anti phospho-ATF-2 (Thr71) Antibody (Cell Signaling, MA).
13. Glutathione S-transferase (GST)–ATF-2 fusion protein (Santa Cruz, CA).
14. SDS-PAGE gel apparatus.
15. 5X SDS gel-loading buffer (*see* **Subheading 2.1.**, **item 5**).
16. Kodak film.
17. [γ-^{32}P]ATP.

2.3. MAPKAP Kinase-2 and MAPKAP Kinase-3 Assays

1. Refrigerated centrifuge
2. PLB (*see* **Subheading 2.1.**, **item 8**).
3. Complete lysis buffer (*see* **Subheading 2.1.**, **item 9**).
4. TBST (*see* **Subheading 2.1.**, **item 10**).

5. Blocking buffer (*see* **Subheading 2.1.**, **item 11**).
6. Washing buffer (*see* **Subheading 2.2.**, **item 6**).
7. Kinase buffer (*see* **Subheading 2.2.**, **item 7**).
8. 1.5 mL screw cap tubes.
9. Protein G-Sepharose (Amersham Pharmacia Biotech, NJ).
10. Control non-immune (rabbit or sheep) IgG (Santa Cruz, CA).
11. Anti-MAPKAP kinase-2 (Upstate Biotechnology, Virginia).
12. Anti-MAPKAP kinase-3 (Upstate Biotechnology, Virginia).
13. Hsp-25 protein (StressGen Laboratories, CA).
14. SDS-PAGE gel apparatus.
15. 5X SDS gel-loading buffer (*see* **Subheading 2.1.**, **item 5**).
16. Kodak film.
17. [γ-^{32}P]ATP.

2.4. Rac1 Activation Assay

1. NETN buffer: 20 mM Tris-HCl, pH 8.0, 100 mM NaCl, 1 mM ethylene diamine tetraacetic acid (EDTA), pH 8.0, 0.5% IGEPAL CA-630.
2. Elution buffer: 10 mM reduced glutathione, 50 mM Tris-HCl, pH 8.0.
3. pGEX vector.
4. pGEX-PBD construct.
5. BL21 (DE3).
6. Ampicilin.
7. Isopropyl-D-thiogalactopyranoside (IPTG).
8. 300 VT Ultrasonic Homogenizer.
9. Titanium Micro Tip 5/32-inch diameter (3.9 mm).
10. Coomassie blue.
11. Glutathione Sepharose 4B (Pharmacia Biotech, NJ).
12. Anti Rac-1 monoclonal antibody (BD Transduction Laboratories, CA).

2.5. Studying of the Role of p38 MAP Kinase on Interferon-Regulated Gene Transcription

1. 6-well plate.
2. 15-mL conical tube.
3. Vector.
4. Vector-p38 AGF construct.
5. ISRE-luciferase construct.
6. Plasmid β-Gal.
7. Superfect (Qiagen, CA).
8. Reporter Lysis Buffer (Promega, WI).
9. Z-Buffer: 60 mM Na$_2$HPO$_4$, 40 mM NaH$_2$PO$_4$, 10 mM KCl, 1 mM MgSO$_4$, 50 mM β-mercaptoethanol (optional), adjust to pH 7.0. Dissolve *o*-nitrophenyl-β-D-galactopyranoside fresh to a final concentration of 4 mg/mL. Store at −20°C.
10. β-Gal stop buffer: 1 M Na$_2$CO$_3$.

11. Luciferase reporter 1000 Assay System (Promega, WI).
12. Disposable cuvettes.
13. Luminometer (TD-20/20 with injector-Turner Designs).
14. Spectrophotometer.

2.6. Studying the Role of the p38 MAPK in the Biological Effects of Interferon on Hematopoiesis, Methylcellulose Colony-Forming Assay

1. Mono-Poly Resolving Medium (Ficoll-Hypaque; MP Biomedicals, OH).
2. MACS Separation columns (Miltenyi Biotech, CA).
3. MACS MultiStand (Miltenyi Biotech, CA).
4. Fluorescein isothiocyanate-conjugated anti-CD34 antibody (Miltenyi Biotech, CA).
5. MethoCult GF H4434 (StemCell Technologies Inc, Vancouver, BC).

3. Methods

Our studies in MAP kinases will be divided into three subsections. These include (1). Our approaches to study the phosphorylation and activation of the p38 MAP kinase, its downstream effectors, and its upstream regulators. (2). The methodologies to study the effect of MAP kinases on interferon-dependent transcriptional activation (3). The experimental approaches to define the role of the p38 MAP kinase pathway in the regulation of normal and malignant hematopoiesis.

3.1. Studying the Phosphorylation and Activation of p38 MAP Kinase and Its Downstream Effector (MAPKAP Kinase-2) and Upstream Regulator G Protein (Rac1)

3.1.1. Immunoblotting to Detect p38 MAP Kinase Phosphorylation

To determine whether the p38 MAPK pathway is activated in response to type I IFN-treatment, cells are incubated in presence or absence of IFNs (10,000 U/mL) for different time periods (*see* **Note 2**).

1. After treatment, for suspension cells centrifuge at $200g$ for 5 min and resuspend the cells in approx 1 mL of cold phosphate-buffered saline (PBS).
2. Wash the cells twice with cold PBS and centrifuge at 4°C for 5 min at $4000g$. For adherent cells, aspirate medium and add 1 to 10 mL of cold PBS, depending on the capacity of the plate, aspirate again and repeat twice. Scrape the cells, collect them in an Eppendorf tube, spin at $4000g$ for 5 min at 4°C.
3. Lyse the cells with complete phosphorylation lysis buffer (*see* **Note 3**).
4. Vortex and keep in ice for 1 h.
5. Centrifuge at $4000g$ for 5 min at 4°C and transfer the supernatant to a new tube (*see* **Note 4**).
6. Determine the protein concentration of the cell lysate by Bradford assay.
7. Analyze sample by 10% SDS-PAGE gel.

8. Incubate membrane with phospho-p38 antibody (dilution 1:1000).
9. Detect the signal by luminescence, using horseradish peroxidase-labeled antibodies (dilution 1:5000; see **Note 5**).
10. To detect differences in protein loading the membrane is erased to remove bound antibodies and reprobed with an anti-p38 antibody (dilution 1:250).

3.1.1.1. Erasing Immunoblots

1. Wash the membrane twice for 5 min in TBST.
2. Incubate the membrane in blocking buffer for 10 min at room temperature.
3. To erase, incubate the membrane for 30 min at 70°C in erasing buffer.
4. Wash the membrane twice for 10 min in TBST, membrane should be incubated with blocking buffer for 1 h prior to reprobe with a new first antibody.

3.1.2. p38 MAP Kinase Assay

This assay is performed to determine whether the kinase activity of p38 MAPK is induced by type I IFN treatment.

Prepare the cell lysate as described in **Subheading 3.1.1.** (*see* **Note 6**). Dilute the lysate in 0.5 to 1.0 mL of lysis buffer to allow a better shaking of solution during the following steps.

3.1.2.1. Preparation of Protein G-Sepharose (*see* **Note 7**)

1. Take 1 mL out of stock solution
2. Remove supernatant (20% ethanol) by gentle centrifugation ($200g$ 2 min).
3. Wash twice with sterile water.
4. Wash twice with sterile PBS.
5. Restore a 50% slurry with PBS.
6. Store at 4°C.

3.1.2.2. Immunoprecipitation

1. Transfer 40 μL of prepared Protein G slurry to a screw cap tube, add your lysate and incubate on a rocker at 4°C for 1 h (*see* **Note 8**).
2. Spin at $8000g$ for 5 min at 4°C and carefully transfer the supernatant to another fresh screw cap tube.
3. Add 5 μg of antibody against p38 MAPK to the precleared lysate
4. Add 5 μg of IgG to the control lysate sample.
5. Add 40 μL of Protein G-Sepharose prepared as indicated by the manufacturer (*see* **Subheading 3.1.2.1.**).
6. Incubate on a rocker at 4°C for either 2 to 3 h or overnight.
7. The immunocomplex is subsequently washed three times with washing buffer, and twice with kinase buffer. Each wash requires a spin of 2 min at $4000g$ at 4°C, during which the supernatant has to be removed carefully.
8. Keep samples on ice until use.
9. Resuspend the beads pellet in 30 μL of kinase buffer containing 5 μg of the exog-

enous p38 substrate that is the GST–ATF-2 fusion protein, and to each sample add 10 μCi of [γ^{32}P]ATP (*see* **Note 9**).
10. Incubation for 20 min at room temperature.
11. Stop the reaction by addition of 5X SDS gel loading buffer.
12. Vortex and boil the sample for 5 min.
13. Immediately cool down in ice.
14. Spin at 10,000g for 5 min.
15. Collect the supernatant and analyze samples by SDS-PAGE gel. The phosphorylated form of ATF-2 can be detected by autoradiography or by immunoblotting with an anti-phospho-ATF-2 antibody (dilution 1:1000).

3.1.3. MAPKAP Kinase-2 and MAPKAP Kinase-3 Assays

Previous studies have identified MAPKAP kinase-2 and MAPKAP kinase-3 as the in vivo substrates for kinase activity of p38 in response to stress and other stimuli (reviewed in **ref. 23**). To determine whether these kinases are also activated downstream of the p38 kinase during engagement of the type I IFN receptor, in vitro kinase assays are performed. Pretreatment of cells with the p38-specific inhibitor SB203580 (10 μ*M*), blocks the activation of MAPKAP kinase-2 and MAPKAP kinase-3 (*see* **Note 10**).

1. After cell treatment and preparation of cell lysates as described in **Subheading 3.1.1.** and after preparation of protein G-Sepharose as explained in **Subheading 3.1.2.**, transfer 40 μL of prepared Protein G slurry to a screw cap tube, add your lysate and incubate on a rocker at 4°C for 1 h (*see* **Note 8**).
2. Spin at 8000g for 5 min at 4°C and carefully transfer the supernatant to another fresh screw cap tube.
3. Add 5 μg of MAPKAP kinase-2 and MAPKAP kinase-3 antibody to the precleared lysate.
4. Add 5 μg of nonimmune IgG to the control lysate sample.
5. Add 40 μL of protein G-Sepharose prepared as indicated by the manufacturer (*see* **Subheading 3.1.2.1.**).
6. Incubate on a rocker at 4°C for either 2–3 h or overnight.

The immunocomplex is subsequently washed three times with washing buffer and twice with kinase buffer. Each wash requires a spin of 2 min at 4000g at 4°C, during which the supernatant has to be removed carefully, especially during the last wash.

7. Keep samples on ice until use.
8. Resuspend the beads in 30 μL of kinase buffer containing 3 μg of Hsp-25 substrate and add 10 μCi of [g-^{32}P]ATP to each sample (*see* **Note 9**).
9. Incubate for 30 min at room temperature.
10. Stop the reaction by the addition of 5X SDS gel loading buffer.
11. Vortex and boil the sample for 5 min.

12. Immediately cool down in ice.
13. Spin at 10,000g for 5 min.
14. Collect the supernatant and analyze samples by SDS-PAGE electrophoresis. Proteins are analyzed by SDS-PAGE, and the phosphorylated form of Hsp-25 is detected by autoradiography.

3.1.4. Rac1 Activation Assay

This assay is to determine whether type I IFNs activate the small GTPase Rac1, which functions as an upstream effector for p38 MAPK. The active form of the GTPase is transient and labile and difficult to measure directly. It is though possible to evaluate Rac1 activation by evaluating binding to GST fusion protein for the binding domain of Pak1. Pak1 binds only to activated GTP bound Rac1. Thus the GST-PBD (Pak1 binding domain) can be used to pull down activated Rac1 from protein lysates, which can then be quantified by immunoblotting. pGEX-PBD is expressed in BL21 strain of *Escherichia coli* as a GST fusion protein (GST-PBD). The GST protein alone is used as an appropriate control.

1. Inoculate glycerol stock or a colony with 20 mL of Luria-Bertani (LB) medium containing 100 µg/mL of ampicillin, grown overnight at 37°C (*see* **Note 11**).
2. Dilute the overnight culture 1:10 into a desired volume of LB medium 100 µg/mL amp.
3. Incubate at 37°C for approx 1 to 2 h until OD_{600} reaches 0.5 to 1.0
4. Induce fusion protein expression by adding 0.1 mM IPTG. Continue incubation for 3 to 4 h at 37°C (*see* **Note 12**).
5. Centrifuge at 5000g for 10 min at room temperature.
6. Resuspend the bacteria pellet in 1 to 20 mL ice-cold NETN buffer containing 1 mM PMSF and protease inhibitors.
7. Aliquot the suspension in a different tube and sonicate (*see* **Note 13**).
8. Pool the samples in 1 tube.
9. Add Triton X-100 to 1% final concentration and rock for 30 min at room temperature (*see* **Note 14**).
10. Centrifuge at 10,000g for 5 min at 4°C.
11. Bacterial extract can now be frozen at –80°C.

Check the production of the GST-PBD by resolving on 12% SDS-PAGE gel and staining with Coomassie blue (*see* **Note 15**).

3.1.4.1. Preparation of Glutathione Sepharose 4B

The following procedure results in a 50% slurry (*see* **Note 16**).

1. Dispense 1.33 mL of the original slurry.
2. Sediment the matrix by centrifugation at 500g for 5 min, carefully decant the supernatant.

3. Wash the glutathione Sepharose 4B with 10 mL of cold PBS. Invert to mix.
4. Sediment the matrix by centrifugation at 500g for 5 min. Decant the supernatant.
5. Add 1 mL of 1X PBS.

3.1.4.2. Purification of GST Proteins

The fusion protein is purified from the supernatant with glutathione-Sepharose 4B.

1. Incubate 50 to 250 µL of 50% slurry glutathione–Sepharose with the bacteria extract.
2. Rock for 2 h at 4°C.
3. Centrifuge the beads at 500g for 5 min at 4°C.
4. Wash three times with PBS.
5. To the sedimented matrix, add 500 µL of elution buffer.
6. Mix gently and incubate at RT (22–25°C) for 10 min to elute the bound material from the matrix.
7. Centrifuge at 500g for 5 min and save the supernatant containing the GST fusion protein.

The purified GST-PAK1 PBD fusion protein interacts with the active form of Rac1. Beads with bound protein are washed, and the amount of Rac1 protein retained is determined by SDS-PAGE.

8. After cell treatment prepare the cell lysates as also described in **Subheading 3.1.1.**, centrifuge the cells at 1000 rpm for 5 min.
9. Resuspend the cells in approx 1 mL of cold PBS.
10. Wash the cells twice with cold PBS and centrifuge at 4°C for 5 min at 4000g.
11. Lyse cells in 500 µL of lysis buffer (*see* **Note 3**).
12. Vortex and keep in ice for 1 h.
13. Centrifuge for 5 min at 4°C and transfer the supernatant to a new tube.
14. Determine the protein concentration of the cell lysates by Bradford assay.
15. For each sample: in a screw cap tube, incubate 50 µL of 50% slurry glutathione–Sepharose beads with 5 µg of GST-PBD.
16. Use another screw cap tube for the control with GST alone.
17. Incubate with gentle agitation for 2 h at 4°C.
18. Centrifuge the beads at 500g for 5 min at 4°C.
19. Wash three times with PLB.
20. Carefully aspirate off supernatant.
21. Add cell lysate to the matrix (*see* **Note 17**).
22. Rock for 1 h at 4°C.
23. Wash four times with washing buffer at 4000g for 2 min.
24. Suspend beads in 30 µL of 1X SDS gel-loading buffer.
25. Vortex and boil the sample for 5 min.
26. Immediately cool down in ice.
27. Spin at 10,000g for 5 min.

28. Collect the supernatant and analyze samples by 12.5% SDS-PAGE.
29. Detect the GST-PBD pull-down with anti Rac-1 antibody (dilution 1:1000).

3.1.5. Study of the Role of p38 MAP Kinase on IFN-Regulated Gene Transcription

We have performed luciferase assays to demonstrate that IFN-dependent gene transcription via IFN-stimulated response elements (ISRE), is inhibited by blocking the activation of p38 MAPK. U2OS cells are transfected with ISRE-luciferase plasmids and a β-galactosidase expression vector (for testing transfection efficiency) using the Superfect transfection reagent as recommended by the manufacturer (Qiagen). To establish the role of p38 in the induction of type I IFN gene transcription via ISRE elements, cells are transfected with a p38AGF construct in which the tyrosine and threonine phosphorylation sites in the TGY motif have been mutated to alanine and phenylalanine, respectively. The p38 AGF exhibits dominant negative effects on the activation of endogenous p38 (*see* **Note 18**).

3.1.5.1. TRANSIENT TRANSFECTION OF ADHERENT CELLS WITH P38 AGF (DOMINANT NEGATIVE MUTANT OF P38) AND EMPTY VECTOR CONTROL

1. Split the cells the day before the transfection, into two different 6-well plates.
2. Seed to each well 2×10^5 cells. The cell number seeded should produce 40 to 80% confluence on the day of transfection.
3. Incubate the cells under their normal growth conditions (37°C and 5% CO_2).
4. On the day of transfection, for each 6-well plate, prepare a different mixture:

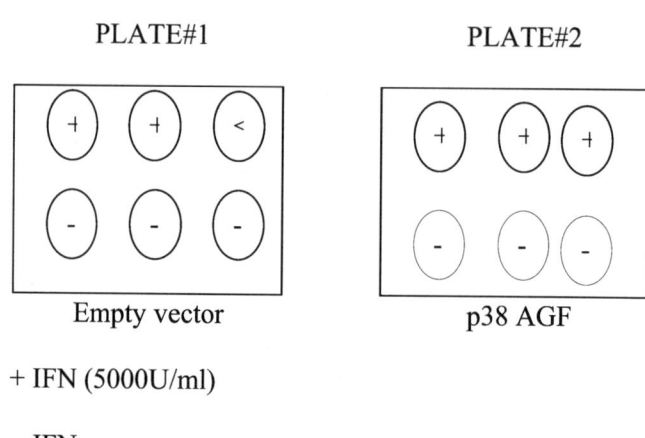

+ IFN (5000U/ml)

− IFN

Take a 15-mL conical tube to make the mix solution (*see* **Note 19**).

Add the following:

	For 1 well	Plate 1 (Volume per plate)	Plate 2 (Volume per plate)
Cell growth medium containing no serum or antibiotics	70 µL	700 µL	700 µL
β-Gal	0.1 µg	0.7 µg	0.7 µg
ISRE	1 µg	7 µg	7 µg
Vector	2 µg	14 µg	None
p38 AGF	2 µg	None	14 µg
SuperFect	3 µL	21 µL	21 µL

5. Mix by pipetting up and down five times;
6. Incubate the mixture for 5 to 10 min at room temperature to allow transfection complex formation.
7. While complex formation takes place, gently aspirate the growth medium from the plate and wash cells twice with 1 mL of PBS.
8. Add 300 µL of cell growth medium containing serum and antibiotics per well.
9. Add 2 mL of growth medium containing serum and antibiotics to the tube containing the transfection complex (*see* **Note 20**). Mix by pipetting up and down twice, and immediately transfer 400 µL to each well.
10. Incubate cells with the transfection complex for 2 to 3 h under their normal growth conditions.
11. Remove medium containing the transfection complex from the cells by gentle aspiration, and wash cells twice with 1 mL of PBS.
12. Add fresh cell growth medium containing serum and antibiotics.
13. Incubate the transfected cells for 36 to 48 h.

After the transient transfection, the cells are incubated with and without IFNs (5000 U/mL) for 6 h, under normal growth conditions. The cells are then harvested and assayed for the luciferase activity.

3.1.5.2. LUCIFERASE ASSAY

1. Remove growth medium from cultured cells.
2. Wash cells in 1 mL of cold PBS, twice.
3. Dispense 400 µL of 1X Reporter lysis buffer into each well.
4. Place on a rocker at room temperature for 20 min.
5. Scrape cells from the dish, and transfer them and the solution to a microcentrifuge tube.
6. Centrifuge at 10,000g for 5min at room temperature and transfer the supernatant to a new tube (*see* **Note 21**).
7. Take 20 µL of cell lysate and measure the light produced by luminometer (TD-20/20 with injector-Turner Designs) using the luciferase reporter 1000 assay system.

3.1.5.3. β-Galactosidase Assay

1. Take 200 µL of cell lysate and transfer to a new microcentrifuge tube.
2. Add 250 µL of Z-buffer.
3. Place at 37°C until the color turns yellow (could be anytime from 0.5–5 h).
4. Stop the reaction by adding 250 µL of β-Gal stop buffer.
5. Read OD at 420 nm (*see* **Note 22**).

3.1.6. Studying of the Role of the p38 MAPK in the Biological Effects of Interferon on Hematopoiesis

Hematopoiesis is the process of development of stem cells into mature red (erythroid) and white (myeloid) cells. This process is tightly regulated by various cytokines that exert both stimulatory and inhibitory control over this process. We have developed assays to study the effects of various cytokines, including interferons, on hematopoiesis, and also have used these assays to study the role of various MAP kinase inhibitors on this process.

3.1.6.1. Expansion of Primary Human Hematopoietic Cells for MAP Kinase Activation Studies

Because the number of $CD34^+$ progenitors derived from bone marrows is limited and not adequate for the performance of MAP kinase activation assays, described earlier with cell lines. To overcome this difficulty, we expand these $CD34^+$-derived erythroid progenitors at the colony-forming units, erythroid (CFU-E) stage of maturation. This expansion/enrichment protocol allows us to perform Map kinase activation experiments in primitive human progenitor cells.

1. Bone marrow aspiration is done in healthy volunteers after informed consent. Mononuclear cells present in the marrow aspirate are separated by Ficoll–Hypaque.
2. $CD34^+$ cells are obtained by positive immunomagnetic bead selection, using Macs columns (Miltenyi Biotech). The mononuclear cells are passed through the columns twice to obtain a purity of 90 to 95% $CD34^+$ cells, which is then confirmed by flow cytometry using fluorescein isothiocyanate-conjugated anti-CD34 antibodies.
3. The $CD34^+$ cells obtained are cultured in a medium (IMDM) containing 15% fetal calf serum, 15% human AB serum, 500 U/mL penicillin, 40 µg/mL streptomycin, 10 ng/mL interleukin-3, 2 U/mL erythropoietin, 50 ng/mL stem cell factor, and 50 ng/mL insulin-like growth factor. The cytokines in this medium promote the differentiation of $CD34^+$ cells and the enrichment of a pure population of CFU-E cells after 7 d of culture. Such cells are subsequently used for signaling studies.
4. Before activation by IFNs, d 7 CFU-E cells are washed twice with IMDM, and in some cases incubated in cytokine-free medium for 4 h. The cells are then stimu-

lated with IFN-α or IFN-β for the indicated times and lysed in phosphorylation lysis buffer, as previously described. Proteins are resolved by SDS-PAGE and immunoblotted with various antibodies for components of MAP kinase signaling pathways, as described in previous sections.

3.1.6.2. Methylcellulose Colony-Forming Assays

1. These assays are also performed using primary human hematopoietic progenitors. Bone marrow mononuclear cells are isolated from bone marrow aspirations from normal healthy volunteers, after obtaining informed consent.
2. The bone marrow aspirate is layered over Ficoll-Hypaque gradient media for the separation of a mononuclear cell layer. The mononuclear cell layer contains the early hematopoietic progenitor population, including CD34$^+$ stem cells.
3. The mononuclear cells are centrifuged and resuspended in IMDM media supplemented with serum and antibiotics. These cells are then used in methylcellulose assays.
4. Commercial methylcellulose, containing a pre-made mixture of cytokines is obtained from Stem Cell Technologies Inc. This is a semisolid media that is mixed at room temperature with 10^4 bone marrow mononuclear cells per milliliter. One milliliter of this mixture media is carefully plated per well in 6 well plates under sterile conditions. Two wells of the 6-well plate are filled with sterile water to ensure adequate humidity so that the cultures do not dry off.
5. After 14 d of culture at 37°C in the incubator the progenitors grow, differentiate and form hematopoietic colonies. There are three main types of colonies that are formed- the erythroid colonies (composed of blast-forming units, frythroid), the myeloid colonies (composed of CFU, granulocytic monocytic) and mixed colonies (formed by the earliest progenitors that can differentiate into both erythroid and myeloid forms). The erythroid blast-forming units, the myeloid (CUF, granulocytic monocytic), and the mixed colonies are counted using an inverted microscope at the end of 14 d of incubation.

In these methylcellulose cultures, cytokines such as IFNs can be added in varying concentrations. If the cytokines are inhibitory to hematopoiesis, then the colony numbers obtained after 14 d are much less than the controls. We have observed that IFNs work well in concentrations ranging from 100 to 1000 U/mL when used in methylcellulose cultures. Hematopoietic cells can also be cultured in the presence of commercially available inhibitors of MAP kinases to test their role in hematopoiesis. The commercially available inhibitors of p38 MAP kinase that we have used are SB203580 and SB202190. We have successfully used these in methylcellulose cultures with interferon and showed that the inhibitory effects of interferons on progenitor colony formation can be reversed in the presence of these inhibitors, which are used at final concentrations at 5 to 10 μ*M*.

4. Notes

1. The kinase buffer has to be prepared fresh for each experiment.
2. Prior the treatment of the cells it may be helpful to starve them for 10 to 14 h to prevent any interference from serum factors on the phosphorylation state of the proteins. Depending on the cell line this may need to be done gradually, reducing the FBS to 2% and then reducing further to serum-free media for a short period of time of 4 to 6 h.
3. Composition of the lysis buffer may vary, depending on the protein kinase of interest. Considering the limited loading volume in a protein gel, it is recommended not to increase the dilution of lysate.
4. For western blotting the cell lysates can be stored at –80°C and analyzed at later times.
5. The membrane may be stored wet, with a preservative, in a refrigerator (2–8°C) after each immunodetection to allow subsequent re-probing.
6. For kinase assays, the lysate should be immediately used after the Bradford protein quantification assay, to ensure maximum enzyme activity.
7. The Protein G-Sepharose is supplied in 20% ethanol as bacteriostatic. The ethanol has to be removed before using the beads, as indicated by the manufacturer. It is recommended to cut the pipet's tip when aspirate Sepharose beads to avoid disruption of the beads. Do not exceed 1-mo storage.
8. It may be appropriate to preclear the lysate to avoid nonspecific protein binding to Protein G-Sepharose beads.
9. To equally distribute the reagents, it is recommended to make a mixture in which to add for each sample: 30 mL of kinase buffer, the p38 exogenous substrate, and the 10 µCi of [$g^{-32}P$]ATP. Distribute the mixture to allow the reaction.
10. The inhibitor is added 1 h before IFN treatment and has to be protected from the light.
11. The transformed bacteria can be stored at –80°C in 15% glycerol of LB medium.
12. The IPTG concentration and the induction period have to be optimized. The addition of IPTG later during the incubation period can minimize the degradation of fusion proteins.
13. During sonication, keep the tube on ice. Complete disruption of 2 g of *E. coli* in 10 mL of solution occurs in 40 s. Excessive sonication can contaminate the fusion protein with other proteins.
14. Triton X-100 is added to prevent the association of fusion protein with the bacterial proteins.
15. It is recommended that a sample in which the fusion protein has not been induced (no IPTG added) be also used as a control. The concentration of the protein can be asserted using BSA as standard.
16. Glutathione Sepharose 4B equilibrated with PBS may be stored at 4°C for up to 1 mo.
17. To allow better shaking it is recommended to use a volume of cell lysate between 0.5 and 1 mL.
18. p38 MAP kinase pathway is activated by IFN treatment and such activation can be blocked by treatment of cells with the specific p38 inhibitors SB203580 and

SB202190. Thus these inhibitors can be used in the luciferase assays instead of the dominant negative mutants of p38 MAPK. In this case, U2OS cells are transiently transfected with ISRE luciferase construct. After 48 h after transfection the cells are incubated with or without IFN-α for 6 h in presence or absence of 10 μM SB203580 at normal growth condition. The inhibitor is added to the culture 30 min prior to IFN-α treatment.

19. Serum and antibiotics present during this step will interfere with complex formation and will significantly decrease transfection efficiency. Prepare enough mix solution for seven wells to allow for pipetting errors.
20. At this stage, serum and antibiotics no longer interfere with complex formation, but significantly enhance the transfection efficiency of SuperFect reagent.
21. After the centrifugation, it is possible to store the supernatant at −80°C.
22. As blank, at 200 μL of 1X reporter lysis add 250 μL of Z-buffer and 250 μL of β-Gal stop buffer.

References

1. Pestka, S., Langer, J. A., Zoon, K. C., and Samuel, C. E. (1987) Interferons and their actions. *Annu. Rev. Biochem.* **56,** 727–777.
2. Verma, A., Deb, D. K., Sassano, A., Uddin, S., Varga, J., Wickrema, A., and Platanias, L. C. (2002) Activation of the p38 mitogen-activated protein kinase mediates the suppressive effects of type I interferons and transforming growth factor-beta on normal hematopoiesis. *J. Biol. Chem.* **277,** 7726–7735.
3. Darnell, J. E., Jr., Kerr, I. M., and Stark, G. R. (1994) Jak-STAT pathways and transcriptional activation in response to IFNs and other extracellular signaling proteins. *Science.* **264,** 1415–1421.
4. Platanias, L. C. and Fish, E. N. (1999) Signaling pathways activated by interferons. *Exp. Hematol.* **27,** 1583–1592.
5. Darnell, J. E., Jr. (1997) Stats and gene regulation. *Science.* **277,** 1630–1635.
6. Darnell, J. E., Jr. (1998) Studies of IFN-induced transcriptional activation uncover the Jak-Stat pathway. *J. Interf. Cyt. Res.* **18,** 549–554.
7. Stark, G. R., Kerr, I. M., Williams, B. R. G., Silverman, R. H., and Screiber, R. D. (1998) How cells respond to interferons. *Annu. Rev. Biochem.* **67,** 227–264.
8. Parmar, S. and Platanias, L. C. (2003) Interferons. Mechanisms of action and clinical applications. *Curr. Opin. Oncol.* **15,** 431–439.
9. Ahmad, S., Alsayed, Y. M., Druker, B. J., and Platanias, L. C. (1997) The type I interferon receptor mediates tyrosine phosphorylation of the CrkL adaptor protein. *J. Biol. Chem.* **272,** 29991–29994.
10. Alsayed, Y., Uddin, S., Ahmad, S., Majchrzak, B., Druker, B. J., Fish, E. N., and Platanias, L. C. (2000) IFN-gamma activates the C3G/Rap1 signaling pathway. *J. Immunol.* **164,** 1800–1806.
11. Fish, E. N., Uddin, S., Korkmaz, M., Majchrzak, B., Druker. B. J., and Platanias, L. C. (1999) Activation of a CrkL-Stat5 signaling complex by type I interferons. *J. Biol. Chem.* **274,** 571–573.

12. Uddin, S., Yenush, L., Sun, X-J, Sweet, M. E., White, M. F., and Platanias, L. C. (1995) Interferon a engages the insulin receptor substrate-1 to associate with the phosphatidylinositol 3'-kinase. *J. Biol. Chem.* **270,** 15938–15941.
13. Platanias, L. C., Uddin, S., Yetter, A., Sun, X-J., and White, M. F.(1996) The type I interferon receptor mediates tyrosine phosphorylation of insulin receptor substrate 2. *J. Biol. Chem.* **271,** 278–282.
14. Uddin, S., Fish, E. N., Sher, D., Gardziola, C., Colamonici, O. R., Kellum, M., et al. (1997) The IRS-pathway operates distinctively from the Stat-pathway in hematopoietic cells and transduces common and distinct signals during engagement of the insulin or IFNa receptors. *Blood.* **90,** 2574–2582.
15. Uddin, S., Fish, E. N., Sher, D. A., Gardziola, C., White, M. F., and Platanias, L. C. (1997) Activation of the phosphatidylinositol 3'-kinase serine kinase by IFNa. *J. Immunol.* **158,** 2390–2397.
16. David, M., Petricoin, E., 3rd, Benjamin, C., Pine, R., Weber, M. J., and Larner, A. C. (1995) Requirement for MAP kinase (ERK2) activity in interferon alpha- and interferon beta-stimulated gene expression through STAT proteins. *Science.* **269,** 1721–1723.
17. Uddin, S., Mazchrzak, B., Woodson, J., Arunkumar, P., Alsayed, Y., Pine, R., et al. (1999) Activation of the p38 map kinase by Type I IFNs. *J. Biol. Chem.* **274,** 30127–30131.
18. Uddin, S., Lekmine, F., Sharma, N., Majchrzak, B., Mayer, I., Young, P. R., et al. (2000) The Rac1/p38 mitogen-activated protein kinase pathway is required for interferon alpha-dependent transcriptional activation but not serine phosphorylation of Stat proteins. *J. Biol. Chem.* **275,** 27634–27640.
19. Mayer, I. A., Verma, A., Grumbach, I. M., Uddin, S., Lekmine, F., Ravandi, F., et al. (2001) The p38 MAPK pathway mediates the growth inhibitory effects of interferon-alpha in BCR-ABL-expressing cells. *J. Biol. Chem.* **276,** 28570–28577.
20. Li, Y., Sassano, A., Majchrzak, B., Deb, D. K., Levy, D. E., Gaestel, M., et al. (2004) Role of p38 alfa Map kinase in type I interferon signaling. *J. Biol. Chem.* **279,** 970–979.
21. Tong, L., Pav, S., White, D. M., Rogers, S., Crane, K. M., Cywin, C. L., et al. (1997) A highly specific inhibitor of human p38 MAP kinase binds in the ATP pocket. *Nat. Struct. Biol.* **4,** 311–316.
22. Kumar, S., McDonnell, P. C., Gum, R. J., Hand, A. T., Lee, J. C., and Young, P. R. (1997) Novel homologues of CSBP/p38 MAP kinase: activation, substrate specificity and sensitivity to inhibition by pyridinyl imidazoles. *Biochem. Biophys. Res. Commun.* **235,** 533–538.
23. Platanias, L.C. (2003) The p38 Map kinase pathway and its role in interferon signaling. *Pharmacol. Ther.* **98,** 129–142.

10

Development of an Interferon-Based Cancer Vaccine Protocol

Application to Several Types of Murine Cancers

W. Robert Fleischmann, Jr. and Tzu G. Wu

Summary

A protocol for the development of cancer vaccines is presented. The protocol is based upon the long-term in vitro treatment of cancer cells with interferon (IFN)-α to create cancer vaccine cells. This protocol has been used to develop cancer vaccines in mice against B16 melanoma, RM-1 prostate cancer, and P388 lymphocytic leukemia. A detailed description of the protocol is presented. Important considerations that are discussed include the method of selection of potential cancer vaccine cells that would make good models for cancer vaccines for human cancers, the effects of in vitro IFN-α treatment concentration on the efficacy of generated cancer vaccine cells, the differential ability of cancer cells to become efficacious cancer vaccine cells in response to IFN-α treatment, the determination of the effectiveness of ultraviolet-light killing of various cancer cell types for generating cancer vaccine cells, and the methods of evaluation of statistical significance of the data obtained. Potential problems also are addressed.

Key Words: Interferon; cancer vaccine; tumor immunity; murine tumor models.

1. Introduction

Cancer is a major cause of morbidity and mortality in the United States and around the world. According to the American Cancer Society Web Site, it is estimated that more than one million Americans will get cancer this year (*1*). Statistics indicate that the lifetime odds of getting cancer in America are one in two for men and one in three for women. This suggests that the approx 40% of Americans will get cancer. More than 20% of deaths among Americans are attributable to cancer, indicating that about 50% will die of their disease. Thus, current treatments with surgery, radiation therapy, chemotherapy, and biological therapy are insufficient to cure many cancer patients. New treatments are needed.

Development of cancer vaccines represents a potentially important new treatment possibility. Cancer vaccines would have the benefit of activating the patient's own immune system to attack the cancer. Several approaches to the development of cancer vaccines have been initiated (for review, see **refs. 2,3**). Clinical studies are now underway to evaluate cancer vaccines based on cancer cells that express granulocytic monocyte-colony-stimulating factor *(4–6)*; cancer cells that express the superantigen, staphylococeal enterotoxin A (SEA) *(7)*; cancer cells *(8)*; or antigen-presenting cells *(9)* that express high levels of tumor antigens; and, injections of tumor antigens with *(10)* or without *(11–13)* cytokines as adjuvants.

Our laboratory has been using another approach to develop cancer vaccines *(14–16)*. Initial studies have been performed with mouse cancer model systems, as models of human cancer. Cancer cells that have been exposed in vitro to long-term (>1 wk) treatment with type I interferon (IFN) appear to undergo physiologic changes that cause them to become better stimulators of the host immune response. If these IFN-treated cancer cells are killed and injected as a whole-cell vaccine, they stimulate the host immune defense to develop an immunity to the parental cancer.

B16 melanoma in the C57Bl/6 mouse has been used as a model for human malignant melanoma *(14,15)*. Vaccination with killed, IFN-treated B16 cells (B16-α cells) provides an efficacious immunity to parental B16 melanoma cells *(15)*. This immunity develops without the use of adjuvant therapy *(15)*. With four vaccinations, 50% of vaccinated mice survive later challenge with parental B16 cells *(15)*. With six vaccinations, approx 90% of vaccinated mice survive later challenge with parental B16 cells *(17)*. It should be noted that injection of killed parental B16 cells is ineffective as a vaccine *(15)*.

The cancer immunity that develops in response to vaccination with killed B16α cells exhibits many features that are to be expected for a vaccine that activates host cancer immunity. The cancer immunity:

- Shows a memory response, protecting 30% of tumor challenge survivors against tumor rechallenge *(15)*;
- Is effective systemically, protecting against tumor challenge at a site distant from the vaccination site *(15)*;
- Is effective against metastases, reducing B16F10 lung metastases by 65% *(15)*;
- Is curative, curing 40 to 50% of mice given a tumor 3 d before initiation of vaccination *(15)*;
- Is tumor-specific, protecting against B16 melanoma but not against syngeneic RM-1 prostate cancer *(17)*; and,
- Requires the function of host macrophages, helper T cells, cytotoxic T cells, and natural killer cells *(16)*.

The vaccination protocol has been extended to other cancer models and to other mouse strains: RM-1 prostate cancer and P388 *(16)*. Long-term, in vitro

IFN treatment has been used to create RM-1α and P388α vaccines. Four to six vaccinations with these vaccines have been shown to protect 20 and 25% of vaccinated mice from later challenge with the respective parental cancer cells. Challenge with the parental cancer cells is otherwise uniformly fatal. These studies indicate that the efficacy of the protocol of long-term in vitro IFN treatment is broadly applicable to various solid cancers and leukemia and is not limited to a specific cancer type.

B16 and RM-1 are syngeneic to C57Bl/6 mice, whereas P388 is syngeneic to DBA/2 mice. These studies indicate that the protocol is likely to be broadly active and is not limited to a specific mouse strain.

Taken together, it would appear that the vaccination protocol, based on long-term IFN treatment of cancer cells, leads to the development of ideal vaccines. First, as whole-cell vaccines, the long-term IFN-treated cancer vaccine cells maintain cell heterogeneity. Second, the vaccine cells can be killed before they are inoculated (an important safety issue) and still trigger host cancer immunity. Third, the vaccine cells can trigger host cancer immunity without the need to employ potentially toxic adjuvants. Fourth, the vaccine cells trigger a potent immune response to the parental tumor that is capable of destroying primary or metastatic cancers. Fifth, the vaccine protocol appears to have broad applicability in the development of vaccines against several different cancers. Although more preclinical work must be accomplished, the vaccination protocol shows considerable promise for applicability to humans.

2. Materials

1. *Sources of non-immunogenic or poorly immunogenic tumor cells:* Murine B16 melanoma cells were obtained from Dr. I. J. Fidler (M.D. Anderson, Houston, TX). RM-1 prostate cancer cells were obtained from Dr. T.C. Thompson (Baylor College of Medicine, Houston, TX). 4T1 breast cancer cells were obtained from Dr. Fred Miller (Michigan Cancer Foundation, Detroit, MI). P388 lymphocytic leukemia cells were obtained from the American type Culture Collection (ATTC, Bethesda, MD).
2. *Growth media:* Two types of growth media were used for cell culture. B16 melanoma cells were grown in Eagle's Minimal Essential Medium (Earle's base, Gibco, Grand Island, NY) supplemented with 10% fetal bovine serum (Intergen, Purchase, NY), 0.22% sodium bicarbonate, 100 U/mL penicillin (Pfizer, New York, NY), 100 µg/mL streptomycin (Pfizer), and 11 µg/mL gentamicin (Invernex, Chagrin Falls, OH *[18]*). RM-1 prostate cancer cells, 4T1 breast cancer cells, and P388 lymphocytic leukemia cells were grown in Dulbecco's Minimal Essential Medium (Gibco) supplemented with fetal bovine serum, sodium bicarbonate, and antibiotics as previously described for the growth medium for B16 melanoma cells *(19,20)*.
3. *Transfer media:* Hanks Balanced Salt Solution (HBSS without calcium and magnesium, Gibco) was used to wash all cells before transfer. HBSS contain-

ing 2 mM ethylene diamine tetraacetic acid (EDTA, Sigma, St. Louis, MO) was used to remove adherent B16 melanoma cells. HBSS containing 4 mM EDTA was used to remove adherent RM-1 prostate cancer cells and 4T1 breast cancer cells. P388 lymphocytic leukemia cells were grown as nonadherent cells.
4. *Inoculation media:* For vaccination and tumor challenge, all cancer cells were suspended in HBSS.
5. *Type I IFNS used for in vitro treatment of tumor cells:* Two type I IFNs have been used in our studies to create cancer vaccine cells: IFN-α and IFN-β.
    a. IFN-α was obtained as rHuIFN-αA/D from Pestka Biomedical Laboratories (New Brunswick, NJ). rHuIFN-αA/D is also known as universal IFN because it can cross species barriers. Indeed, its activity on many species of animal cells is comparable to that of IFN-α or IFN-β made in those species of animal cells. rHuIFN-αA/D was reported to have a titer of 1×10^6 and a specific activity of 1.17×10^8 U/mg of protein. In our hands, using mouse reference standard G002-904-511, the batch of rHuIFN-αA/D employed had a titer of 8×10^4 International Reference Units/mL (IRU/mL).
    b. MuIFN-β was obtained from Access Biomedical Diagnostic and Research Laboratories, Inc. (San Diego, CA).

3. Methods

3.1. Overview of the Protocol for Production of Vaccine Cells by In Vitro Treatment With IFN

Parental cancer cells of the selected type are grown in vitro in the presence of type I IFN for at least 1 wk. These long-term IFN-treated cells are designated α-cells or β-cells, to indicate the type I IFN to which they have been exposed. Prior to inoculation as a vaccine, the cells are inactivated by ultraviolet (UV) light or by γ-irradiation. The inactivated vaccine cells are injected into mice (without adjuvant therapy). Four to six vaccinations may be required to establish cancer immunity. Each step in this protocol must be performed with care.

3.2. Selection of Tumor Cells That Are Nonimmunogenic or Poorly Immunogenic

Human cancers are nonimmunogenic or poorly immunogenic. Thus, it is important to select a mouse cancer model that is non-immunogenic or poorly immunogenic, so it will serve as a good model for human cancer. To demonstrate that a cancer cell line is non-immunogenic or poorly immunogenic, the parental cancer cells should be grown in culture, killed by UV light or γ-irradiation, and injected into syngeneic mice as a vaccine. At least four to six vaccinations should be given, as it takes that many vaccinations for long-term IFN-treated cancer vaccine cells to trigger host cancer immunity. **Table 1** presents the data for representative experiments employing B16 melanoma, RM-1 prostate cancer, P388 lymphocytic leukemia, and 4T1 breast cancer in which

Table 1
Efficacy of the Vaccination Protocol Against B16 Melanoma, RM-1 Prostate Cancer, P388 Lymphocytic Leukemia, and 4T1 Breast Cancer

Vaccination cell type[a]	Tumor challenge	Number of vaccinations	Day of death[b] Mean ± SE	Number of survivors (90 d)	% Mice protected[c]
1. None	B16	(HBSS)	14.4 ± 0.8	0/19	0%
2. B16	B16	4	15.3 ± 3.7	0/19	0%
3. B16-α	B16	4	27.1 ± 4.9	6/18	33%
4. None	B16	(HBSS)	14.9 ± 0.4	0/20	0%
5. B16-α	B16	4	56.1 ± 5.8	10/20	50%
6. B16-α	B16	6	49.7 ± 9.9	15/18	83%
7. None	RM-1	(HBSS)	12.9 ± 0.5	0/19	0%
8. RM-1	RM-1	4	16.0 ± 1.5	0/15	0%
9. RM-1α	RM-1	4	17.6 ± 1.5	0/17	0%
10. None	RM-1	(HBSS)	14.0 ± 0.3	0/24	0%
11. RM-1	RM-1	6	19.7 ± 0.7	0/23	0%
12. RM-1α	RM-1	6	20.1 ± 0.9	4/20	20%
13. None	P388	(HBSS)	24.0 ± 0.3	0/19	0%
14. P388	P388	4	25.6 ± 0.4	0/18	0%
15. P388-α	P388	4	32.6 ± 1.8	4/16	25%
16. None	4T1	(HBSS)	21.8 ± 1.0	0/20	0%
17. 4T1	4T1	4	22.7 ± 1.1	0/19	0%
18. 4T1-α	4T1	4	33.9 ± 1.7	1/18	6%

[a]C57Bl/6 mice were vaccinated once a week for 4 or 6 wk, as specified, with 10^6 inactivated cells of the cell type indicated. After the last vaccination (on d 0), the mice were challenged with an i.p. injection of 10^6 live B16 cells or of 10^5 live RM-1, P388, or 4T1 cells. Control mice received only mock vaccinations with carrier (HBSS).

[b]Survivors are excluded.

[c]Fisher exact probability test for the % mice protected: group 1 vs group 3, $p = 0.0013$; group 4 vs group 5, $p = 0.00022$; group 4 vs group 6, $p = 0.0001$; group 5 vs group 6, $p = 0.028$; group 10 vs group 12, $p = 0.036$; group 13 vs group 15, $p = 0.035$; group 16 vs group 18, $p = NS$.

mice were inoculated four or six times with carrier, killed parental cells, and killed long-term IFN-treated vaccine cells. The mice were then challenged with live parental cells. The number of survivors and the day of death of mice that died were noted.

Examination of the data for B16 melanoma show that, with four vaccinations with parental B16 cells, there were no survivors and there was no increase in the survival time relative to injection with carrier alone (line 2 vs line 1). Similarly, the data for P388 lymphocytic leukemia show that, with four vaccinations with parental P388 cells, there were no survivors and there was no increase in survival time relative to injection with carrier alone (line 14 vs line 13). On the other hand, with four vaccinations with the B16α vaccine cells (line 3) and with four vaccinations with P388α vaccine cells (line 15), there were 33% and 25% survivors, respectively, and a significant increase in the survival time of those mice that died. These results indicate the B16 melanoma and P388 lymphocytic leukemia cells are not immunogenic or very poorly immunogenic.

Examination of the data for RM-1 prostate cancer cells shows that, with six vaccinations with parental RM-1 cells, there were no survivors but that there was a slight but significant increase in the survival time relative to injection with carrier alone (line 11 vs line 10). With six vaccinations with the RM-1α vaccine cells (line 12), there were 20% survivors and a significant increase in the survival time of those mice that died. These results indicate that the RM-1 parental cells are poorly immunogenic. They also indicate that the RM-1α vaccine is not as effective a vaccine on a per vaccination basis as B16α and P388α vaccine cells (*see* **Note 1**).

3.3. Differential Efficacy of Cancer Vaccine Cells Treated With Different Concentrations of IFN

The efficacy of cancer vaccine cells is dependent upon the concentration of IFN in which the vaccine cells are grown. Thus, it is necessary to determine the IFN treatment concentration that gives the best vaccine efficacy. The data shown in **Table 2** and **Fig. 1** illustrate this point. B16-α cells grown in different concentrations of IFN exhibited different vaccine efficacies. Vaccinations with killed B16-α vaccine cells grown in 300 IRU/mL, 1,000 IRU/mL, 3,000 IRU/mL, and 10,000 IRU/mL were able to protect 21%, 30%, 60%, and 21% of mice from challenge with parental B16 cells, respectively. Thus, B16-α cells grown in 3000 IRU/mL showed greatest efficacy as a vaccine (*see* **Note 2**).

3.4. Differential Ability of Different Cancer Cells To Become Efficacious Cancer Vaccine Cells in Response to IFN Treatment

As shown in **Table 1**, B16-α melanoma vaccine cells and P388-α lymphocytic leukemia vaccine cells have about the same ability to serve as cancer vaccine cells. It can be seen that four vaccinations with B16-α vaccine cells provide a significant protective effect, ranging in the two experiments from 33% (line 3) to 50% (line 5) of the mice protected. (Parenthetically, it should be noted that 33% survival was observed in experiments before the vaccination protocol became optimized; 50 to 60% survival is routine for the optimized vaccine protocol.) Six vaccinations provide an even greater protective effect (83%, line 6). For P388α vaccine cells, four vaccinations provide a protective effect to 25% of the mice (line 15), about the same protective effect as was seen for four vaccinations with B16-α vaccine cells.

Table 2
Comparative Efficacies of Vaccinations Using Inactivated B16α Cells Grown in Various Concentrations of IFN-α.

Vaccination cell type[a]	Concentration of IFN-α in culture (IRU/mL)	Day of death[b] Mean ± SE	Number of survivors (90 d)	% Mice protected[c]
1. None	None	16.2 ± 0.6	0/20	0%
2. B16α	300	26.9 ± 2.8	4/19	21%
3. B16α	1,000	36.6 ± 4.0	6/20	30%
4. B16α	3,000	42.8 ± 7.0	12/20	60%
5. B16α	10,000	45.9 ± 3.7	4/19	21%

[a]C57Bl/6 mice were vaccinated with 10^6 inactivated B16 or B16-a cells on days -21, -14, -7 and 0 prior to i.p. challenge with 10^6 live B16 cells on day 0. Control mice received only mock vaccinations with carrier (HBSS).
[b]Survivors are excluded.
[c]Fisher exact probability test for the % mice protected: group 1 vs 2: $p = 0.047$; group 1 vs 3: $p = 0.010$; group 1 vs 4: $p < 0.0001$; group 1 vs 5: $p = 0.047$.
Reprinted with permission from **ref. 15**.

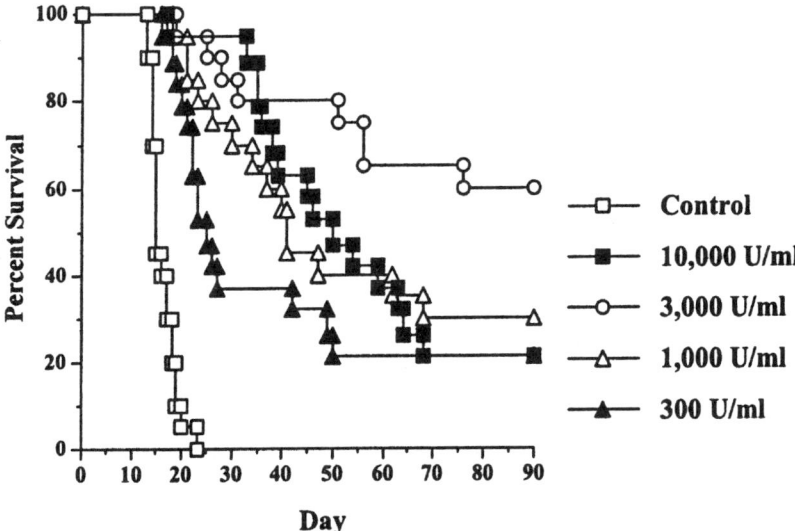

Fig. 1. Effect of in vitro IFN-α treatment concentration. Mice were inoculated i.p. on days −21, −14, −7, and 0 with 10^6 inactivated B16-α cells. The inactivated B16-α cells were pretreated for more than 14 d with 300, 1000, 3000, or 10,000 IRU/mL of IFN-α. Control mice were inoculated with the carrier (HBSS). On day 0, all mice were challenged i.p. with 10^6 live B16 cells. The graph plots the combined data of two experiments as cumulative survival vs day after tumor inoculation. Day of death was noted. (Reprinted with permission from **ref. 15**.)

However, RM-1α prostate vaccine cells and 4T1-α breast cancer vaccine cells have less of an ability than B16-α and P388-α vaccine cells to serve as a cancer vaccine, given the same IFN treatment. For RM-1α vaccine cells, four vaccinations does not protect mice from dying when challenged with live RM-1 cells (line 9). Six vaccinations with RM-1α vaccine cells were required to provide a significant protective effect (line 12). For 4T1-α vaccine cells, four vaccinations provided a marginal protective effect, with only 1 of 18 mice surviving challenge with live 4T1 cells (line 18). Thus, different cancer cells have differential abilities to respond to a given IFN treatment to become cancer vaccines.

It has been long recognized that different cell lines express different relative levels of sensitivity to IFNs *(24,25)*. As previously described for **Fig. 1** and **Table 2**, the ability of B16-α vaccine cells to serve as effective vaccines appears to depend upon the concentration of IFN used to create the B16-α vaccine cells. Thus, it is possible that cancer cell lines that are relatively resistant to IFN might not be good candidates for a cancer vaccine.

To test this possibility, the relative sensitivities of the different cancer cells to IFN were tested. As shown in **Fig. 2**, B16, RM-1, and 4T1 cancer cells had approximately equal sensitivities to IFN treatment. As seen in **Table 1**, four vaccinations with B16-α vaccine cells are efficacious, whereas four vaccinations with RM-1α vaccine cells and with 4T1-α vaccine cells are not efficacious. Thus, whereas all three cell types have equal sensitivity to IFN as measured by IFN's antiproliferative effect, they have different abilities to respond to the IFN as measured by its ability to create efficacious vaccine cells.

However, a number of different IFN activities can be measured and a given cell line might be relatively sensitive to IFN's antiviral activity but might be relatively resistant to IFN's antiproliferative activity *(26,27)*. To date, it is not known which IFN activity correlates with the ability of the cancer cells to respond well to IFN treatment to serve as an efficacious vaccine. Thus, the relative vaccine efficacy of each tumor cell type, with a given IFN treatment, must be empirically determined.

3.5. Determination of UV-Light Sensitivity of the Cancer Cells

Injection of live cells during the vaccinations can give rise to tumor formation. Because live cells should not be injected during vaccination, it is necessary to effectively kill the vaccine cells. Different cancer cell lines express differential levels of sensitivity to killing by UV light. The effectiveness of UV-light killing can be quantitatively measured by cloning the cancer cells at the end of the UV light exposure period. Briefly, monolayers or suspensions of cancer cells in plastic culture dishes are placed at a defined distance below a

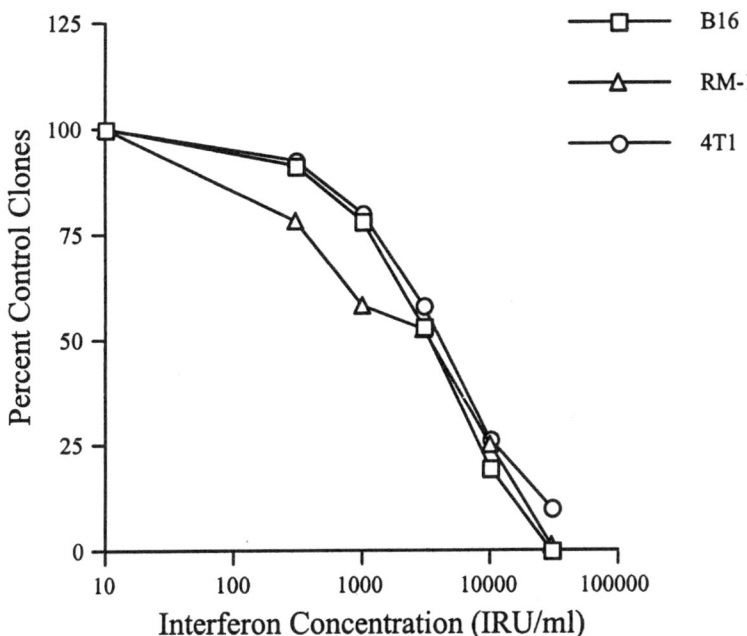

Fig. 2. Relative sensitivities of cancer cells to the antiproliferative effects of IFN-α. B16 melanoma, RM-1 prostate cancer, and 4T1 breast cancer cells were cloned in the presence of varying concentrations of IFN-α. The cells were plated at 600 cells/60-mm tissue culture dish. After 7 d of incubation, 100 to 200 clones developed. The clones were stained with crystal violet (1 in 20% methanol) and counted using a binocular dissecting microscope. The data are presented as percent clones vs interferon concentration.

germicidal UV light and the lid of the culture dish is removed for a defined period of time. The cells in the culture dishes are then counted and cloned. The number of clones that develop after 7 d of incubation is a measure of the percent surviving cancer cells with different levels of exposure to UV light.

As shown in **Fig. 3**, the number of viable B16 cells (measured by their ability to form clones) can be reduced to less than one viable cell in 10^6 cells by exposure to UV-light for 16 min (cells exposed to a 15 watt germicidal lamp at a distance of 35 cm). For the same UV-light treatment, it requires about 1000 minutes of UV-light exposure to reduce RM-1 clones to one viable cell in 10^6 cells. If the distance from the UV-light is reduced to 26 cm, the number of viable RM-1 cells can be reduced to less than one viable cell in 10^6 cells with a 16-min exposure. Thus, B16 cells are much more sensitive to UV killing than are RM-1 cells (*see* **Note 3**).

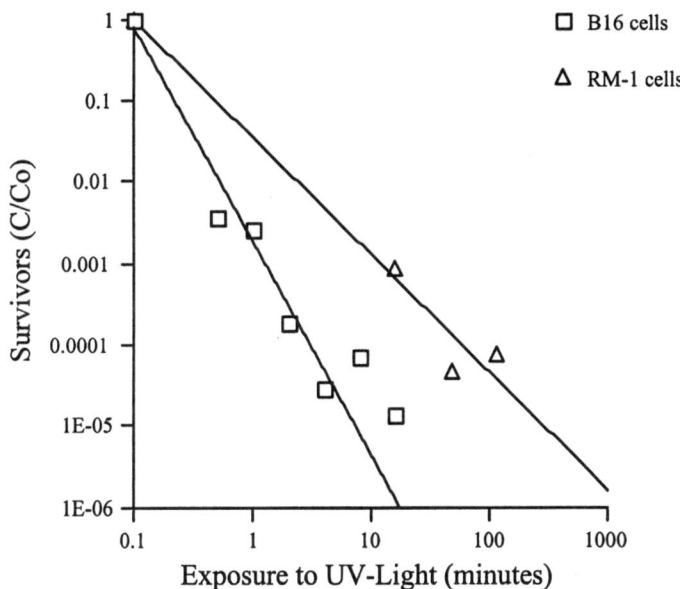

Fig. 3. Differential ultraviolet(UV) light sensitivities of B16 melanoma and RM-1 prostate cancer cells. Petri dishes of suspensions of B16 melanoma and RM-1 prostate cancer cells in HBSS and EDTA were placed under a 15 watt UV light. The lids of the Petri dishes were removed for the indicated time periods. The cells were removed from the Petri dishes, counted and plated under cloning conditions. After 7 d of incubation, the clones were stained with crystal violet (1 in 20% methanol) and counted using a binocular dissecting microscope. The data are plotted as Survivors vs Exposure to UV light.

3.6. Procedure for Growing and Preparing Vaccine Cells for Injection Into Mice

3.6.1. Growth of the Parental and Vaccine Cancer Cells

All cells were grown in plastic tissue culture dishes that were maintained in a humidified incubator (NAPCO, Portland, OR) at 37°C with 5% CO_2. All cells were passaged two times weekly and were split at least 1:4. Parental cells were grown in the appropriate growth medium. Vaccine cells were grown in the appropriate growth medium plus 3000 IRU/mL of IFN.

To passage the parental B16 and vaccine B16-α melanoma cells, the adherent cells were washed once with Hank's Balanced Salt Solution (HBSS, Gibco) and removed from the plates by incubation in 2 mM ethylenediaminetetraacetic acid (EDTA, Sigma, St. Louis, MO) in phosphate-buffered saline (PBS) for 5 min. The cells were centrifuged in a clinical centrifuge, resuspended in HBSS, centrifuged again, and resuspended in growth medium. The cells were plated on tissue culture dishes of the appropriate size.

To passage the parental RM-1 and vaccine RM-1α prostate cancer cells, the adherent cells were washed once with HBSS and removed from the plates for passaging by incubation in 4 mM EDTA in PBS for 5 min. The cells were centrifuged in a clinical centrifuge, resuspended in HBSS, centrifuged again, and resuspended in growth medium. The cells were plated on tissue culture dishes of the appropriate size.

To passage the parental 4T1 and vaccine 4T1-α breast cancer cells, the adherent cells were washed once with HBSS and removed from the plates for passaging by incubation in 4 mM EDTA in PBS for 5 min. The cells were centrifuged in a clinical centrifuge, resuspended in HBSS, centrifuged again, and resuspended in growth medium. The cells were plated on tissue culture dishes of the appropriate size.

To passage the parental P388 and vaccine P388-α lymphocytic leukemia cells, the nonadherent cells were centrifuged in a clinical centrifuge, resuspended in HBSS, centrifuged again, and resuspended in growth medium. The cells were plated on tissue culture dishes of the appropriate size.

3.6.2. Preparation of the Parental and Vaccine Cancer Cells for Injection

Monolayers or suspensions of vaccine cancer cells were exposed to UV-light as indicated above. Following UV-light exposure, the cells were washed three times with HBSS to eliminate any residual bovine fetal serum and IFN supplemented in the growth medium. Then, the cells were removed from the tissue culture dishes (using the appropriate method described above for each cell line), washed with HBSS to remove EDTA, resuspended in HBSS for vaccine preparation, and counted in a hemocytometer. The cell count was adjusted to 10^7 cells/mL by dilution in HBSS. The cell preparations were maintained as uniform suspensions by frequent agitation. For preparation of killed parental cells for use as a vaccine control, the cell preparations were made by the same procedure. For preparation of live parental cells for use as a challenge, the cell preparations were made by the same procedure, without exposure to UV-light.

3.6.3. Injection of Parental and Vaccine Cancer Cells

The appropriate cell suspensions were carried to the animal room to inject the mice. For each experiment, there were 10 mice per group, housed 5 mice per cage. Using one cell suspension preparation, 5 mice for each group were injected with the cells as follows. After, agitation of the cell suspension, a volume of 0.6 mL was drawn into a 1-mL syringe. Then, 0.1 mL of cell suspension was injected into the peritoneal cavity of each of the 5 mice of the group,

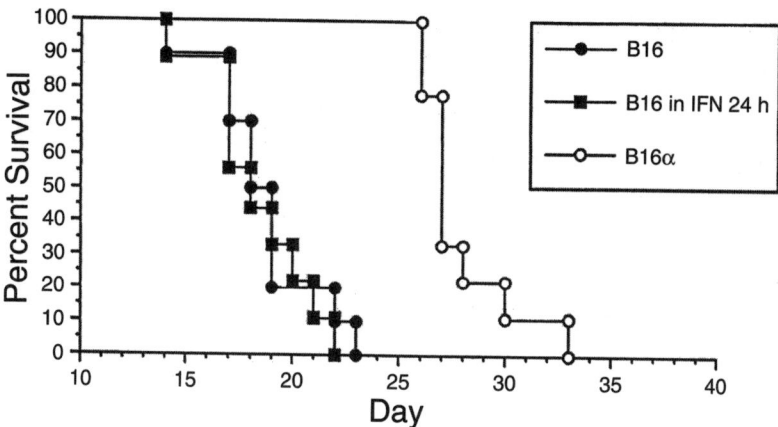

Fig. 4. Effect of duration of in vitro IFN-α treatment on survival time of mice. Female C57Bl/6 mice were divided into groups of 9 or 10 mice and inoculated i.p. with 10^6 untreated B16 melanoma cells, 10^6 B16 melanoma cells treated in vitro with 10,000 U/mL IFN-α for 24 h, or 10^6 B16 melanoma cells treated in vitro with 10,000 U/mL of IFN-α for ≤14 d (B16-α cells). The graph plots the data as percent survival with time. (Reprinted with permission from **ref. 14**.)

with agitation of the contents of the syringe between injections. Note that injection of 0.1 mL of a 10^7 cells/mL suspension resulted in an injection of 10^6 cells per mouse. A total of four or six vaccinations with killed vaccine cells or killed parental cancer cells were given at 1-wk intervals. Challenge with live parental cancer cells was given as soon as possible on the same day as the last vaccination (*see* **Note 4**).

3.7. Determination of the Cancer Vaccine Efficacy

After challenge with live parental cancer cells, the mice are monitored for day of death or day of moribundity. The data may be expressed in tabular form as percent survivors (as shown in **Tables 1** and **2**). The statistical significance of comparative measurements of percent survivors for various groups can be obtained with Student's *t* test or the Fisher's exact probability test. The data may be expressed as survival curves that indicate the number of survivors on each day after challenge with live parental cells (as shown in **Figs. 1** and **4**). The statistical significance of comparative survival curves for various groups can be determined with the Log-rank (Mantel-Cox) statistical analysis.

4. Notes

1. The goal of animal cancer studies is to mimic as closely as possible the characteristics of human cancers. Experiments using mouse cancer cells that are immuno-

genic for vaccine studies may well show successful vaccination characteristics. However, they are unlikely to provide useful information about human cancers. If injection of killed parental cancer cells of a given cancer type is seen to lead to survivors or greatly enhanced survival times following challenge with the parental cancer cell, this would be indicative of an innate immunogenicity of the cancer cell in question. The given cancer cell should not be used for vaccination studies.

2. Cancer vaccine cells are generated by treatment of tumor cells with IFN. The duration of in vitro IFN treatment is an important parameter in the generation of efficacious vaccine cells. In early studies, mice injected with B16α cells demonstrated an increased survival time relative to mice injected with B16 cells (**Fig. 4** *[14]*). The ability of mice to show an increased survival time with B16-α injection was an early demonstration of the immunogenicity of B16α cells. In these same studies, it was shown that in vitro treatment of B16 cells with IFN for 24 h did not lead to an enhanced survival time, indicating that B16 cells treated with IFN for 24 h did not demonstrate immunogenicity. Thus, B16 cells treated with IFN for 24 h were judged not to be suitable for the generation of an efficacious vaccine. It has been noted that cancer cells grown in vitro in IFN for an extended period of time lose their vigor. They begin to exhibit a slower growth rate and begin to die. This negative effect of growth in IFN is observed when cancer cells have been grown for more than two months in the IFN. Thus, for generation of efficacious, viable vaccine cells, cancer cells are maintained in IFN for 1 to 8 wk. Then, new cultures of vaccine cells are initiated.

3. As shown above, RM-1α prostate cancer cells are relatively more resistant to killing by UV light than B16-α melanoma cells. With increasing dosages of UV light (achieved by decreasing the distance between the UV light source and the cell monolayer), the RM-1 cells become sticky and subject to clumping. Clumping of the cells makes it difficult to achieve an accurate count of the cells in a hemocytometer, and makes it difficult to assure injection of the correct number of cells per injection. Further, clumping of the cells makes it difficult to inject essentially identical numbers of cells into each mouse. One solution to the problem of clumping of RM-1α cells involved maintaining the cells as non-adherent cells by plating them on non-tissue culture dishes *(17)* in HBSS plus 4% EDTA during the duration of UV light exposure. With this precaution, clumping was greatly reduced or eliminated and the RM-1 cells could be completely killed by exposure to UV-light at a distance of 26 cm for 16 min *(17)*. Another potential solution involved γ-irradiation (10^4 rads) of the RM-1 cells *(17)*.

4. As indicated above, each experiment had 10 mice in a group, housed 5 mice per cage. It was possible that the cells in the cell suspension might lyse during the period of time from their preparation to the last injection. To minimize the effect of such lysis, if it occurred, only one set of five mice in each group was injected with a given preparation of single-cell suspension. Another single-cell suspension was prepared for injection of the second set of five mice in each group. Furthermore, the order of injection of the groups during the first round of injec-

tions was noted. The order of injection of the groups during the second round of injections was reversed. At the end of the experiment, the data from the first five mice and from the second five mice were compared. If the data for the first five mice and second five mice of the first and last groups injected were different, it would indicate that significant cell lysis had occurred during the injection period. This should be monitored. However, using the technique described, no differences were noted.

References

1. American Cancer Society home page: www.cancer.org/docroot/home/index.asp
2. Jafee, E. M. (1999) Immunotherapy of cancer. *Ann. NY Acad. Sci.* **886,** 67–72.
3. Nabel, G. J. (2004) Genetic, cellular and immune approaches to disease therapy: past and future. *Nat. Med.* **10,** 135–141.
4. Thomas, M. C., Greten, T. F., Pardoll, D. M., and Jaffee, E. M. (1998) Enhanced tumor protection by granulocyte-macrophage colony-stimulating factor expression at the site of an allogeneic vaccine. *Hum. Gene Ther.* **9,** 835–843.
5. Dranoff G. (2003) GM-CSF-secreting melanoma vaccines. *Oncogene* **22,** 3188–3192.
6. Nemunaitis, J. and Nemunaitis, J. (2003) Granulocyte-macrophage colony-stimulating factor gene-transfected autologous tumor cell vaccine: focus on non-small-cell lung cancer. *Clin. Lung Cancer* **5,** 148–157.
7. Ma, W., Yu, H., Wang, Q., Jin, H., Solheim, J., and Labhasetwar, V. (2004) A novel approach for cancer immunotherapy: tumor cells with anchored superantigen SEA generate effective antitumor immunity. *J. Clin. Immunol.* **24,** 294–301.
8. Liao, X., Li, Y., Bonini, C., Nair, S., Gilboa, E., Greenberg, P. D., and Yee, C. (2004) Transfection of RNA encoding tumor antigens following maturation of dendritic cells leads to prolonged presentation of antigen and the generation of high-affinity tumor-reactive cytotoxic T lymphocytes. *Mol. Ther.* **9,** 757–764.
9. Hsueh, E. C., Essner, R., Foshag, L. J., Ollila, D. W., Gammon, G., O'Day, S. J., et al. (2002) Prolonged survival after complete resection of disseminated melanoma and active immunotherapy with a therapeutic cancer vaccine. *J. Clin. Oncol.* **20,** 4549–4554.
10. Salem, M. L., Kadima, A. N., Zhou, Y., Nguyen, C. L., Rubinstein, M. P., Demcheva, M., et al. (2004) Paracrine release of IL-12 stimulates IFN-gamma production and dramatically enhances the antigen-specific T cell response after vaccination with a novel peptide-based cancer vaccine. *J. Immunol.* **172,** 5159–5167.
11. Slingluff, C. L. Jr., Petroni, G. R., Yamshchikov, G. V., Barnd, D. L., Eastham, S., Galavotti, H., et al. (2003) Clinical and immunological results of a randomized Phase II Trial of vaccination using four melanoma peptides either administered in granulocyte-macrophage colony-stimulating factor in adjuvant or pulsed on dendritic cells. *J. Clin. Oncol.* **21,** 4016–4026.

12. Maraskovsky, E., Sjolander, S., Drane, D. P., Schnurr, M., Le, T. T., Mateo, L., et al. (2004) NY-ESO-1 protein formulated in ISCOMATRIX adjuvant is a potent anticancer vaccine inducing both humoral and CD8+ t-cell-mediated immunity and protection against NY-ESO-1+ tumors. *Clin. Cancer Res.* **10**, 2879–2890.
13. Sinibaldi-Vallebona, P., Rasi, G., Pierimarchi, P., Bernard, P., Guarino, E., Guadagni, F., and Garaci, E. (2004) Vaccination with a synthetic nonapeptide expressed in human tumors prevents colorectal cancer liver metastases in syngeneic rats. *Int. J. Cancer* **110**, 70–75.
14. Fleischmann, C. M., Wu, T. Y., and Fleischmann, W. R. Jr. (1997) B16 melanoma cells exposed in vitro to long-term IFN-α treatment (B16α cells) as activators of host cell tumor immunity in mice. *J. Interferon Cytokine Res.* **17**, 37–43.
15. Wu, T. Y. and Fleischmann, W. R. Jr. (1998) Efficacy of B16 melanoma cells exposed in vitro to long-term IFN-α treatment (B16α cells) as a tumor vaccine in mice. *J. Interferon Cytokine Res.* **18**, 829–839.
16. Wu, T. Y. and Fleischmann, W. R. Jr. (2001) Murine B16 melanoma vaccination-induced tumor immunity: identification of specific immune cells and functions involved. *J. Interferon Cytokine Res.* **21**, 1117–1127.
17. Wu, T. Y. and Fleischmann, W. R. Jr. Unpublished observations.
18. Fidler, I. J. (1973) Selection of successive tumor lines for metastasis. *Nature New Biol.* **242**, 148–149.
19. Thompson, T. C., Southgate, J., Kitchener, G., and Land, H. (1989) Multi-stage carcinogenesis induced by ras and myc oncogenes in a reconstituted organ. *Cell* **56**, 917–930.
20. Baley, P. A., Yoshida, K., Qian, W., Sehgal, I., and Thompson, T. C. (1995) Progression to androgen insensitivity in a novel *in vitro* mouse model for prostate cancer. *J. Steroid Biochem. Mol. Biol.* **52**, 403–413.
21. Coveney, E., Clary, B., Philip, R., and Lyerly, K. (1996) Active immunotherapy with transiently transfected cytokine-secreting tumor cells inhibits breast cancer metastases in tumor-bearing animals. *Surgery* **120**, 265–273.
22. Morecki, S., Lubina-Salomon, A., Slavin, S., and Nagler, A. (1998) Cytokine gene transduction into non-immunogeneic murine tumor cells. *Cytokines Cell. Mol. Ther.* **4**, 87–94.
23. Ozer. H. L. (1966) Purine pyrophosphorylase as a selective genetic marker in a mouse lymphoma, P388, in cell culture. *J. Cell Physiol.* **68**, 61–68.
24. Evinger, M., Rubinstein, M., and Pestka, S. (1981) Antiproliferative and antiviral activities of human leukocyte interferons. *Arch. Biochem. Biophys.* **210**, 319–329.
25. Ortaldo, J. R., Mantovani, A., Hobbs, D., Rubinstein, M., Pestka, S., and Herberman, R. B. (1983) Effects of several species of human leukocyte interferon on cytotoxic activity of NK cells and monocytes. *Int. J. Cancer* **31**, 285–289.
26. Rehberg, E., Kelder, B., Hoal, E. G., and Pestka, S. (1982) Specific molecular activities of recombinant and hybrid leukocyte interferons. *J. Biol. Chem.* **257**, 11,497–11,502

27. Ortaldo, J. R., Mason, A., Rehberg, E., Kelder, B., Harvey, C., Oscheroff, P., et al. (1983) Augmentation of NK activity with recombinant and hybrid recombinant human leukocyte interferons, in *The Biology of the Interferon System* (DeMaeyer E. and Schellekens, H., eds.), Elsevier Science Publishers B. V., Amsterdam, Netherlands, pp. 353–358.

11

Type I Interferons as Regulators of the Differentiation/Activation of Human Dendritic Cells

Methods for the Evaluation of IFN-Induced Effects

Stefano M. Santini, Caterina Lapenta, and Filippo Belardelli

Summary

Recent studies have revealed that type I interferons (IFNs) are powerful inducers of the differentiation and activation of dendritic cells (DCs). These findings emphasize the importance of these cytokines in linking innate and adaptive immunity, suggesting that effects of type I IFN on DCs can play a role in the antitumor and antiviral activity observed in some IFN-treated patients. Thus, the evaluation of the effects of IFN on the differentiation/activation of DCs has become an important approach for testing novel biologically important IFN activities, and the description of some reference methods are urgently needed. In this chapter, we describe some methods for testing the effects of IFNs on the differentiation and activation of human DCs from the peripheral blood monocytes and for the characterization of the DCs generated after IFN treatment.

Key Words: IFN; dendritic cells; differentiation; activation; immune response; antibodies; CD8 T lymphocytes; SCID mice.

1. Introduction

An ensemble of recent studies have revealed that type I interferon (IFN) can exert a potent immune adjuvant activity as revealed by a remarkable enhancement of both humoral and cellular immune response to reference antigens in mice *(1,2)*. These findings are consistent with recently published reports showing that these cytokines can play an important role in inducing the differentiation and activation of both mouse *(3)* and human *(4–9)* dendritic cells (DCs). Altogether, these results have underscored the importance of type I IFN in linking innate and adaptive immune response by acting on special types of DC precursors, thus inducing their rapid differentiation into highly active antigen-presenting cells (APCs) *(10,11)*. In particular, we have recently shown that a 3-d

From: *Methods in Molecular Medicine, Vol. 116: Interferon Methods and Protocols*
Edited by: D. J. J. Carr © Humana Press Inc., Totowa, NJ

treatment of monocytes with type I IFN, in the presence of granulocytic monocyte colony-stimulating factor (GM-CSF) used as survival factor, results in a marked differentiation into partially mature DCs, characterized by high functional activities in vitro as well as in vivo *(5,7,9)*. These results are in agreement with studies from other groups (*4,6,8*; for a review, *see* **ref. 11** and references therein). Thus, because the biological importance of the IFN effects on DCs and their possible relevance for the clinical use of these cytokines have recently been acknowledged in the field of IFN research *(10,11)*, the definition of some reference methods for testing these novel IFN activities in vitro as well as in vivo has become an essential requirement for allowing a reliable comparison of the activity of IFN preparations and for the interpretation of results generated in different laboratories. Of note, we have found that the in vitro and in vivo functional activity of the monocyte-derived DCs generated in the presence of IFN was definitively superior to that of the immature DCs generated by the standard protocol based on the use of interleukin (IL)-4 and GM-CSF *(5,7,9)*, further emphasizing the biological importance of these IFN-induced effects.

In this chapter, we describe some main methods for testing the effects of IFNs on the differentiation and activation of human DCs generated from peripheral blood monocytes and for the characterization of the DCs obtained after IFN treatment (named as "IFN-DCs"). We discuss the specific features of the IFN-DCs in view of the recent knowledge on the heterogeneicity of in vivo DC subsets and taking into account the influence that different experimental conditions may exert on the phenotype and function of the DCs generated after IFN treatment.

2. Materials

2.1. Preparation of Monocytes for the DC Differentiation Assay

These are the materials needed for the enrichment or purification of blood monocytes from blood or buffy coats:

1. Ficoll Biocoll separating solution (density 1.077; Biochrom KG, Berlin, Germany).
2. For positive immunoselection, we recommend Immunomagnetic CD14 Microbeads by Miltenyi Biotec GmbH (Germany).
3. Immunoselection buffer: phosphate-buffered saline (PBS), pH 7.2, supplemented with 0.5% bovine serum albumin (or human albumin or autologous plasma) and 2 mM ethylene diamine tetraacetic acid.

2.2. Cell Culture Media and Cytokines

1. Depending on the experimental purposes (*see* **Note 2**), the following culture media are recommended: RPMI 1640 Medium (Gibco BRL, Gaithersburg, MD) to be

used with fetal bovine serum (FBS) or AIM-V Medium (Gibco BRL, Gaithersburg, MD) to be used with autologous serum or plasma.
2. The cytokines used for monocyte-DC differentiation are as follows: (a) GM-CSF: (R&D Systems or (Peprotech, Rocky Hill, NJ) and (b) Natural IFN-α (Alfa-Wasserman), IFN-α2b (Schering-Plough), IFN-β (Peprotec or Serono). These are the IFN preparation mostly used in our studies. However, any IFN preparation can be tested using dosages and experimental conditions recommended subsequently.

2.3. Immunostaining and Flow Cytometry

The following monoclonal antibodies (MAbs) are recommended for immunofluorescent staining of IFN-DCs: anti-CD14, CD11c, CD54, CD80, and HLA-DR (Becton Dickinson, San Jose CA) and CD1a, CD40, CD86, and CD83 (Pharmingen, San Diego CA).

2.4. In Vitro Migration Assay

1. 24-well transwell cell culture chambers (Costar, Corning, NY) are used.
2. The chemokines used for the in vitro migration assays are: RANTES, MIP1-α, or MIP1-β from R&D System (Abingdon, UK) and MIP3-α and MIP3-β from Peprotech (Rocky Hill, NJ).

2.5. Severe Combined Immunodeficient (SCID) Mice for the In Vivo Testing of the Functional Activity of Monocyte-Derived DCs Generated in the Presence of IFNs

1. SCID (CB17 scid/scid) female mice (Harlan, Nossan, Italy) are preferably used at 4 wk of age and kept under specific pathogen-free conditions.
2. SCID mice must be housed in microisolator cages and all food, water, and bedding must be autoclaved before use.

3. Methods

3.1. Evaluation of the Effects of IFN on the Differentiation of DCs From Monocytes

The generation of human DCs can be achieved by treatment of myeloid precursors $CD14^+$ monocytes derived from peripheral blood with type I IFN and GM-CSF (5). Several type I IFNs can be used to induce DC differentiation; the optimal IFN concentrations for DC differentiation must be determined by testing dilutions ranging from 500 to 10,000 IU/mL and is selected as the dose capable of promoting high levels of expression of DC differentiation/activation antigens, with minimal toxicity and consequent cell death (see **Note 1**). The IFN-induced effects on blood monocytes can be demonstrated both phenotypically and functionally.

3.1.1. Preparation of Monocytes and Cytokine Treatment

CD14$^+$ monocytes can be enriched or purified from whole blood or buffy coats by different methods (*see* **Subheading 2.1.** for the materials).

1. Start with freshly drawn human blood or buffy coat, treated with an anti-coagulant (e.g., heparin, ethylene dimaine tetraacetic acid, citrate, acid citrate dextrose anticoagulant or citrate phosphate dextrose).
2. Dilute buffy coats with 2 to 4 volumes of calcium/magnesium free PBS. Fresh whole blood should be diluted with one volume of PBS.
3. Purify peripheral blood mononuclear cells (PBMCs) by Ficoll density gradient centrifugation.
4. Wash extensively with calcium/magnesium free PBS.
5. To eliminate contaminating platelets, carefully resuspend the cell pellet in 50 mL of PBS and centrifuge at 200g for 10 to 15 min at 20°C. Carefully remove the supernatant completely. Repeat this last washing step. Most of the platelets will remain in the supernatant upon centrifugation at 200g.
6. Resuspend the cells in complete RPMI 1640 medium supplemented with 10% fetal calf serum (FCS) at a concentration of 5×10^6 cells /mL in culture flask or dish.
7. Place in a cell incubator at 37°C for 2 h.
8. Collect the supernatant containing nonadherent cells (lymphocytes, NK cells)
9. Wash extensively with cold PBS.
10. The adherent fraction is mostly represented by monocytes

Alternatively, monocytes can be purified by positive or negative immunomagnetic labeling and selection. For positive selection of CD14$^+$ monocytes, start from **step 5**. Resuspend the cells in immunoselection buffer, add antibody-conjugated magnetic microbeads, and proceed as recommended by the manufacturer.

Monocytes should be plated at the concentration of 2.0×10^6 cells/mL in complete medium as RPMI 1640 supplemented with 2 mM glutamine, 50 µg penicillin, 10 µg/mL streptomycin and 10% fetal bovine serum, containing 500 IU/mL of GM-CSF and type I IFN from 500 to 10,000 IU/mL (*see* **Note 2**). Materials are listed in **Subheading 2.2.** If the purpose of the experimental work is to generate preclinical data for the use of IFN-DCs in clinical trials, clinically graded medium (AIM-V) and other suitable reagents must be used (*see* **Note 2**).

3.1.2. Phenotypic Characterization of Monocyte-Derived IFN-DCs

Exposure of blood monocytes to type I IFN in conjunction with GM-CSF results in marked phenotypic changes within 3 d *(5)*. The easiest method to monitor these changes is to evaluate the modulation of selected membrane marker expression by FACS analysis (*see* **Note 3**). The antibody panel used to characterize IFN-DCs is reported in **Subheading 2.3.**, whereas examples of FACS profiles are shown in **Fig. 1**.

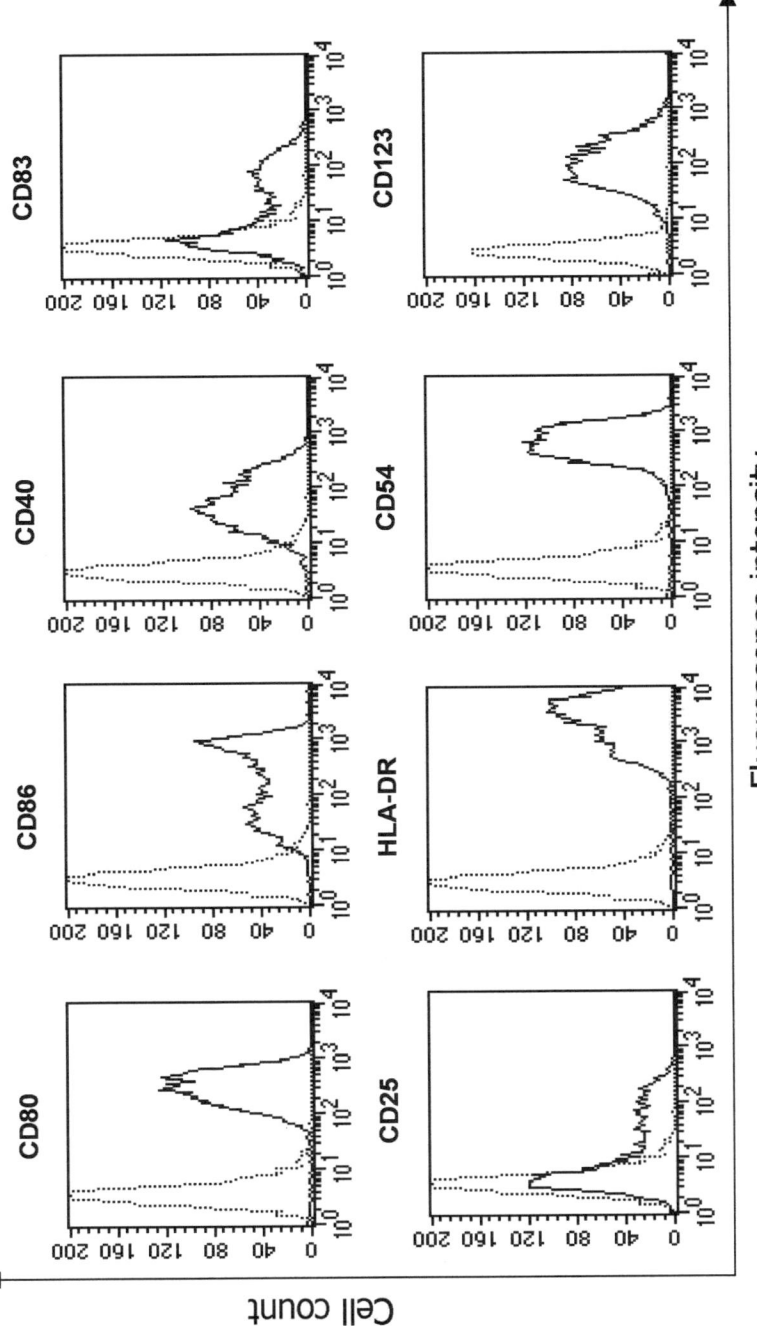

Fig. 1. Phenotypic profile of IFN-DCs obtained by exposure of blood monocytes to 500 IU/mL GM-CSF and 10,000 IU natural IFN-α for 3 d. Fluorescence-activated cell sorting analysis suggests the presence of a more mature subpopulation of IFN-DCs.

1. Wash DCs in PBS containing 2% human serum (see **Note 4**).
2. Resuspend the cells in 50 µL of PBS containing 2% human serum.
3. Add the appropriate fluorochrome-conjugated MAbs to relevant antigens and incubate for 30 min at 4°C.
4. Wash DCs in PBS containing 2% human serum.
5. Resuspend in 500 µL of PBS.
6. Collect and analyze data by flow cytometry. Gate electronically the DC population according to light scatter properties in order to exclude cell debris and contaminating lymphocytes.

3.2. Functional Characterization of Monocyte-Derived IFN-DCs by In Vitro Assays

The effect of type I IFN on the differentiation/activation of monocyte-derived DCs needs also to be evaluated at functional level. In fact, phenotypic changes are paralleled by enhancement of immune-stimulating properties of IFN-DCs *(5,7,9)*. Moreover, IFN-DCs have been shown to retain a specific pattern of chemokine and cytokine production. As an example, Mip3-β, IP-10, and DC-CK1 genes have been shown to induced in IFN-DCs *(7)*; of note, these cells also express significant levels of IL-15, whose release in the culture supernatants is augmented by LPS stimulation together with IL-12 production *(5)*. Cytokine production is easily assayed by commercial ELISA kits or by reverse-transcription polymerase chain reaction.

3.2.1. Mixed Lymphocyte Reaction

The simplest way to test IFN-DC functionality is the *allogenic* "mixed lymphocyte reaction" (MLR) assay *(5)*. IFN-DCs exhibit an enhanced allostimulatory capacity (MLR). Allogeneic PBLs are efficiently stimulated at a stimulator/responder ratio of 1:10, 1:20, and 1:40.

1. Seed monocyte-depleted PBLs seeded into 96-well plates (Costar, Cambridge, MA) at 10^5 cells per well.
2. Add purified allogeneic DCs (from 5×10^1 to 5×10^3) to each well in triplicate.
3. After 5 d, add 1 µCi of methyl-^{3}H-Thymidine (Amersham) to each well
4. Continue incubation for an additional 18 h.
5. Collected cells by a cell harvester and measure thymidine uptake by β liquid scintillation counting.

3.2.2. Induction of Primary Response to Reference Antigens and Proliferation Assay

Although allogenic MLR represents a rapid assay for DC functional activity, the effects of type IFN on DC differentiation/activation should also be tested by evaluating the capability to induce a primary response, which is a peculiar feature of professional APCs.

3.2.2.1. Preparation of the Immunogen

IFN-DCs can be efficiently loaded with peptides *(12)*, pulsed with recombinant proteins, apoptotic bodies, or cell lysates (unpublished data). Herein, we describe the procedure mostly used in our laboratory, which is based on the use of chemically inactivated HIV-1 as immunogen *(5,9)*.

HIV-1 is inactivated by AT-2 following a procedure described by Rossio et al. *(13)*; Prepare a stock solution of AT-2 (Sigma, St. Louis, MO) 500 mM in dimethyl sulfoxide (Aldrich, Milwaukee, WI) The solution is prepared and added directly to virus to produce the desired AT-2 concentration.

Clarify virus by centrifugation of the supernatants of infected PBMC cultures at 400 g for 30 min.

1. Treat virus preparations with 2 mM AT-2 for 1 h at 37°C. At the conclusion of the inactivating procedures, treatment agent is removed by ultrafiltration with a centrifugal filtration device with a 500-kDa cut-off (*see* **Subheading 2.4.**)
2. Inactivated virus can be kept on ice until used (within 2 h) or stored at –140°C for subsequent use.

3.2.2.2. DC Loading With AT-2 Inactivated HIV-1

1. Wash twice the IFN-DCs with culture medium without serum.
2. Resuspend the cells in a small volume of culture medium supplemented with 10% FCS or 2% human AB serum or 2% autologous plasma.
3. Load IFN-DCs with 100 ng (p24 titrated by enzyme-linked immunosorbent assay [ELISA]) inactivated virus/ 3×10^6 cells and incubate for 2 h at 37°C.
4. Wash three times with serum free culture medium.
5. Antigen-loaded IFN-DCs are used immediately or frozen in liquid nitrogen before use. Cells are resuspended in 90%FCS–10% dimethyl sulfoxide. Alternatively, the cells can be frozen in 50% AIM-V medium, 40%/autologous serum,10% dimethyl sulfoxide.

3.2.2.3. Proliferation Assay

1. Stimulate PBLs with autologous inactivated virus-loaded IFN-DCs at E/S ratio of 4:1 into triplicate wells.
2. Add 25 IU/mL of IL-2 after 3 d of culture.
3. Restimulate the PBLs with virus-pulsed DCs at a 7-d interval for 2 wk; add 25 IU/mL of IL-2, 3 d after each stimulation.
4. After 6 d from the last stimulation, add 1 µCi of methyl-^{3}H-thymidine to each well and continue incubation for additional 18 h.
5. Collect the cells by cell harvesting and determine thymidine uptake by beta liquid scintillation counting.

3.2.2.4. Enzyme-Linked Immunospot (ELISPOT) Assay

ELISPOT assays are performed according to the manufacturer's instructions (Euroclone or Becton-Dickinson). We briefly describe the main steps.

1. Coat the plates with anti-IFN-γ or anti Granzyme-B capture antibodies.
2. Perform a blocking step to avoid nonspecific binding.
3. Restimulate overnight the PBLs from primary cultures with IFN-DCs pulsed with inactivated HIV-1, at a E/S ratio from 1:1 to 1:4. Add to triplicate wells and incubate for 18 h at 37°C in a 5% CO_2 humidified incubator.
4. Proceed for detection step and enumerate spots using an automatic analyzer.

3.3. Functional Characterization of Monocyte-Derived IFN-DCs by In Vivo Assays

SCID mice reconstituted with human PBL (Hu-PBL-SCID mice) have been widely used for in vivo studies on the effects of certain human pathogens (especially HIV-1) on cells of the human immune system *(14–17)*. In particular, we have shown that the hu-PBL-SCID mouse is a valuable model to assess the efficacy of newly generated APCs to induce human cellular and humoral response in vivo *(5,9)*. In fact, this xenochimeric model suffers from the lack of functional antigen presenting cellular compartment, which is rapidly lost after reconstitution of immunodeficient SCID mice with human PBMCs and antigen priming is restored by supplying human autologous APCs. Antigen-pulsed IFN-DCs are injected intraperitoneally (i.p.) into SCID mice previously reconstituted with autologous PBMCs.

3.3.1. Evaluation of the Capability of Antigen-Pulsed IFN-DCs to Generate an Antibody Response in the hu-PBL-SCID Mouse Model

We have developed a vaccination protocol in the xenochimeric Hu-PBL-SCID mouse model *(9)*. In our studies, we evaluate the capability of DCs pulsed with aldrithiol-2 (AT-2)-inactivated HIV-1 in inducing a human immune response in SCID mice reconstituted with human PBL (Hu-PBL-SCID mice).

Hu-PBLs are obtained from the peripheral blood of healthy donors screened for HIV-1 and hepatitis prior to donation. The hu-PBLs are obtained by Ficoll density gradient centrifugation. Resuspend 20 to 30 millions of PBLs in 0.5 mL of RPMI 1640 medium and inject into the peritoneum of recipient mice. Three days after reconstitution with human PBLs, hu-PBL-SCID mice are injected i.p. with 2.5×10^6 autologous DCs, pulsed 2 h at 37°C with AT-2-inactivated HIV-1 (100 ng of p24). Mice are boosted with the inactivated virus-pulsed autologous DCs on d 7 and then subjected to a final vaccination boost consisting of AT-2-inactivated HIV alone (100 ng of p24) on d 14. The immunization schedule is schematically described in **Fig. 2**.

3.3.1.1. ELISA for Human Immunoglobulins

IFN-DCs are potent stimulators of antibody production *(5,9)*. This can be evaluated directly in the immunized hu-PBL-SCID mice. Sera can be collected and tested for antibodies to HIV-1 using a commercial ELISA kit detecting

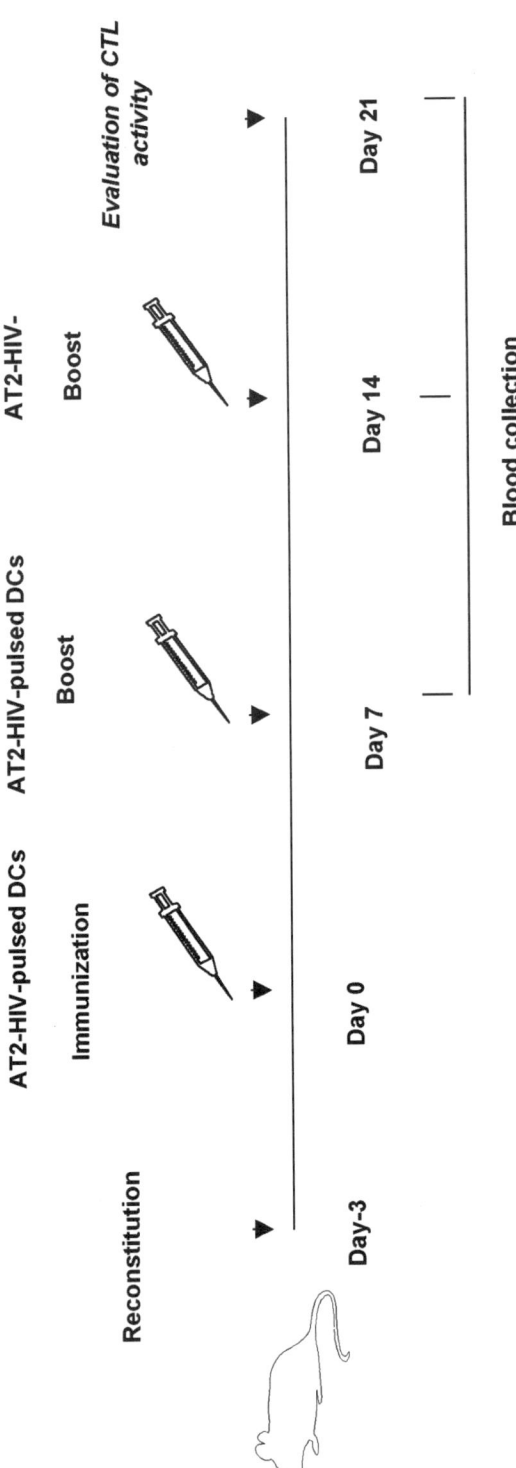

Fig. 2. Vaccination protocol of hu-PBL-SCID mice for testing the in vivo activity of DCs generated in the presence of IFN. Xeno-chimeric mice are vaccinated with human autologous IFN-DCs, and given two boost immunizations at 7-d intervals. Second boost immunization is performed with free inactivated HIV-1 injected intraperitoneally.

human IgG, IgM and IgA specific to a series of envelope and core HIV-1 peptides (Abbott Murex HIV-1.2.O). However, it is possible to set up a sensitive ELISA system to quantitate human total immunoglobulins (Igs), IgM, IgG1, and IgG4 immunoglobulins for detection of specific anti-HIV antibodies directed to specific peptides, e.g., ERYLKDQQLLGIWGCSGKLIC and ELDKWAS HIV-1 gp41. Sera from nonimmunized hu-PBL-SCID mice should be used as negative controls of all the ELISA determinations. The cutoff value can be calculated as the mean absorbance value of all the control sera plus 0.100 A. Sera showing A_{490} values higher than this threshold are considered positive for anti-HIV antibodies.

ELISA is a widely used test whose detailed description can be easily found in manuals and commercial kit instructions. Briefly:

1. Coat the plate with the diluted antigen (5 mg/mL).
2. Incubate at 4°C overnight.
3. Wash the unbound antigen off the plate, fill the wells with distilled water, and wash with PBS-Triton two times.
4. Block nonspecific binding by adding of 5% BSA/PBS.
5. Incubate for 30 to 60 min at room temperature.
6. Wash plate as reported in **step 3**.
7. Add serially diluted mouse sera to appropriate wells; include a positive control and sera from negative control mice. Incubate for 1 h at room temperature.
8. Repeat washing step.
9. Prepare appropriate dilution of the second step conjugated-antibody to detect human total Igs, IgM, IgG1, and IgG4 immunoglobulins in the sera of the xenochimeras. Add 100 µL of second step antibody to wells and incubate for 1 h.
10. Repeat the washing step.
11. Add 100 µL of substrate to well and incubate at room temperature for 60 min.
12. Add stopping solution if appropriate.
13. Read plates on an ELISA plate reader.

3.3.1.2. WESTERN BLOT

Sera from hu-PBL-SCID mice immunized with AT-2/HIV-1-pulsed DCs can be assayed by a commercial Western blot kit (Cambridge Biotech HIV Western blot Kit, Rockville, MD *[9]*). Briefly, incubate individual nitrocellulose strips overnight with different mouse serum samples (diluted 1:20) or with human positive or negative control sera (diluted 1:1,000 and usually provided by the manufacturer). Include sera from non-immunized hu-PBL-SCID mice as experimental negative controls. Visualize human Igs specifically bound to HIV-1 proteins by incubation with substrate chromogen after the addition of biotin-conjugated goat anti-human IgG and streptavidin-conjugated horseradish peroxidase as recommended by the manufacturer.

IFN and Dendritic Cell Differentiation

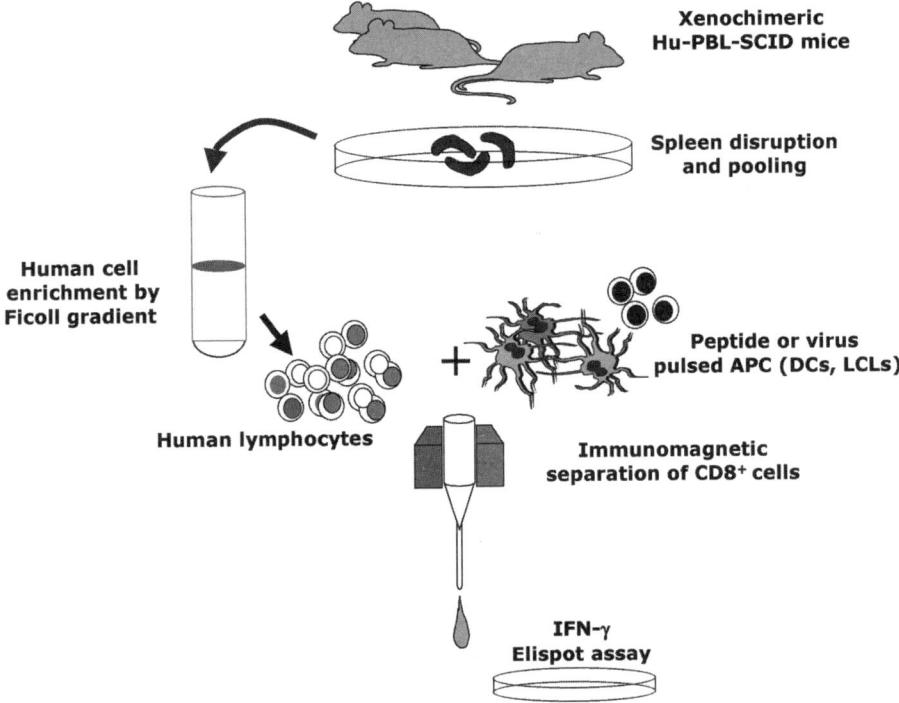

Fig. 3. Testing of in vivo capability of IFN-DCs to induce the generation of antigen-specific CD8 T-cell responses starting from purification of human CD8 cells from hu-PBL-SCID mice. Cells from spleens or peritoneal washings are pooled and enriched by Ficoll density centrifugation and immunoselected with magnetic beads. Cells are then processed for testing the generation of human $CD8^+$ T cells against HIV antigens as illustrated in the figure and described in the text.

3.3.2. Evaluation of the Capability of Antigen-Pulsed IFN-DCs to Induce the Generation of Antigen-Specific $CD8^+$ T Cells in the hu-PBL-SCID Mouse Model

Human cells can be recovered from either the spleen or peritoneal washings of hu-PBL-SCID mice of each group and pooled (three or four mice per group) for testing the presence of human antigen-specific $CD8^+$ T cells. A scheme of the procedure is described in **Fig. 3**.

3.3.2.1. ENRICHMENT OF HUMAN CELLS FROM CELLULAR POOLS

1. Collect cells from the peritoneal cavity or spleen.
2. Pass cell suspension trough a cell strainer to eliminate debris or connective tissue and wash twice in RPMI 1640 medium.

3. Resuspend the cells in 2 mL of RPMI 1640 medium 10% FCS.
4. Overlay cell suspension on 2 mL Ficoll cushion (for human use) in a 5 mL polystyrene tube (Falcon 352054 from Becton-Dickinson is suitable).
5. Density gradient centrifugation is carried out at 400 g for 20 min.
6. Collect the cell ring and wash twice with PBS.

3.3.2.2. ELISPOT ASSAY FOR IFN-γ AND GRANZYME-B PRODUCTION

Enriched human lymphocytes are stimulated with autologous IFN-DCs pulsed with AT-2 inactivated HIV-1 at a ratio E/S 4:1. After 2 d, supplement culture with 25 IU/ of IL-2. After 5 to 7 d, $CD8^+$ T cells are positively selected by MACS Micro Beads (Miltenyi Biotec GmbH) and assayed in ELISPOT for human IFN-γ or Granzyme-B production as described in **Subheading 3.2.2.4.** (ELISPOT assay).

3.4. Evaluation of the Migratory Properties of IFN-DCs

IFN-DCs are also characterized by an enhanced migratory behavior, which can be demonstrated in vitro as well as in vivo *(7)*.

3.4.1. In Vitro Chemotaxis Assay

Cell migration is performed in 24-well Transwell cell culture chamber (Costar, Corning, NY) as described previously *(18,19)*.

1. Load 5×10^5 cells in the upper chamber compartment of a 24-well Transwell cell culture chamber of 8-μm pore size in triplicate, see materials described in **Subheading 2.4.**
2. Dilute RANTES, MIP1-α, or MIP1-β (500 ng/mL; R&D System), MIP3-α, and MIP3-β (100 ng/mL; Peprotech, Rocky Hill, NJ) in serum-free medium and add them to the lower compartment. The lower compartment of control chambers contains medium alone.
3. After 2 h of incubation at 37°C, collect and count the cells that have migrated through pores size in the lower compartment.

3.4.2. In Vivo Migration of DCs After Injection Into SCID Mice

Migration of DCs after injection into SCID mice is evaluated as follows.

1. Inject 2×10^6 DCs intravenously or subcutaneously into SCID mice.
2. After 4 h, sacrifice the mice and collect skin, lymph nodes, and spleen.
3. Extract deoxyribonucleic acid (DNA) from each organ and determine the presence of human sequences by DNA–polymerase chain reaction by using specific primers for the HLA-DQα *(20)*.

4. Notes

1. Depending on the IFN source and dose, the IFN-induced DC differentiation may be associated with a certain percentage of monocyte/DC death. At 3 d, cellular

Table 1
Expression of Selected Membrane Markers Associated With IFN-DC Differentiation in RPMI 1640 Supplemented With FBS

Marker	Percentage ± SD	MFI ± SD
CD40	96 ± 11	87 ± 15
CD80	91 ± 10	175 ± 83
CD86	79 ± 20	254 ± 105
CD83	25 ± 14	52 ± 6
CD25	23 ± 12	50 ± 10
HLA-DR	96 ± 3	2060 ± 467
CD54	95 ± 4	641 ± 113
CD14	36 ± 18	60 ± 12
CD1a	41 ± 17	105 ± 21

yield may vary from 50 to 70%; very few trypan blue-stainable cells can be observed in cultures, suggesting an efficient phagocytic or scavenging activity.

2. The choice of different culture media has different outcomes on DC phenotype. RPMI 1640 can be substituted by clinical grade media, such as AIM-V (GIBCO) supplemented with 2% human AB serum or autologous plasma. It is worth noting that substitution of FBS with human serum deeply influences the final DC phenotype, exerting major effects on CD1a and CD83 expression, which becomes poorly observed or even undetectable. IFN promotes early cell detachment from substrate, which can be seen within 24 h of culture in RPMI 1640 media in the presence of FCS, while the use of AIM-V and autologous plasma or AB serum results in a prolonged cell adhesion to the substrate. Type I IFN also promotes DC clumping in large cellular masses, which can be detected especially in the presence of FBS. The size of cellular clumps is also affected by the presence of contaminating lymphocytes, which seem to be strongly involved in clump formation. On the whole, the differentiation of monocytes into DCs can be deeply influenced by the presence of others cells; of special note, the direct differentiation of DCs from total PBMCs or in the presence of contaminating lymphocytes results in higher expression of co-stimulatory molecules and DC maturation markers (21).

3. A 3-d exposure of blood monocytes to IFN-α results in a dramatic upregulation of the co-stimulatory molecules CD80 and CD86, as well as of CD40 and HLA-DR. IFN-DCs maintain intermediate levels of CD123 expression, higher than those expressed by DCs from IL-4 treated monocytes but lower than those expressed by plasmacytoid DCs (see **Table 1**). Differently from classical DCs generated from monocytes in the presence of IL-4 and GM-CSF, a significant percentage of IFN-DCs retains CD14 expression, while CD1a is expressed by a low percentage of cells. However, these characteristics do not affect or impair the functional activity of IFN-DCs.

Despite the majority of DCs generated in the presence of type I IFN displays features of immature DCs, markers of activated DCs, such as CD83 and CD25, can be demonstrated in a variable percentage of the cells, together with very high levels of expression of costimulatory molecules (see **Table 1**). The expression of DC maturation markers (CD83 and CD25) and higher levels of costimulatory molecules by IFN-DCs strongly depend on the presence of contaminating cells. In fact, it has been found that generation of IFN-DCs from total PBMCs cultures results in higher percentages of cells displaying the phenotype of mature DCs. In particular, it has been demonstrated the importance of DC-NK cell interaction *(21)*.

4. Like monocytes, IFN-DCs are likely to to show a non-specific binding of antibodies via Fc receptors. Appropriate saturation with human serum or Fc-blocking reagents improves the specificity of antibody staining.

References

1. Le Bon, A., Schiavoni, G., D'Agostino, G., Gresser, I., Belardelli, F., and Tough, D. F. (2001) Type I interferons potently enhance humoral immunity and can promote isotype switching by stimulating dendritic cells in vivo. *Immunity* **14**, 461–470.
2. Proietti, E., Bracci, L., Puzelli, S., Di Pucchio, T., Sestili, P., De Vincenti, E., et al. (2002) Type I IFN as a natural adjuvant for a protective immune response: lessons from the influenza vaccine model. *J. Immunol.* **169**, 375–383.
3. Montoya, M., Schiavoni, G., Mattei, F., Gresser, I., Belardelli, F., Borrow, P., and Tough, D. F. (2002) Type I interferons produced by dendritic cells promote their phenotypic and functional activation. *Blood* **99**, 3263–3271.
4. Paquette, R. L., Hsu, N. C., Kiertscher, S. M., Park, A. N., Tran, L., Roth, M. D., et al (1998) Interferon-alpha and granulocyte-macrophage colony-stimulating factor differentiate peripheral blood monocytes into potent antigen-presenting cells. *J. Leukoc. Biol.* **64**, 358–367.
5. Santini, S. M., Lapenta, C., Logozzi, M., Parlato, S., Spada, M., Di Pucchio, T., and Belardelli F. (2000) Type I interferon as a powerful adjuvant for monocyte-derived dendritic cell development and activity in vitro and in Hu-PBL-SCID mice. *J. Exp. Med.* **191**, 1777–1788.
6. Blanco, P., Palucka, A. K., Gill, M., Pascual, V., and Banchereau, J. (2001). Induction of Dendritic Cell Differentiation by IFN-α in Systemic Lupus Erythematosus. *Science* **294**, 1540–1543.
7. Parlato, S., Santini S. M., Lapenta, C., Di Pucchio T., Logozzi, M., Spada, M., et al. (2001) Expression of CCR-7, MIP-3beta, and Th-1 chemokines in type I IFN-induced monocyte-derived dendritic cells: importance for the rapid acquisition of potent migratory and functional activities. *Blood* **98**, 3022–3029.
8. Buelens, C., Bartholome, E. J., Amraoui, Z., Boutriaux, M., Salmon, I., Thielemans, K., et al. (2002). Interleukin-3 and interferon beta cooperate to induce differentiation of monocytes into dendritic cells with potent helper T-cell stimulatory properties. *Blood* **99**, 993–998.
9. Lapenta, C., Santini, S. M., Logozzi, M., Spada, M., Andreotti, M., Di Pucchio, T., et al. (2003) Potent immune response against HIV-1 and protection from virus

challenge in hu-PBL-SCID mice immunized with inactivated virus-pulsed dendritic cells generated in the presence of IFN-alpha. *J. Exp. Med.* **198**, 361–367.
10. Belardelli, F. and Ferrantini, M. (2002) Cytokines as a link between innate and adaptive antitumor immunity. *Trends Immunol.* **23**, 201–208.
11. Santini, S. M., Di Pucchio, T., Lapenta, C., Parlato, S., Logozzi, M., and Belardelli, F. (2002) The natural alliance between type I interferon and dendritic cells and its role in linking innate and adaptive immunity. *J. Interferon. Cytokine Res.* **22**, 1071–1080.
12. Santodonato, L., D'Agostino, G., Nisini, R., Mariotti, S., Monque, D. M., Spada, M., et al. (2003) Monocyte-derived dendritic cells generated after a short-term culture with IFN-alpha and granulocyte-macrophage colony-stimulating factor stimulate a potent Epstein-Barr virus-specific CD8+ T cell response. *J. Immunol.* **170**, 5195–5202.
13. Rossio, J. L., Esser, M. T., Suryanarayana, K., Schneider, D. K., Bess, J. W. Jr, Vasquez, G. M., et al. (1998) Inactivation of human immunodeficiency virus type 1 infectivity with preservation of conformational and functional integrity of virion surface proteins. *J. Virol.* **72**, 7992–8001.
14. Mosier, D. E., Gulizia, R. J., Baird, S. M., and Wilson, D. B. (1988) Transfer of a functional human immune system to mice with severe combined immunodeficiency. *Nature* **335**, 256–259.
15. Bosma, M. J. and Carroll, A. M. (1991) The SCID mouse mutant: definition, characterization, and potential uses. *Annu. Rev. Immunol.* **9**, 323–350.
16. Mosier, D. E., Gulizia, R. J., Baird, S. M., Wilson, D. B., Spector, D. H., and Spector, S. A. (1991) Human immunodeficiency virus infection of human-PBL-SCID mice. *Science* **251**, 791–794.
17. Rizza, P., Santini, S. M., Logozzi, M. A., Lapenta, C., Sestili, P., Gherardi, G., et al. (1996) T-cell dysfunctions in hu-PBL-SCID mice infected with human immunodeficiency virus (HIV) shortly after reconstitution: in vivo effects of HIV on highly activated human immune cells. *J. Virol.* **70**, 7958–7964.
18. Sato, K., Kawasaki, H., Nagayama, H., Enomoto, M., Morimotom, C., Tadokoro, K., et al. (2000) TGF-beta 1 reciprocally controls chemotaxis of human peripheral blood monocyte-derived dendritic cells via chemokine receptors. *J. Immunol.* **164**, 2285–2295.
19. Sato, K., Kawasaki, H., Nagayama, H., Serizawa, R., Ikeda, J., Morimoto, C., et al. (1999) CC chemokine receptors, CCR-1 and CCR-3, are potentially involved in antigen-presenting cell function of human peripheral blood monocyte-derived dendritic cells. *Blood* **93**, 34–42.
20. Locardi, C., Puddu, P., Ferrantini, M., Parlanti, E., Sestili, P., Varano, F., and Belardelli, F. (1992) Persistent infection of normal mice with human immunodeficiency virus. *J. Virol.* **66**, 1649–1654.
21. Tosi, D., Valenti, R., Cova, A., Sovena, G., Huber, V., Pilla, L., et al. (2004) Role of cross-talk between IFN-alpha-induced monocyte-derived dendritic cells and NK cells in priming CD8+ T cell responses against human tumor antigens. *J. Immunol.* **172**, 5363–5370.

12

Flow Cytometric Techniques for Studying Plasmacytoid Dendritic Cells in Mixed Populations

Stacey L. Olshalsky and Patricia Fitzgerald-Bocarsly

Summary

Plasmacytoid dendritic cells (PDCs) are the natural interferon (IFN-α)-producing cells in human peripheral blood that produce vast quantities of IFN-α in response to viral infection and other stimuli. PDCs are a rare cell type, making up less than 0.5% of peripheral blood mononuclear cells. To date, these cells have not been successfully cultured in vitro and are very sensitive to selection via magnetic bead labeling, making them very difficult to study as a purified population. Therefore, our laboratory has developed techniques to study PDCs in mixed populations. Using flow cytometry to label specific cell-surface markers, PDCs can be easily identified from other peripheral blood mononuclear cells or in mononuclear cell suspensions of lymphoid tissue. PDCs can also be permeabilized and stained for intracellular proteins or cytokines. Using surface and intracellular flow cytometry, phenotypic and functional aspects can be combined to accurately study PDCs in a mixed population of cells.

Key Words: Plasmacytoid dendritic cells; IFN-α; IRF-7; intracellular flow cytometry.

1. Introduction

Plasmacytoid dendritic cells (PDCs) are a unique and rare population of cells found in the peripheral blood and lymphoid organs of humans and are key players in the innate immune system. These cells are known to be identical to the natural interferon-α (IFN-α)-producing cells in peripheral blood and have also been found in bone marrow, spleen, tonsils, and lymph nodes (*1–4*, and our unpublished data), as well as in some nonlymphoid tissues in pathological conditions *(5,6)*. PDCs produce large quantities of IFN-α (as much as 2–5 pg/cell) in response to a wide array of stimuli, including enveloped viruses, some bacteria, CpG-containing deoxyribonucleic acid (DNA), and members of the imidazoquindine family of synthetic compounds *(7–14)*. The remarkable ability of PDC to produce IFN-α and a variety of chemokines, such as MIP-1α, MIP-1β, IP-10, and MCP-1 *(15,16)*, allows these cells to have a large impact on a developing immune response. Depending on the stimulus, PDCs can induce either a Th1 or Th2 type response. Viral stimulation of PDCs leads to IFN-α production, which in turn stimulates naïve T cells to produce the Th1 cytokine, IFN-γ *(17)*. In contrast, interleukin (IL)-3- and CD40 ligand-stimulated PDCs induce T cells to produce IL-4, IL-5, and IL-10, which are typical Th2 cytokines *(3)*. PDCs also play an important role in the ability of natural killer (NK) cells to lyse infected target cells *(18,19)*. Our laboratory has shown that the chemokines secreted by virally stimulated PDCs allow for the recruitment of NK cells and activated T cells, demonstrating important roles in directing both innate and adaptive immune responses *(15)*.

PDCs can be identified by their cell surface markers; PDCs are lineage negative, HLA-DR$^+$, CD11c$^-$, and CD123^{bight} (IL-3 receptor; Fig. 1A *[1,20]*). They also express the recently identified blood dendritic cell antigens, BDCA-2 and BDCA-4 *(21)*. BDCA-2 has been identified as a C-type lectin and may be involved in antigen uptake by PDCs *(22)*. BDCA-4 has been found to be identical to neuropilin-1, a neuronal receptor for axon guidance factors, and its function on PDCs has yet to be elucidated *(23)*. In peripheral blood, PDCs are the only cells that express BDCA-2 and BDCA-4. BDCA-2 is downregulated on PDCs as they are cultured or matured. BDCA-4 has been found to be upregulated in PDCs upon culture; however, it is also upregulated on myeloid DC within 48 h of in vitro culture *(21)*.

Because of their infrequency, PDCs can be very challenging to study, making up only 0.1 to 0.5% of all peripheral blood mononuclear cells (PBMCs) *[24–27]*). In addition, PDCs cannot be cultured in vitro in the absence of cytokines, such as IL-3, tumor necrosis factor-α, or IFN-α. However, these cytokines, while keeping PDCs alive, also induce their maturation, thereby affecting their phenotype and function *(28–30)*. Therefore, in order to study these cells, PBMCs must be freshly harvested from the blood of donors at the commencement of each experiment. Classical methods to study IFN-α production by PDC include the enzyme-linked immunospot (i.e., ELISPOT) assay, the enzyme-linked immunosorbent assay (ELISA), or the IFN bioassay *(24,31,32)*. Traditionally, PBMCs are used in these assays. Because PDCs are the primary cells in peripheral blood that produce IFN-α in response to stimulation with herpes simplex virus (HSV), most IFN-α detected in these assays is assumed to be produced by PDCs. However, when PBMCs are stimulated with other viruses, such as Sendai virus or HIV, both monocytes and PDCs respond, making it impossible to determine the source of IFN-α using these assays *(7)*.

PDCs can be isolated from PBMCs using antibody-conjugated magnetic beads *(33)*. In one protocol, the first step is a negative isolation in which PBMCs are labeled with antibody-conjugated microbeads against CD3,

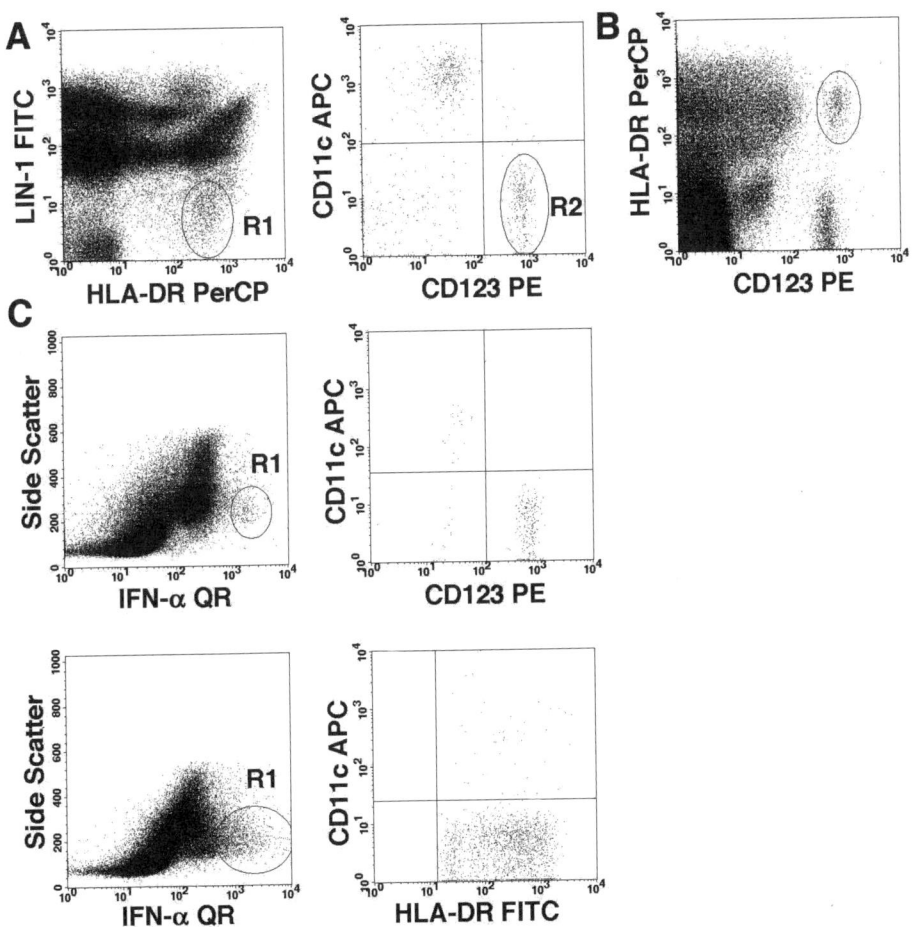

Fig. 1. Plasmacytoid dendritic cell phenotype. (**A**) PBMCs were isolated from the blood of healthy donors and surfaced stained using anti-Lin-1-FITC, anti-HLA-DR-PerCP, anti-CD123-PE, and anti-CD11c-APC antibodies. PDCs are gated as LIN-1$^-$ and HLA-DR$^+$ (R1) and CD123$^+$ and CD11c$^-$ (R2). (**B**) The PDC population also can be gated on from PBMCs by surface staining for CD123 and HLA-DR. (**C**) PBMCs were stimulated with HSV-1 at an m.o.i. = 1 for 6 h at 37°C. The cells were surface stained with the PDC markers CD123-PE and CD11c-APC (top row) or HLA-DR-FITC and CD11c-APC (bottom row) followed by intracellular staining for IFN-α. The phenotype of the IFN-α-producing cells was determined by first gating on the IFN-positive cells as seen in a scatter plot of IFN vs side scatter (left panels, R1). The IFN-positive cells are shown to be CD123$^+$, HLA-DR$^+$, and CD11c$^-$ (right panels).

CD11b, and CD16 to deplete T cells, monocytes, and NK cells, respectively. The cell suspension is run through a magnetic column; microbead-labeled cells remain in the column, whereas any unlabeled cells freely flow through. A partially purified population containing mostly DCs and B cells is recovered. This is followed by a positive selection step in which these negatively selected cells are labeled with anti-CD4 conjugated microbeads. The CD4+ DCs will remain in the column, whereas any unlabeled cells flow through. The purified DCs can then be flushed from the column. The positively selected DCs are typically greater than 95% pure. The recent identification of the PDCs' unique cell surface markers, BDCA-2 and BDCA-4, have allowed for the creation of a one-step positive selection procedure for the enrichment of PDCs. However, during our work using these purified PDC, we discovered that crosslinking a variety of cell surface markers, such as CD4, BDCA-2, and BDCA-4 as well as others, with antibody and microbeads on the surface of these cells leads to the downregulation of IFN-α production in response to viral stimulation (Olshalsky et al., submitted for publication). This phenomenon also has been reported by others who have shown that ligation with BDCA-2 antibody leads to inhibition of IFN-α production by PDCs in response to stimulation with influenza virus and CpG-containing DNA *(22,34)*. This sensitivity to cell surface receptor ligation, which probably exists to prevent over-activation of the cells as they communicate with other cell types via cognate receptors, creates a huge problem in studying functional aspects of PDCs in a purified setting.

Because of the many roadblocks encountered during the study of PDCs, our laboratory has focused on flow cytometric techniques to study PDCs in mixed populations of cells. By using specific combinations of surface stains, we can gate on PDCs and confidently identify them within the PBMC population. In addition to overcoming functional alterations in positively selected PDCs, the flow cytometric techniques can be performed using relatively small numbers of cells, making phenotypic and functional studies possible using patient samples that are quite small. Experiments in our laboratory have shown that PDCs can be identified from PBMCs using only two colors, thereby leaving two open channels for analysis of other cell surface markers when using standard four-color fluorescence-activated cell-sorting (FACS) analysis (**Figs, 1B, 2B–G**). Along with using flow cytometry to identify PDCs and their cell surface markers, it can also be used to investigate cytokine production by these cells. A Golgi blocker, such as Brefeldin A, is added to the cells after stimulation to prevent secretion of cytokine. The cells can then be permeabilized to stain intracellular protein. This intracellular flow cytometry procedure also can be used to study PDC transcription factors. We have used this procedure to successfully stain for interferon regulatory factors, IRF-3 and IRF-7, which are well-known transcription factors involved in IFN-α production by PDCs *(35–*

37). Using this method, we determined that PDCs express high constitutive levels of IRF-7, which is even further upregulated in response to stimulation with HSV (**Fig. 3C** *[37,38]*). In addition, flow cytometry allows for the examination of multiple factors simultaneously. For example, PDCs can be stained for IFN-α and IRF-7 in the same experiment (**Fig. 3D**). The recent development of antibodies directed against signaling molecules allows for the identification of signaling events via flow cytometry. Using an antibody specific for phosphorylated tyrosine (Santa Cruz Biotechnology Inc., Santa Cruz, CA), we have been able to detect signaling in PDCs following crosslinking of various cell-surface receptors (Olshalsky et al., submitted for publication).

2. Materials

All reagents are stored at 4°C unless otherwise stated.

2.1. PDC Phenotyping

1. 0.1% bovine serum albumin (BSA) in 1xPBS, sterile filtered.
2. Human serum, heat-inactivated.
3. PDC phenotyping antibodies: FITC-, PE-, PerCP-, APC-conjugated HLA-DR, CD123 (BD Biosciences, San Diego, CA), BDCA-2 and BDCA-4 (Miltenyi Biotec, Auburn, CA).
4. 1X phosphate-buffered saline (PBS).

2.2. Intracellular Flow Cytometry

1. HSV-1 strain 2931 (Note: Any other wild-type strain of HSV or other IFN-α inducers such as other enveloped virus, CpG DNA, etc., may be used to stimulate PDCs).
2. 10% fetal calf serum (FCS) in RPMI (10% RPMI).
3. Wash buffer: 2% FCS in 1X PBS, sterile filtered.
4. Permeabilization Buffer: 0.5% Saponin in wash buffer, sterile filtered (make fresh every 2 wk).
5. Brefeldin A (BFA) 10 mg/mL stock solution in ethanol (store at –20°C).
6. 1% paraformaldehyde in 1X PBS (make fresh every month).
7. Human serum, heat-inactivated.
8. Biotinylated anti-human IFN-α antibody clone MMHA-2 (PBL Biomedical Laboratories, Piscataway, NJ). (Note: Antibody was purchased unconjugated and was biotinylated using *N*-hydroxysuccinimide biotin; Sigma.)
9. Streptavidin-conjugated Quantum Red (light sensitive; Sigma).

3. Methods

The methods below describe standard protocols for cell surface staining (**Subheading 3.1.**) and intracellular staining (**Subheading 3.2.**) of PBMCs for flow cytometry.

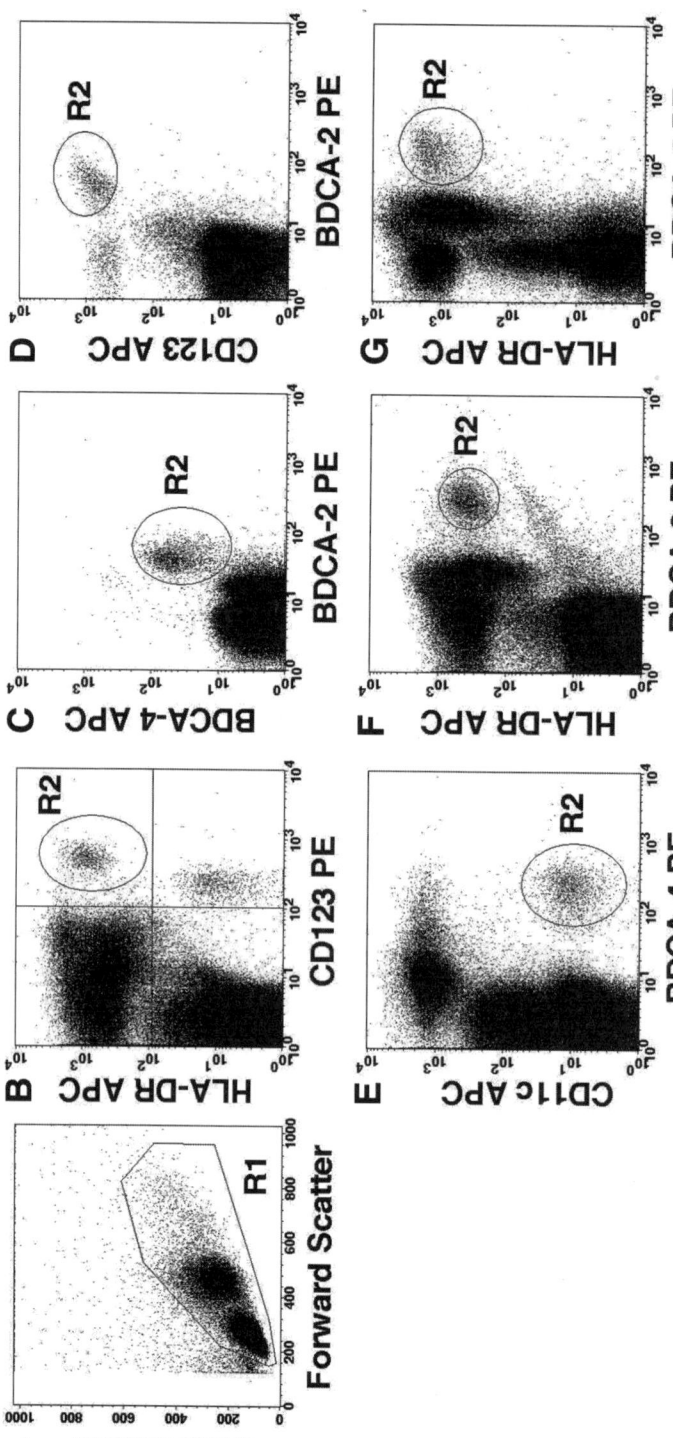

Fig. 2. Several combinations of surface markers can be used to gate on plasmacytoid dendritic cells within PBMCs. PBMCs were purified from the whole blood of a healthy donor. (A) Forward scatter vs side scatter was used to gate on the PBMC population (R1). (B–G) The gate R1 was then used to produce the scatter plots using PDC-specific stains. The gate R2 was used to define the PDC population. Cells were stained with the following: (B) anti-CD123-PE and anti-HLA-DR-APC antibodies, (C) anti-BDCA-2-PE and anti-BDCA-4-APC antibodies, (D) anti-BDCA-2-PE and anti-CD123-APC antibodies, (E) anti-BDCA-4-PE and anti-CD11c-APC antibodies, (F) anti-BDCA-2-PE and anti-HLA-DR-APC antibodies, and (G) anti-BDCA-4-PE and anti-HLA-DR-APC antibodies. PDC are defined as R1*R2.

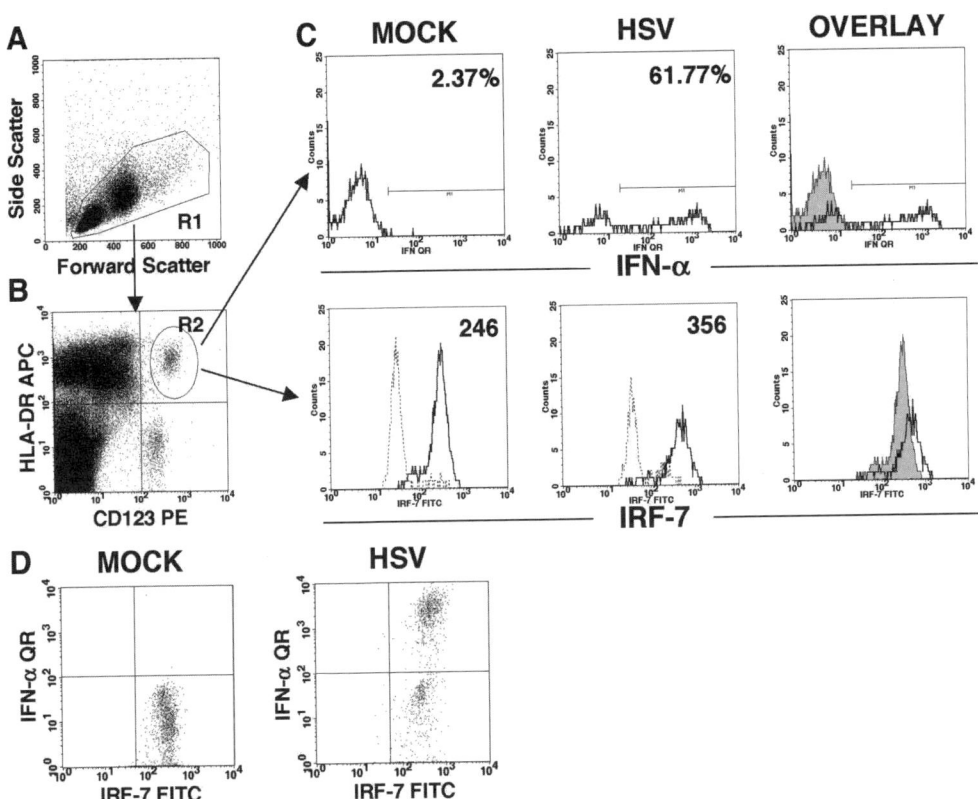

Fig. 3. IFN-α production and IRF-7 expression by HSV-stimulated plasmacytoid dendritic cells as determined by intracellular flow cytometry. PBMCs were mock (filled line) or HSV (m.o.i. = 1) (solid line) stimulated for 6 h at 37°C. Cells were stained for PDC surface markers followed by intracellular flow cytometry for IFN-α and IRF-7 (rabbit IgG isotype control, dashed line). (**A**) Forward vs side scatter was used to gate on PBMCs (R1). (**B**) From the gate R1, the expression of HLA-DR and CD123 was examined. The double positive population was gated as PDC (R2). (**C**) The combination of R1 and R2 (R1*R2) was used to examine IFN-α production (top row) and IRF-7 expression (bottom row). The number of IFN-α producing PDCs is shown as a percentage in the upper right hand corner (top row). The mean fluorescence intensity (MFI) of IRF-7 expressed by PDCs is shown in the upper right hand corner (bottom row). (**D**) A scatter plot can be used to examine IFN-α and IRF-7 simultaneously.

3.1. PDC Phenotyping

1. Begin with 1×10^6 PBMCs per condition in 12×75-mm polystyrene snap cap tubes.
2. Wash cells by adding cold 0.1% BSA in 1X PBS and spin in cold centrifuge for 8 to 10 min at 1200 rpm ($425g$).

3. Pour off supernatant and disrupt pellet.
4. Add 5 μL of heat-inactivated human serum to each tube.
5. Add 5 μL of each fluorochrome-conjugated antibody in the dark, keeping tubes cold.
6. Cover with foil and incubate 20 min at 4°C.
7. Wash in cold 1X PBS and spin down in cold centrifuge.
8. Pour off supernatant and disrupt pellet.
9. Fix in 300 μL of PBS containing 1% paraformaldehyde.
10. Store covered at 4°C until acquired by FACS.

3.2. Intracellular Flow Cytometry for IFN-α

1. Begin with PBMCs at a concentration of 2×10^6 cells/1 mL 10% RPMI.
2. Stimulate cells with HSV at an multiplicity of infection (m.o.i.) = 1.
3. Incubate 4 h at 37°C with 5% CO_2.
4. Add Brefeldin A to tubes at a final concentration of 5 μg/mL (*see* **Note 1**).
5. Incubate 2 h at 37°C with 5% CO_2.
6. Wash cells in 0.1% BSA in 1X PBS and surface stain as described above.
7. Fix with 500 μL of 1% paraformaldehyde and store at 4°C overnight.
8. Wash with wash buffer, pour off supernatant and disrupt pellet.
9. Resuspend cells in 500 μL of permeabilization buffer and incubate for 15 min at room temperature (RT) (*see* **Notes 2** and **3**).
10. Centrifuge to pellet cells, pour off supernatant and resuspend pellet.
11. Add 5 μL of heat-inactivated human serum and incubate 10 min at RT.
12. Add anti-human IFN-α antibody (200 ng) to each tube and incubate 30 min at RT.
13. Wash two times in permeabilization buffer.
14. Disrupt pellet and add 8 μL of Streptavidin QR. Incubate 30 min at RT.
15. Wash once in permeabilization buffer.
16. Wash once in wash buffer.
17. Wash once in 1X PBS.
18. Fix with 300 μL of PBS containing 1% paraformaldehyde and store at 4°C until ready to acquire by FACS.

3.3. FACS Analysis

Data can be analyzed using CellQuest software (BD Biosciences). In order to gate on PDCs, 300,000 events should be acquired for each sample. The first step in the analysis is to draw a scatter plot of the PBMC looking at side scatter versus forward scatter. Using the free-forming gate tool, make a gate around the PBMC population. This gate will be gate 1 (G1) or region 1 (R1) (**Fig. 3A**). To gate on the PDCs within the PBMC population, make a new scatter that will be HLA-DR versus CD123 (or whatever markers you are using to gate on PDC) using the cells in R1. The double positive population is the PDCs (**Fig. 3B**). Make a gate around this population, R2. Now a gate can be made that combines R1 and R2 (G3 = R1*R2). In order to examine other factors in the PDC population the gate should be set on G3. To look at IFN-α production by the PDC, make a histogram using G3 as the gate (**Fig. 3C**).

1. Acquire 300,000 events for each sample.
2. Gate on PBMC using side scatter versus forward scatter. This will be R1. (**Fig. 3A**)
3. From R1 draw a scatter plot CD123 vs. HLA-DR. (**Fig. 3B**)
4. Gate on the double positive PDC. This will be R2. (**Fig. 3B**)
5. In the gate list make G1 = R1*R2. This is the PDC population for further analysis.
6. Use histogram to look at IFN, IRF-7, etc. within the PDC population (G1) (**Fig. 3C**; *see* **Notes 3–7**).

4. Notes

1. The addition of Brefeldin A is only necessary when looking at a secreted product. It is not necessary when staining for transcription factors or other intracellular proteins, and may, in fact be detrimental to the expression of IRF-7. BFA should be added during the last 2 to 4 h of incubation. Longer incubation with BFA leads to cell toxicity.
2. After addition of permeabilization buffer, cells will be slippery. Take caution when dumping supernatant. If loss of cells becomes a problem, the supernatants may be aspirated after centrifugation. Also, the cells are fragile after permeabilization. The cell pellet should be disrupted gently.
3. When looking at a protein that is found primarily in the cytoplasm, saponin is a sufficient detergent for permeabilization. However, saponin does not work well to permeabilize the nuclear membrane. If a protein is nuclear, another detergent, such as Triton-X, should be used for permeabilization.
4. For IRF-7 staining, add rabbit anti-human IRF-7 antibody (400 ng) (Santa Cruz Biotechnology Inc., Santa Cruz, CA). For secondary antibody, add 5 μL of goat anti-rabbit IgG antibody-FITC conjugate (BD-Pharmingen).
5. Any colors can be substituted with other colors as necessary for individual experiments. For example, Streptavidin-conjugated PE may be used instead of Streptavidin-conjugated QR.
6. Surface staining and intracellular staining may be performed consecutively, however, cells must be fixed overnight before being permeabilized.
7. Individual blood donors are different and may display slightly different PDC phenotypic profiles. For example, a minority of individuals does not have a distinct HLA-DR+/CD123+ PDC population. This may create problems when attempting to gate on a pure PDC population. If this is a recurring problem, a third marker, such as CD11c, may be included to help distinguish the PDC population. Conversely, another combination of markers may be used such as BDCA-2/BDCA-4, CD123/BDCA-2, or BDCA-4/CD11c. Also, the PDC population may move after stimulation, so it is important to make sure your PDCs stay within your gate for each condition. In some instances, it may be necessary to make a new PDC gate for every condition (i.e., mock, HSV, etc.).

References

1. Siegal, F., Kadowaki, N., Shodell, M., Fitzgerald-Bocarsly, P., Shah, K., Ho, S., et al. (1999) The nature of the principal type 1 interferon-producing cells in human blood. *Science* **284**, 1835–1837.
2. Cella, M., Jarrossay, D., Facchetti, F., Alebardi, O., Nakajima, H., Lanzavecchia, A., and Colonna, M. (1999) Plasmacytoid monocytes migrate to inflamed lymph nodes and produce large amounts of type I interferon. *Nat. Med.* **5**, 919–923.
3. Grouard, G., Rissoan, M., Filguiera, L., Durand, I., Banchereau, J., and Liu, J. (1997) The enigmatic plasmacytoid T cells develop into dendritic cells with interleukin-3 and CD40 ligand. *J. Exp. Med.* **185**, 1101–1111.
4. Fitzgerald-Bocarsly, P. (2002) Natural IFN-alpha producing cells: The plasmacytoid dendritic cells. *BioTechniques* **33**, S16–S29.
5. Sellati, T. J., Waldrop, S. L., Salazar, J. C., Bergstresser, P. R., Picker, L., and Radolf, J. D. (2001) The cutaneous response in humans to *Treponema pallidum* lipoprotein analogues involves cellular elements of both innate and adaptive immunity. *J. Immunol.* **166**, 4131–4140.
6. Jahnsen, F., Lund-Johansen, F., Dunne, J., Farkas, L., Haye, R., and Brandtzaeg, P. (2000) Experimentally induced recruitment of plasmacytoid (CD123high) dendritic cells in human nasal allergy. *J. Immunol.* **165**, 4062–4068.
7. Feldman, S. B., M. Ferraro, H. M. Zheng, N. Patel, S. Gould-Fogerite, and P. Fitzgerald-Bocarsly. (1994) Viral induction of low frequency interferon-alpha producing cells. *Virology* **204**, 1.
8. Svensson, H., Cederblad, B., Lindahl, M., and Alm, G. (1996) Stimulation of natural interferon-α/β-producing cells by *Staphylococcus aureus*. *J. Interferon Cytokine Res.* **16**, 7–16.
9. Remoli, M. E., Giacomini, E., Lutfalla, G., Dondi, E., Orefici, G., Battistini, A., et al. (2002) Selective expression of type I IFN genes in human dendritic cells infected with *Mycobacterium tuberculosis*. *J. Immunol.* **169**, 366–374.
10. Gibson, S. J., Imbertson, L. M., Wagner, T. L., Testerman, T. L., Reiter, M. J., Miller, R. L., et al. (1995) Cellular requirements for cytokine production in response to the immunomodulators imiquimod and S-27609. *J. Interferon Cytokine Res.* **15**, 537–545.
11. Kadowaki, N., Antonenko, S., and Liu, Y. J. (2001) Distinct CpG DNA and polyinosinic-polycytidylic acid double-stranded RNA, respectively, stimulate CD11c- type 2 dendritic cell precursors and CD11c+ dendritic cells to produce type I IFN. *J. Immunol.* **166**, 2291–2295.
12. Kadowaki, N., Ho, S., Antonenko, S., Malefyt, R. W., Kastelein, R. A., Bazan, F., and Liu, Y. J. (2001) Subsets of human dendritic cell precursors express different toll-like receptors and respond to different microbial antigens. *J. Exp. Med.* **194**, 863–869.
13. Krug, A., Rothenfusser, S., Hornung, V., Jahrsdorfer, B., Blackwell, S., Ballas, Z. K., et al. (2001) Identification of CpG oligonucleotide sequences with high induction of IFN-alpha/beta in plasmacytoid dendritic cells. *Eur. J. Immunol.* **31**, 2154–2163.

14. Krug, A., Towarowski, A., Britsch, S., Rothenfusser, S., Hornung, V., Bals, R., et al. (2001) Toll-like receptor expression reveals CpG DNA as a unique microbial stimulus for plasmacytoid dendritic cells which synergizes with CD40 ligand to induce high amounts of IL-12. *Eur. J. Immunol.* **31**, 3026–3037.
15. Megjugorac, N., Young, H., Amrute, S., Olshalsky, S., and Fitzgerald-Bocarsly, P. (2004) Virally stimulated plasmacytoid dendritic cells produce chemokines and induce migration of T and NK cells. *J. Leuk. Biol.* **75**, 504–514.
16. Penna, G., Sozzani, S., and Adorini, L. (2001) Cutting Edge: Selective usage of chemokine receptors by plasmacytoid dendritic cells. *J. Immunol.* **167**, 1862–1866.
17. Cella, M., Facchetti, F., Lanzavecchia, A., and Colonna, M. (2000) Plasmacytoid dendritic cells activated by influenza virus and CD40L drive a potent TH1 polarization. *Nat. Immunol.* **1**, 305–310.
18. Bandyopadhyay, S., Perussia, B., Trinchieri, G., Miller, D. S., and Starr, S. (1986) Requirement for HLA-DR$^+$ accessory cells in natural killing of cytomegalovirus-infected fibroblasts. *J. Exp. Med.* **164**, 180–195.
19. Fitzgerald-Bocarsly, P., Feldman, M., Curl, S., Schnell, J., and Denny, T. (1989) Positively selected Leu-11a (CD16$^+$) cells require the presence of accessory cells or factors for the lysis of HSV-infected fibroblasts but not HSV-infected Raji. *J. Immunol.* **143**, 1318–1326.
20. Svensson, H., Johannisson, A., Nikkila, T., Alm, G. V., and Cederblad, B. (1996) The cell surface phenotype of human natural interferon-a producing cells as determined by flow cytometry. *Scand. J. Immunol.* **44**, 164–172.
21. Dzionek, A., Fuchs, A., Schmidt, P., Cremer, S., Zysk, M., Miltenyi, S., Buck, D. W., and Schmitz, J. (2000) BDCA-2, BDCA-3, and BDCA-4: three markers for distinct subsets of dendritic cells in human peripheral blood. *J. Immunol.* **165**, 6037–6046.
22. Dzionek, A., Sohma, Y., Nagafune, J., Cella, M., Colonna, M., Facchetti, F., et al. (2001) BDCA-2, a novel plasmacytoid dendritic cell-specific type II c-type lectin, mediates antigen capture and is a potent inhibitor of interferon alpha/beta induction. *J. Exp. Med.* **194**, 1823–1834.
23. Dzionek, A., Inagaki, Y., Okawa, K., Nagafune, J., Rock, J., Sohma, Y., et al. (2002) Plasmacytoid dendritic cells: From specific surface markers to specific cellular functions. *Hum. Immunol.* **63**, 1133–1148.
24. Cederblad, B. and Alm, G. (1990) Infrequent but efficient interferon-α-producing human mononuclear leukocytes induced by herpes simplex virus in vitro studies by immunoplaque and limiting dilution assays. *J. Interferon Res.* **10**, 65–73.
25. Feldman, S., Stein, D., Amrute, S., Denny, T., Garcia, Z., Kloser, P., et al. (2001) Decreased interferon-α production in HIV-infected patients correlates with numerical and functional deficiencies in circulating type 2 dendritic cell precursors. *Clin. Immunol.* **101**, 201–210.
26. Soumelis, V., Scott, I., Gheyas, F., Bouhour, D., Cozon, G., Cotte, L., et al. (2001) Depletion of circulating natural type 1 interferon-producing cells in HIV-infected AIDS patients. *Blood* **98**, 906–912.

27. Chehimi, J., Campbell, D. E., Azzoni, L., Bacheller, E., Papasavvas, G., Jerandi, K., et al. (2002) Persistent decreases in blood plasmacytoid dendritic cell number and function despite effective highly active antiretroviral therapy and increased blood myeloid dendritic cells in HIV-infected individuals. *J. Immunol.* **168,** 4796–4801.
28. Kadowaki, N., Antonenko, S., Lau, J. Y., and Liu, Y. J. (2000) Natural interferon alpha/beta-producing cells link innate and adaptive immunity. *J. Exp. Med.* **192,** 219–226.
29. Ito, T., Amakawa, R., Inaba, M., Ikehara, S., Inaba, K., and Fukuhara, S. (2001) Differential regulation of human blood dendritic cell subsets by IFNs. *J. Immunol.* **166,** 2961–2969.
30. Kohrgruber, N., Halanek, N., Groger, M., Winter, D., Rappersberger, K., Schmitt-Egenolf, M., et al. (1999) Survival, maturation, and function of CD11c- and CD11c+ peripheral blood dendritic cells are differentially regulated by cytokines. *J. Immunol.* **163,** 3250–3259.
31. Howell, D., Feldman, S., Kloser, P., and Fitzgerald-Bocarsly, P. (1994) Decreased frequency of natural interferon producing cells in peripheral blood of patients with the acquired immune deficiency syndrome. *Clin. Immunol. Immunopath.* **71,** 223–230.
32. Feldman, S. B., Milone, M. C., Kloser, P., and Fitzgerald-Bocarsly, P. (1995) Functional deficiencies in two distinct IFN-α producing cell populations in PBMC from human immunodeficiency virus seropositive patients. *J. Leuk. Biol.* **57,** 214–220.
33. Ferbas, J. J., Toso, J. F., Logar, A. J., Navratil, J. S., and Rinaldo, C. R. (1994) CD4+ blood dendritic cells are potent producers of IFN-α in response to in vitro HIV-1 infection. *J. Immunol.* **152,** 4649—4662.
34. Kerkmann, M., Rothenfusser, S., Hornung, V., Towarowski, A., Wagner, M., Sarris, A., et al. (2003) Activation with CpG-A and CpG-B oligonucleotides reveals two distinct regulatory pathways of type I IFN synthesis in human plasmacytoid dendritic cells. *J. Immunol.* **170,** 4465–4474.
35. Sato, M., Suemori, H., Hata, N., Asagiri, M., Ogasawara, K., Nakao, K., et al. (2000) Distinct and essential roles of transcription factors IRF-3 and IRF-7 in response to viruses for IFN-alpha/beta gene induction. *Immunity* **13,** 539–548.
36. Barnes, B. J., Lubyova, B., and Pitha, P. (2002) On the role of interferon regulatory factors in host defense. *J. Interferon Cytokine Res.* **22,** 59–71.
37. Izaguirre, A., Barnes, B. J., Amrute, S., Yeow, W. S., Megjugorac, N., Dai, J., et al. (2003) Comparative analysis of IRF and IFN-alpha expression in human plasmacytoid and monocyte-derived dendritic cells. *J. Leuk. Biol.* **74,** 1125–1138.
38. Dai, J. H., Megjugorac, N., Amrute, S., and Fitzgerald-Bocarsly, P. (2004) Regulation of IRF-7 and IFN-alpha production by enveloped virus and LPS in human plasmacytoid dendritic cells. *J. Immunol.* **173,** 1535–1548.

13

Analysis of Anti-Interferon Properties of the Herpes Simplex Virus Type I ICP0 Protein

Karen Mossman

Summary

A defining hallmark of the type 1 interferons (IFNs) is their ability to interfere with virus replication. As such, viruses have evolved diverse mechanisms to subvert the antiviral effects of interferons. Herpes simplex virus type 1 (HSV-1) is a large deoxyribonucleic acid virus best known for its ability to cause cold sores in infected individuals. In cultured cells, HSV-1 is relatively resistant to the effects of IFNs. Plaque reduction assays were used to determine that the immediate early HSV-1 gene product ICP0 functions in part to ensure successful replication in the presence of an IFN-induced antiviral response. Northern blot analysis showed that in the absence of ICP0, HSV-1 transcript accumulation is significantly decreased. Finally, nuclear run-on assays demonstrated that ICP0 functions to overcome IFN-induced blocks to virus transcription. The methods used in these studies are described in detail in this section.

Key Words: Interferon; herpes simplex virus; ICP0; antiviral; innate; immune response; plaque reduction; Northern blot; nuclear run-on.

1. Introduction

Interferons (IFNs) initially were discovered based on their ability to interfere with virus replication *(1)*. Although it is now clear that both type 1 (IFN-α/β) and type 2 (IFN-γ) IFNs are multifunctional cytokines, antiviral defense and initiation of the innate immune response remain the major functions of IFN-α/β *(2)*. As such, many viruses have evolved strategies to block IFN production or its antiviral activities *(3,4)*. Large deoxyribonucleic acid (DNA) viruses such as herpes simplex virus type 1 (HSV-1) are relatively resistant to the effects of IFN in cultured cells *(5)*. To explore the basis for the relative resistance of HSV-1 to IFN in cell culture, we examined the effects of mutations that alter known regulatory proteins on the sensitivity to IFN-α in a plaque reduction assay *(6)*. In this assay, cells are pretreated with IFN to establish an antiviral state before infection with virus. Each virus mutant is then

From: *Methods in Molecular Medicine, Vol. 116: Interferon Methods and Protocols*
Edited by: D. J. J. Carr © Humana Press Inc., Totowa, NJ

tested for its ability to produce plaques, indicative of productive infection, in cells that are pretreated with IFN vs cells left untreated. Using this approach, we discovered that HSV-1 mutants lacking ICP0, an immediate early regulatory protein *(7)*, were hypersensitive to the effects of IFN *(6)*. Northern blot analysis of RNA transcript accumulation demonstrated that HSV-1 ICP0 mutants fail to accumulate significant levels of viral transcripts in cells pretreated with IFN. In order to distinguish between a defect in transcription, pre messenger ribonucleic acid (mRNA) processing or mRNA stability, nuclear run-on assays were performed to investigate the efficiency of transcription of HSV-1 genes in mutants lacking ICP0 after treatment with IFN *(8)*. Nuclear run-on assays, also referred to as transcriptional run-on assays, measure the level of RNA polymerases traversing a specific gene at a given time in cells subjected to an experimental condition, such as viral infection *(9)*. Because initiation of transcription is extremely inefficient in isolated nuclei, transcriptional activity of a target gene can be measured by incubating isolated nuclei with [^{32}P]uridine triphosphate (UTP) and allowing the radiolabeled UTP to incorporate into nascent RNA transcripts by RNA polymerases that were in the process of transcribing the target gene at the time of nuclei harvest. Radiolabeled RNA molecules are then purified and hybridized to membranes containing immobilized DNA from the target gene to determine the transcriptional activity of that gene *(10)*. This approach demonstrated that one function of ICP0 is to overcome an IFN-induced block to virus transcription. Similar findings were subsequently reported by a second group *(11)*. Recently, we also have found that ICP0 subverts IFN-independent innate immune responses initiated after the entry of HSV-1 particles into susceptible cells *(12,13)*. Thus, ICP0 plays a key role in establishing a productive HSV-1 infection by blocking IFN-dependent and -independent cellular antiviral responses.

2. Materials

1. Tissue culture cells and appropriate medium.
2. Tissue culture dishes (six-well, 60-mm dishes).
3. Recombinant IFN, reconstitute at 1000 U/µL (1000X stock), and freeze in small aliquots at –80°C to avoid repeated freeze–thaw cycles.
4. Pooled human serum (Sigma), store in aliquots at –20°C.
5. 1% methylcellulose solution (autoclave 2% methylcellulose in H$_2$O and allow to cool [solution will be clumpy until completely cooled], add equal volume 2X media and serum to 5%); solution will be viscous.
6. Methanol (store at room temperature).
7. Giemsa stain (Sigma). Prepare a fresh 1X solution in H$_2$O before use.
8. Trizol (Invitrogen) or other commercial kit for harvesting total cellular RNA.
9. Diethylpyrocarbonate (DEPC). Solution is toxic and should be handled with care in a fume hood.

10. 10X MOPS: 200 mM MOPS, pH 7.0, 20 mM sodium acetate, 10 mM ethylene diamine tetraacetic acid (EDTA), pH 8.0, DEPC. Treat and autoclave before use; light sensitive.
11. Oligo-labeling buffer: 300 mM, pH 8.0, 30 mM MgCl$_2$, 65 mM 2-mercaptoethanol, 125 µM each dGTP, dATP, and dTTP, 1.3 M HEPES, pH 6.6; aliquot and store at $-20°C$.
12. Random primer (sequence NNNNNN). Aliquot and store at $-20°C$ to avoid freeze–thaw cycles.
13. Bovine serum albumin (BSA), 10 mg/mL stock (often sold with restriction enzymes and buffers).
14. Formaldehyde, solution is toxic and should be handled with care in a fume hood.
15. Formamide, reagent-grade, aliquot and freeze at $-80°C$ immediately upon opening.
16. Radionucleotides [α-^{32}P]dCTP and [^{32}P]UTP (10 µCi/µL stocks); use protocols in place at each institution for handling of radioactive compounds.
17. TE: 10 mM Tris-HCL, pH 8.0; 1 mM EDTA.
18. Phenol–chloroform. Caution should be taken when handling.
19. Enzymes (DNase I, RNase A, Klenow, proteinase K).
20. 10% sodium dodecyl sulfate (SDS), wear mask when preparing this solution, filter sterilize.
21. Sephadex G-50 columns, commercially available.
22. Reticulocyte Saline Buffer (RSB): 10 mM NaCl, 10 mM Tris-HCl, pH 7.4, 5 mM MgCl$_2$.
23. Nonidet-P40 (NP-40).
24. Nuclear freezing buffer: 50 mM Tris-HCl, pH 8.0, 5 mM MgCl$_2$, 40% glycerol, 0.5 mM dithiothreitol; make fresh using sterile glycerol.
25. 5X run-on buffer: 25 mM Tris-HCl, pH 8.0, 12.5 mM MgCl$_2$, 770 mM KCl, 12.5 mM each ATP, CTP, and GTP; make fresh in DEPC-treated H$_2$O.
26. 10X SET: 10% SDS; 100 mM Tris-HCl, pH 7.5, 50 mM EDTA.
27. 10X SSC: 1.5 M NaCl, 150 mM sodium citrate.
28. ExpressHyb (Clontech). Church buffer: 1% BSA, 1 mM EDTA, 7% SDS made in 0.5 M phosphate buffer.
29. Phosphate-buffered saline (PBS): 137 mM NaCl, 2.7 mM KCl, 10 mM Na$_2$HPO$_4$, 2 mM KH$_2$PO$_4$, autoclave to sterilize.
30. NH$_4$OAc, transfer RNA, isopropanol.
31. Transfer membrane, preferably nitrocellulose for nucleic acid transfer.
32. Tubes (screw capped tubes with O-rings, 50-mL and 15-mL conical).
33. Ultraviolet (UV) crosslinker.
34. Hybridization oven and bottles.
35. Plastic wrap, X-ray film and cassettes with intensifying screens

3. Methods

The methods outlined here describe (1) plaque reduction assays, (2) Northern blot hybridizations, and (3) nuclear run-on analyses that were used to determine that the HSV-1 ICP0 protein overcomes IFN-induced blocks to virus transcription. The methods are described in a general fashion such that they can be used with a variety of virus recombinants under different experimental parameters.

3.1. Plaque Reduction Assay

The large DNA virus HSV-1 is relatively resistant to the antiviral effects of IFN in cultured cells *(5)*. To determine whether this resistant phenotype depends on a specific regulatory protein, the effects of mutations that alter known virus regulators were examined in a plaque reduction assay (**Fig. 1**). Wild-type HSV-1 (strain KOS) along with mutants bearing lesions in the genes encoding ICP0, ICP22, UL13, vhs, and VP16 were used *(6)*. However, any virus that forms foci or plaques in cultured cells can be used in this assay. It is important to remember, however, that most IFN is species specific, thus an appropriate source of IFN (species matched or universal) should be selected for each experimental situation.

1. Seed cultured cells into wells of a six-well plate at a density of approx 2 to 3×10^5 cells per well, in the presence or absence of 1000 U of IFN per milliliter. For each virus to be tested, two six-well plates are required (one –IFN and one +IFN).
2. 16 h later, prepare six serial 10-fold dilutions of 1 mL each, for each virus to be tested, in the appropriate media minus serum (*see* **Note 1**).
3. Remove media from two six-well plates (one –IFN and one +IFN). Beginning with the highest dilution (i.e., least amount of virus), add 400 µL of each dilution to one well of each plate. Repeat for each virus to be tested.
4. Return plates to incubator and rock every 10 min for 1 h. After the 1-h infection, remove the virus innoculum and replace with either medium containing 1% human serum (for HSV-1) or 1% methylcellulose solution (for other viruses).
5. Once plaques are visible, remove media and fix cells with methanol (2 mL per well) at room temperature for 5 min. Remove methanol and add 5 mL of 1X Giemsa per well.
6. Once cells are stained (>2 h), remove Giemsa, rinse plates thoroughly with water, and count plaques. Determine the viral titer from each plate.
7. To determine the IFN-mediated fold reduction in plaque formation of each virus mutant, divide the viral titer in the absence versus presence of IFN-α pretreatment.

3.2. Northern Blot Hybridization

Once ICP0 mutant viruses were identified as being hypersensitive to IFN, based on a significant fold reduction in plaque formation, the next step was to determine the stage of the virus replication cycle that was negatively regulated by IFN. Northern blot hybridization *(14)* was used to examine the accumulation of viral transcripts in IFN-treated and control cells at various times postinfection with wild type and ICP0 mutant viruses.

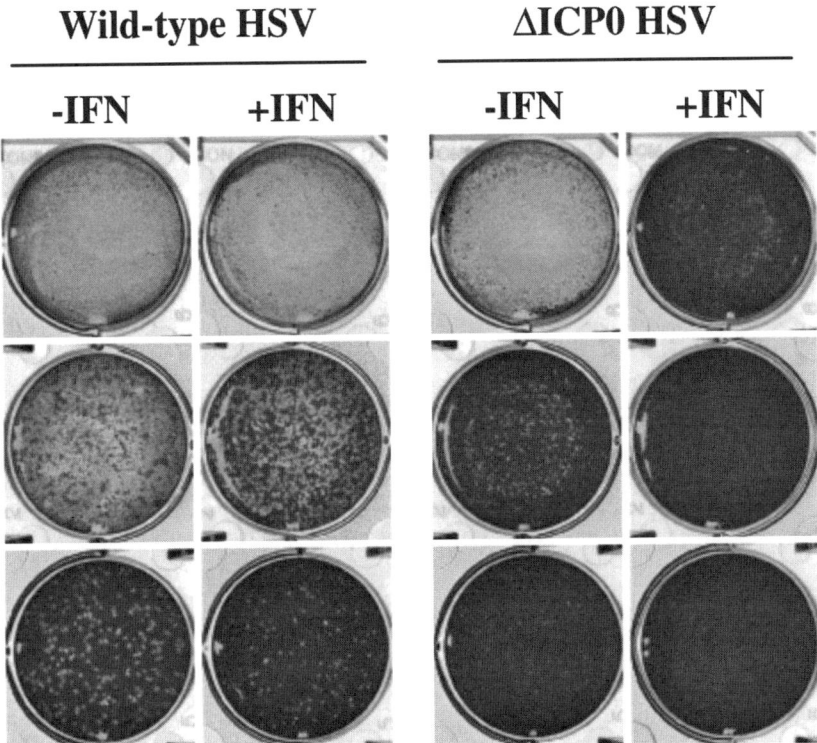

Fig. 1. Investigation of IFN sensitivity using a plaque reduction assay. Vero cells were mock treated or pretreated with human universal interferon prior to infection with 10-fold serial dilutions of wild-type or ICP0 mutant herpes simplex viruses. Cells were fixed and stained 2 d after infection.

3.2.1. Preparation of Total RNA

1. Seed cultured cells into 60-mm dishes at a density of approx 5×10^5 cells per well, in the presence or absence of 1000 U of IFN per milliliter. To seed the correct number of dishes, determine the number of time points required per virus and multiply by two (± IFN). Seed one extra dish for counting cells before infection.
2. 16 h later, count cells and determine the amount of each virus stock required for a multiplicity of infection of five plaque-forming units per cell. Add 1 mL of total innoculum per plate and infect for 1 h, followed by replacement of complete media.
3. At the predetermined times after infection, harvest total RNA using Trizol (Invitrogen) or another commercially available RNA retrieval kit, as per manufacturer's specifications.

3.2.2. Gel Electrophoresis and Transfer of RNA

1. Prepare agarose gels for electrophoresis. Gels are prepared in 1X MOPS and contain 2% formaldehyde. The running buffer is 1X MOPS (*see* **Note 2**).
2. Prepare RNA for gel electrophoresis by mixing 5 µg of total RNA with 3 µL of 10X MOPS, 15 µL of formamide, 5 µL of formaldehyde, and DEPC-treated H_2O to reach a final volume of 30 µL (*see* **Note 3**). Heat samples to 55°C for 15 min, place on ice for 5 min, load, and run gel.
3. To transfer RNA from the gel to a membrane, use either a semi-dry transfer apparatus, as per manufacturer's instructions, or set up a capillary transfer (*see* **Note 4**).

3.2.3. Preparation of Radiolabeled Probe

1. Determine the optimum DNA sequences required for probe to detect the transcripts of choice. Purified plasmid DNA fragments or PCR products work well.
2. Mix approx 150 ng of probe DNA with 200 ng of random primer and H_2O in a total volume of 34 µL. Incubate at 95°C for 10 min and immediately place on ice for 5 min.
3. Add 7 µL of oligo-labeling buffer, 20 µg of BSA, 50 of µCi [α-^{32}P]dCTP, and 5 units Klenow enzyme in a final volume of 50 µL (*see* **Note 5**). Incubate at 37°C for 30 min.
4. Add 50 µL of TE, pH 8.0, and 100 µL of phenol:chloroform. Vortex tube and centrifuge at maximum speed for 5 min.
5. To separate labeled probe from unincorporated nucleotides, apply aqueous phase to a Sephadex G-50 column and elute as per manufacturer's specifications.

3.2.4. Hybridization and Detection

There are many different methods of hybridization *(14)*. We prefer using ExpressHyb (Clonetech), as the procedure is rapid (total time 2.5 h) and the blots are clean. We also use Church buffer, although this procedure is lengthy in comparison (requires overnight hybridization).

1. Pre-heat ExpressHyb solution to 68°C to completely dissolve. (The solution at room temperature is very viscous and often forms a white precipitate.)
2. Prehybridize membrane for 30 min at 68°C in hybridization bottles containing O-rings.
3. Heat probe to 95°C for 5 min. Immediately add 2×10^6 cpm of probe per mL ExpressHyb, directly into hybridization solution, taking care not to touch the membrane directly with the probe. Hybridize for 1 h at 68°C.
4. Remove probe and wash membrane in a generous quantity of 2X SSC and 0.05% SDS for 30 min at room temperature with two changes of solution. Repeat procedure with 0.1X SSC and 0.1% SDS at 50°C.
5. Remove the blot with forceps, wrap in plastic wrap and expose to X-ray film at −70°C using intensifying screens.

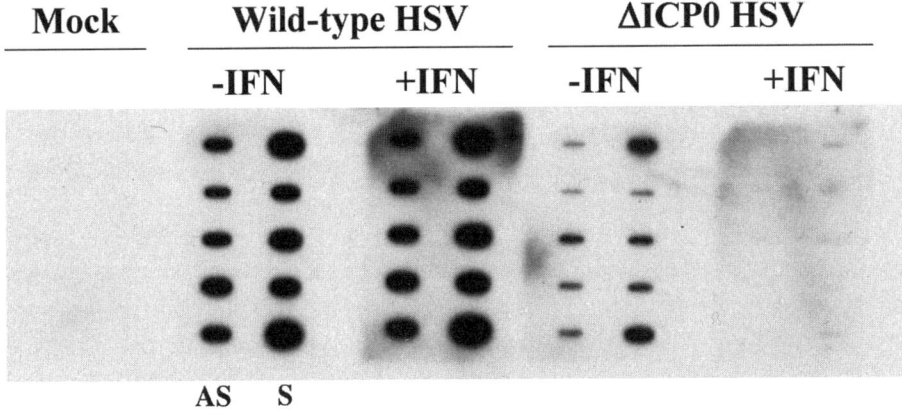

Fig. 2. Investigation of the effects of IFN on viral transcription using a nuclear run on assay. Vero cells were mock treated or pretreated with human universal interferon before infection with wild-type or ICP0 mutant herpes simplex viruses. Nuclei were harvested 6 h after infection and transcripts associated with RNA polymerases were elongated in the presence of radiolabeled UTP. Labeled RNA species were hybridized to membranes containing both sense (S) and antisense (AS) single-stranded DNA probes representing various herpes simplex virus genes.

3.3. Nuclear Run-On Assays

The failure of ICP0 mutants to accumulate viral mRNA in IFN-treated Vero cells was consistent with a defect in transcription, pre-mRNA processing or mRNA stability. Nuclear run-on assays were performed to delineate whether ICP0 regulates viral gene transcription in the presence of IFN (**Fig. 2**).

3.3.1. Isolation of Nuclei

1. Seed 1 to 2×10^7 cells per experimental condition and treat with or without 1000 U of IFN per milliliter for 16 h.
2. Remove media and infect cells as outlined in **Subheading 3.1.** (*see* **Note 6**).
3. Six hours after infection, remove media and rinse well with ice-cold PBS. All solutions should be ice cold in subsequent steps.
4. Add 5 mL of PBS to each plate, scrape the cells off of the plate, and transfer to a 50-mL conical tube on ice. Add a further 5 mL of PBS to the plate to collect residual cells and add to the tube.
5. Pellet cells at 1000 rpm for 10 min at 4°C, discard supernatant, and resuspend cell pellet in 20 mL of RSB.
6. Re-pellet cells at 1000 rpm for 10 min at 4°C, discard supernatant, and resuspend cell pellet in 2 mL of RSB. Once fully resuspended, add 18 mL of RSB containing 0.5% NP40 and pipet vigorously to ensure outer membranes are lysed (*see* **Note 7**).

7. Pellet nuclei at 2100 rpm for 5 min at 4°C, remove supernatant and do a further quick spin to bring down any residual liquid containing NP40. Ensure that all liquid is removed from the nuclear pellet.
8. Resuspend nuclear pellet in 105 µL of nuclear freezing buffer, transfer to screw-capped tubes with O-rings and store at –70°C.

3.3.2. Preparation of Slot Blots for Hybridization

We were extremely fortunate to receive single-stranded (ss)DNA from Dr. Charlotte Spencer (University of Alberta) for these studies. If both sense and antisense transcripts are to be investigated, then ssDNA representing both strands of a given gene must be utilized. Cloning vectors such as pBluescript II (Stratagene) are phagemids (plasmids with a phage origin) that enable the rescue of both the sense and non-sense strand of a given DNA sequence. If the orientation of transcription is not an issue, then dsDNA probes can be used. In this case, the cDNA or gene of interest is denatured using NaOH and NaCl before use (11). It must be noted, however, that many DNA viruses transcribe both strands of their genome, requiring the use of ssDNA probes.

1. Prepare slot blot apparatus according to manufacturer's instructions. The use of a charged membrane is suggested.
2. Apply 200 µL of DNA in 1X SSC to each slot (5 µg dsDNA or 1 µg ssDNA).
3. Wash the blots by applying 300 µL 1X SSC to each slot. Repeat.
4. Remove the blot from the apparatus and UV crosslink while filter is still wet. Mark the filters on one corner to identify the correct side and orientation. The blots are now ready for use, and can be stored for several weeks wrapped in plastic wrap (*see* **Note 8**).

3.3.3. Preparation of Nuclei and Hybridization

1. To 105 µL of thawed nuclei, add 30 µL of 5X run-on buffer and 15 µL of ^{32}P-UTP (10 µCi/µL stock; *see* **Note 9**).
2. Vortex and incubate at 30°C for 30 min with gentle shaking of tubes every 10 min.
3. To each sample, add 10 µL of DNase I, vortex and incubate for 5 min at 30°C. Repeat with a further addition of 5 µL of DNase I.
4. Add 18 µL 10X SET buffer and 50 µg of proteinase K per sample and incubate at 45°C for 45 min.
5. To stop the reaction, add 180 µL of phenol:chloroform, vortex well, and centrifuge at 12,000*g* for 5 min.
6. Remove the aqueous phase, place in a new screw capped tube and add 100 µL of 7.5 M NH$_4$OAc, 2.5 µL of carrier transfer RNA, and 300 µL of isopropanol. Place in dry ice or a –80°C freezer for 20 min to precipitate. Spin at 12,000*g* for 15 min to pellet RNA.
7. Resuspend pellet in 50 µL of TE, apply to a Sephadex G-50 spin column, and elute as per manufacturer's instructions.

8. Prehybridize filters containing DNA in 1-mL Church buffer at 65°C.
9. Add labeled RNA to the filters and hybridize at 65°C for 36 to 48 h (*see* **Note 10**).
10. To wash filters:
    a. Wash twice at room temperature with 0.1% SDS and 1X SSC for 5 min each time.
    b. Wash once in RNase wash buffer (2 µg/mL RNase A in 2X SSC) for 30 min at room temperature.
    c. Wash twice in 0.1% SDS and 1X SSC for 5 min each time at room temperature.
    d. Wash twice in 0.1% SDS and 0.1X SSC for 30 min each time at 65°C.
11. Wrap filters in plastic wrap and expose to film at −70°C for 2 to 5 d.

4. Notes

1. The 10-fold dilution series chosen depends on the titer of each virus stock. For example, dilutions of 10^{-1} to 10^{-6} are appropriate for virus stocks with titers of approximately 10^7 pfu/mL (typical of ICP0 mutants on Vero cells) whereas dilutions of 10^{-4} to 10^{-9} are appropriate for virus stocks with titers of approx 10^{10} pfu/mL (typical of wild type HSV-1).
2. To avoid using excessive amounts of formaldehyde, a known carcinogen, the running buffer is devoid of formaldehyde. As such, the gel must be run fairly quickly to avoid diffusion of formaldehyde from the gel into the running buffer. We typically run our gels at 100 to 150 volts for 1 to 2 h.
3. Caution should be taken when working with RNA because of the abundance of RNases *(14)*. 10X MOPS and H_2O should be DEPC-treated before use by adding 1 mL of DEPC per liter of solution and incubating for more than 1 h at 37°C followed by autoclaving. Formaldehyde should be opened in the fume hood. If formamide turns yellow in color, it must be deionized before use. To avoid ionization of formamide, purchase reagent-grade formamide, aliquot into small amounts immediately upon opening of a new bottle and freeze aliquots at −80°C until further use.
4. Although a semidry transfer apparatus will transfer the RNA to a membrane very quickly (i.e., within 30–45 min), we have found that this method requires supervision of the procedure because the gel will shrink during the transfer process, requiring tightening of the apparatus at regular intervals. We prefer to use capillary transfer, even though this requires at least 8 h for successful transfer. To set up a capillary transfer, place a pipet tip box into a larger container filled with 10X SSC. On top of the tip box, place a glass plate large enough to hold the gel. Over top of the glass plate, place two layers of Whatman paper long enough to reach into the 10X SSC. Ensure that this "wick" is completely wet with buffer and devoid of bubbles between the layers. Place the gel face down on the wick and again remove any bubbles between the layers. Surround the gel completely with plastic wrap or old pieces of X-ray film to ensure that subsequent layers of paper do not touch the wick or underlying buffer. On top of the gel, layer the membrane followed by two pieces of Whatman paper, all of which are precut to the size of

the gel and pre-soaked in buffer. Finally, place a 2- to 3-inch stack of paper towels on top, followed by a weight to hold the transfer in place. We use old ICN catalogs for this purpose.
5. Caution should be taken when working with radioactivity and all steps should be performed according to procedures outlined in each institution's radiation safety guidelines. To eliminate accidental contamination, screw-capped tubes with O-rings are recommended. In addition, radioactive nucleotides are available spiked with a colored dye for easy detection.
6. Because ICP0 mutants replicate poorly in Vero cells, particularly in the presence of IFN, the multiplicity of infection was increased from 5 to 20 plaque-forming units per cell for the mutants. At the lower multiplicity of infection, we found that the run-on signal was very low and difficult to quantitate. Thus, depending on the mutant to be tested and the cell line involved, increasing the multiplicity of infection may assist in obtaining useable data.
7. RSB is a hypotonic buffer, which causes the cells to swell. Subsequent pellets will be very loose, thus caution is required when removing supernatants. In addition, before NP40 is added to the cells, ensure that the cell pellet is well resuspended in RSB. This will prevent clumping of cells and nuclei.
8. After the successful application of DNA to the membrane, ensure that the slot blot apparatus is appropriately cleaned. Place apparatus in a glass dish and soak in 1 N of HCl for 20 to 30 min. Thoroughly rinse apparatus in distilled H_2O and allow it to dry. If RNA is applied to a membrane, simply soak apparatus in 1 N of NaOH as opposed to HCl. Take care to wear gloves when working with these solutions.
9. This procedure uses a large quantity of ^{32}P (150 µCi per sample). Care should be taken throughout the procedure. Tube containing O-rings should be used for all steps. Depending on the number of samples to be tested within each experiment, ring detectors for monitoring exposure levels may be required, depending on the radiation safety protocols of each institution.
10. To hybridize filters with a minimal amount of hybridization buffer (1 mL), filters were placed in 15-mL conical tubes that were then placed in standard glass hybridization tubes. Since conical tube lids do not generally contain O-rings, we initially experienced frequent leakage of the radioactive hybridization solution, particularly during the wash steps. Changing the lids after each step in the procedure significantly reduced the amount of leakage from the conical tubes.

References

1. Isaacs, A. and Lindenmann, J. (1957) Virus interference. I. The interferon. *Proc. R. Soc. London Serv. B.* **147,** 258–267.
2. Stark, G. R., Kerr, I. M., Williams, B. R. G., Silverman, R. H., and Schreiber, R. D. (1998). How cells respond to interferons. *Annu. Rev. Biochem.* **67,** 227–264.
3. Goodbourne, S., Didcock, L., and Randall, R. E. (2000) Interferons: cell signalling, immune modulation, antiviral responses and virus countermeasures. *J. Gen. Virol.* **81,** 2341–2364.

4. Sen, G. C. (2001) Viruses and interferon. *Ann. Rev. Microbiol.* **55,** 255–281.
5. Mossman, K. L. (2002) Activation and inhibition of virus and interferon: the herpesvirus story. *Viral Immunol.* **15,** 3–15.
6. Mossman, K. L., Saffran, H. A., and Smiley, J. R. (2000) Herpes simplex virus ICP0 mutants are hypersensitive to interferon. *J. Virol.* **74,** 2052–2056.
7. Everett, R. D. (2000) ICP0, a regulator of herpes simplex virus during lytic and latent infection. *Bioessays* **22,** 761–70.
8. Mossman, K. L. and Smiley, J. R. (2002) Herpes Simplex Virus ICP0 and ICP34.5 counteract distinct interferon-induced barriers to virus replication. *J. Virol.* **76,** 1995–1998.
9. Sambrook, J. and Russell, D. W. (2001) Transcriptional run-on assays, in *Molecular Cloning: A Laboratory Manual*, vol. 3. Cold Spring Harbor Laboratory Press, Cold Spring Harbor, New York, pp. 17.23–17.29.
10. Srivastava, R. A. and Schonfeld, G. (1998) Measurements of rate of transcription in isolated nuclei by nuclear "run-off" assay. *Methods Mol. Biol.* **86,** 201–207.
11. Harle, P., Sainz, B., Jr., Carr, D. J., and Halford, W. P. (2002) The immediate-early protein, ICP0, is essential for the resistance of herpes simplex virus to interferon-alpha/beta. *Virology* **293,** 295–304.
12. Collins, S. E., Noyce, R. S., and Mossman, K. L. (2004) The innate cellular response to virus particle entry requires IRF3 but not virus replication. *J. Virol.* **78,** 1706–1717.
13. Lin, R., Noyce, R. S.,Collins, S. E., Everett, R. D., and Mossman, K. L. (2004) The herpes simplex virus ICP0 RING finger domain inhibits IRF3- and IRF7-mediated activation of interferon-stimulated genes. *J. Virol.* **78,** 1675–1684.
14. Sambrook, J. and Russell, D. W. (2001) Northern hybridization, in –*Molecular Cloning: A Laboratory Manual*, Third ed, vol. 1. Cold Spring Harbor Laboratory Press, Cold Spring Harbor, New York, pp. 7.42–7.45.

14

Interferon Subtype Gene Therapy for Regulating Cytomegalovirus Disease

Cassandra M. James, Emmalene J. Bartlett, Josephine P. Mansfield, and Vanessa S. Cull

Summary

Delivery of type I interferon (IFN) subtypes by intramuscular inoculation of mice with a recombinant mammalian expression vector encoding IFN stimulates the immune response. Such immunomodulation drives towards a Th1-like response. The degree of stimulation of the immune response was influenced by several parameters of the naked deoxyribonucleic acid (DNA) vaccination protocol. Pretreatment of mice with bupivacaine increased transgene expression *in situ*. The specific subtype gene of type I IFN, the DNA concentration, the combined use of two or more subtypes, and the timing of the DNA immunisations were all found to influence the level of efficacy of IFN gene therapy in a mouse model for cytomegalovirus (CMV) infection and disease. In addition, adjuvant therapy, using type I IFN genes, for DNA virus vaccination (CMV glycoprotein B) enhanced viral-specific immunity and reduced the severity of myocarditis in mice. Thus, type I IFN gene therapy has potent adjuvant properties when delivered as DNA and can be used to regulate virus infection and disease via pleiotropic actions in the stimulation of immune responses.

Key Words: Interferon; gene therapy, cytomegalovirus (CMV), DNA, expression vector.

1. Introduction

The herpes virus, cytomegalovirus (CMV) causes persistent, recurrent, and latent infections. Myocarditis, an often fatal disease characterized by cellular inflammation of the heart, can be triggered by previous CMV infection *(1)*. The disease has an acute viral phase followed by a chronic postviral autoimmune phase. Recent developments in herpes virus vaccines incorporate recombinant deoxyribonucleic acid (DNA) plasmid constructs, which are safer than live infectious virus vaccines *(2)*. The transfection of DNA constructs in vivo allows the appropriate cytosolic synthesis and processing of the transgene antigen in the mammalian cell *(3)*. Presentation of the transgene product occurs via major histocompatibility complex class I and class II pathways and elicits both humoral and cell-mediated immune responses *(4)*. The innate cytokines, type I interferons (IFNs), are important in shaping the antiviral immune response because they form a pivotal link between innate and adaptive immunity *(5)*. Thus, IFN-α/β subtypes make a powerful tool for immunotherapy. Use of the IFN gene therapy and co-immunization of IFN with a DNA vaccine, composed of the viral glycoprotein B (gB) gene of CMV, has been our focus in treating CMV infection and disease. This chapter describes the techniques for optimal delivery of IFN gene therapy alone or in combination with viral DNA vaccination for improved protection using a mouse model for CMV.

Multiple type I IFN subtypes with pleiotropic properties occur in both humans and mice *(6)*. There are more than 12 human and murine IFN-α subtypes, with a single IFN-β subtype in each species. However, only limited IFN subtypes (frequently HuIFN-α2a) are licensed for treatment of virus infections, cancers, and chronic disorders. Knowledge of the biological properties of other subtypes for alternative treatment of disease will expand the therapeutic use of IFN. Gene therapy with IFN subtypes that are encoded by a mammalian expression vector provides an avenue to examine the role of individual IFN subtypes. We have uzed the mammalian expression vector, pkCMVint.polyLi, which contains the HCMV IE-1 promoter/enhancer element and intron A, with the SV40 polyadenylation signal. Individual IFN constructs were made with murine IFN subtype gene inserts, including the 69-nucleotide signal sequence upstream of the first cysteine codon. All inserts were sequenced in both directions to ensure complete integrity. We have made the novel discovery that specific subtypes of murine IFN delivered as naked DNA therapy have differential activities in vivo, involving regulation of anti-viral *(7–13)*, anti-leukemic *(14)*, and anti-inflammatory responses *(15–17)*.

Functional differences of the most efficacious IFN-α6, -α9, and -β subtypes involved antiviral effects, homing of inflammatory T cells to the heart, switching of antibody isotype, enhanced apoptosis, inhibition of cell proliferation, and differential activation of signal transducers and activators of transcription (STAT) molecules. Because IFN subtypes showed differential activation of intracellular transcriptional factors, it is possible that distinct signalling pathways exist. Differences in biological function also have been identified in the human IFN family. IFN-α21 showed higher efficacy in stimulating phosphorylation of STAT1 in human T cells than IFN-α1 and IFN-α2 *(18)*.

In our model for CMV myocarditis, we have found expression of IFN-α *(IFNA)* genes, after intramuscular inoculation of 200 μg naked DNA, to be effective in reducing murine CMV (MCMV) replication in mice. Analysis of individual specific IFN subtypes within the multigene family showed differential efficacy. Characterization of a large panel of seven individual IFN subtype

IFN Gene Therapy

DNA constructs (*IFNA1*, *A2*, *A4*, *A5*, *A6*, *A9*, and *B*) revealed that *IFNA6* treatment was superior in inhibiting MCMV replication. Treatment with *IFNA6*, *A9*, or *B*, but not *IFNA1*, *A2*, *A4*, or *A5* regulated the severity of disease in both acute and chronic phases of myocarditis. Furthermore, treatment with select combinations of efficacious IFN subtypes demonstrated synergy.

We also have investigated the use of IFN gene therapy with viral DNA vaccines encoding MCMV gB. The combined *gB/IFNA6/IFNB* DNA vaccine was superior to the *gB* DNA vaccine alone in inducing protective immunity to MCMV. Acute myocarditis was preferentially reduced with either *IFNA9* or *IFNB* but not with *IFNA6* coimmunization with *gB* DNA vaccine. However, *IFNA6*, *IFNA9*, and *IFNB* markedly reduced chronic myocarditis in *gB*-vaccinated mice challenged with MCMV. Thus select type I IFN subtype DNA vaccination may orchestrate a favorable immune response in the host to combat viral infection and subsequent postviral autoimmunity.

2. Materials
2.1. Reagents and Supplies for Gene Delivery

1. DNA vaccines: The MCMV gB gene, 2874-bp fragment from pBR322.gB (generously provided by Dr T. Scalzo, University of Western Australia), was subcloned into the *Bam*HI site of the expression vector, pkCMVint.polyLi (generously provided by VICAL Int., CA). Seven individual IFN constructs were made using the pkCMVint.polyLi vector with the murine type I IFN-α1, -α2, -α4, -α5, -α6, -α9, or -β gene inserts, including the 69 nucleotide signal sequence upstream of the first cysteine codon (*[16], see* **Notes 1** and **2**).
   Notes have been renumbered to align with their citations in the notes.
2. Animals: Specific pathogen-free inbred male BALB/c mice of 4 wk of age were supplied by the Animal Resources Centre (Murdoch, Western Australia, Australia). We routinely use 5-wk-old mice for immunization of DNA 5 d after bupivacaine treatment for improved uptake and expression of DNA (*see* **Note 3**).
3. Virus: Prepare the K181 Perth strain of MCMV (originally obtained from Dr. D. J. Lang, Duke University, Durham, NC) as a salivary gland homogenate by passage through 3-wk-old female BALB/c mice and store in liquid nitrogen until use.
4. General Reagent:
   a. Tris-buffered phenol: Thaw phenol at 65°C. Add 0.1% v/v 8-hydroxyquinolone and extract with 1 M Tris, pH 8.0, by stirring overnight. Change buffer three times over a 24-h period or until pH of the aqueous phase is more than 7.6. Extract once more with 0.1 M Tris, pH 8.0, and store under equilibrium buffer at 4°C in the dark.
   b. Phenol: Chloroform:isoamyl alcohol (25:24:1): Add an equal volume of chloroform /isoamyl alcohol (24:1 v/v) to Tris-buffered phenol and store under 0.1 M Tris, pH 8.0, at 4°C in the dark.
   c. Isopropanol.

d. Ethanol.
e. RNase, DNase-free.
f. Sodium acetate.
g. Insulin syringes: Ultra-fine needle, 31-gage (0.33 mm × 12.7mm) with a 0.5-mL barrel volume.
h. Marcain (0.5% bupivacaine).
i. Pyrogen-free saline (0.9% sodium chloride).
j. Sterile gauze (autoclave).

2.2. General Buffers for DNA Preparation

1. Terrific Broth; Solution A: 1.3% w/v Bacto Tryptone (BDH), 2.7% w/v yeast Extract, 0.4% v/v glycerol; Solution B: 719 mM K_2HPO_4, 169 mM KH_2PO_4. Autoclave Solution A and Solution B separately. Combine the two solutions at a ratio of 9:1, respectively. Add the antibiotic kanamycin at 10 µg/mL.
2. TEG swelling buffer: 25 mM Tris-HCl, pH 8.0, 10 mM ethylene diamine tetraacetic acid, 0.9% glucose (w/v). Store at 4°C.
3. Lysis buffer: 0.2 M NaOH, 1% v/v sodium dodecyl sulfate. Prepare fresh prior to use.
4. High-Salt Neutralization buffer: 2.5 M potassium acetate, 5% formic acid (v/v).
5. LiCl solution: 5 M LiCl, 1% w/v MOPS (w/v), pH to 8.0. Store at 4°C.
6. TAE buffer [50X]: 2 M Tris-HCl, 5.7% v/v glacial acetic acid, 0.05 M ethylene diamine tetraacetic acid, pH to 8.0.

2.3. Reagents for Plaque Assay

1. RPMI: 1.04% w/v Rosewell Park Memorial Institute medium 1640 (Gibco BRL Life Technologies, NY), 24 mM $NaHCO_3$, and 1% v/v penicillin/streptomycin solution in sterile H_2O, pH to 7.2, filter sterilize, and store at 4°C.
2. Methyl cellulose overlay: Autoclave 3.5% w/v methyl cellulose (4000 centipoises, Sigma, MO) in ultrapure H_2O, and shake until solution dissolves and allow to cool to room temperature. Add equal volume of 2X RPMI and 1% v/v fetal calf serum (FCS). If preferred, a sterile magnetic flea may be used to assist further mixing at 4°C. Store at 4°C.
3. Methylene blue/formaldehyde Stain: 0.5% w/v Methylene blue solution stirred overnight and filtered through 3MM Whatmann paper. Add 10% v/v formaldehyde.
4. Bouin's Fluid: 23.8% v/v Formaldehyde (40% stock), 4.8% v/v glacial acetic acid, and 71.4% picric acid. Store in a safety cabinet.

3. Methods

3.1. Preparation of DNA Constructs

1. Clone IFN subtype genes and the full-length gB MCMV gene into the mammalian expression vector, pkCMVint.polyLi (VICAL, San Diego, CA) as previously described *(9,16)*.

IFN Gene Therapy

2. Prepare bacterial cultures containing the required plasmid by inoculating a loopful of transformed bacteria from glycerol stock into 1 L of Terrific Broth (containing 10 µg/mL kanamycin). Incubate overnight at 37°C with shaking.
3. Centrifuge at 2500g at 4°C for 10 min and discard supernatant.
4. Resuspend pellet in 50 mL of TEG swelling buffer at 4°C.
5. Add 100 mL of lysis buffer and incubate on ice for 10 min.
6. Add 75 mL of high salt neutralization buffer and shake suspension until a white precipitate forms. Centrifuge at 2500g, 4°C, 10 min.
7. Pour the supernatant through four layers of sterile gauze and add an equal volume of cold isopropanol. Centrifuge at 2500g, 4°C, 10min.
8. Discard the supernatant and resuspend the pellet in 20 mL of double-deionized H_2O (dd H_2O). Transfer the solution to a polypropylene tube.
9. Add 20 mL of LiCl solution at 4°C, mix and stand on ice for 10 min. Centrifuge at 2500g, 4°C, 15min. Transfer the supernatant to a fresh polypropylene tube and discard pellet.
10. Extract the supernatant with an equal volume of phenol/chloroform/isoamyl alcohol. Centrifuge at 1800g, 20°C, 5 min.
11. Transfer the aqueous phase to a polypropylene tube and add 40 mL of cold isopropanol. Mix by inversion. Centrifuge at 2500g, 4°C, 10 min. Discard the supernatant.
12. Briefly air-dry the pellet and dissolve in 0.4 mL of ddH_2O. Transfer to an Eppendorf tube.
13. Add 4 µL of RNase and incubate at 37°C for 15 min.
14. Add 40 µL of 3 M sodium acetate (pH 4.8) and 1 mL of ethanol. Leave on dry ice for 15min (or at –20°C overnight). Centrifuge at 13,000g for 30 min at 20°C.
15. Wash pellet with 1 mL of 70% ethanol and centrifuge at 13,000g for 5 min at 20°C.
16. Briefly dry pellet and resuspend in ddH_2O.
17. Read OD at 260 nm and 280 nm.
18. Check DNA integrity by agarose gel electrophoresis and determine concentration by spectrophotometric analysis (*see* **Note 4**).

3.2. Delivery of DNA Constructs In Vivo

1. Restrain mice (4-wk-old male BALB/c) by grasping the skin behind the ears with the thumb and index finger and holding the tail underneath the smallest finger to stretch the body. Spray the fur on the legs with 70% ethanol to enable clear identification of the tibialis anterior (TA) muscle for intramuscular inoculation.
2. Inoculate 20 µL of 0.5% bupivacaine bilaterally via TA muscles (**Fig. 1**, *see* **Note 3**).
3. Five days later, inoculate DNA constructs (200 µg/mouse) by the intramuscular route (**Fig. 1**, *see* **Notes 5–7**). Dilute DNA in a 50-µL volume of sterile pyrogen-free 0.09% saline (4 µg/µL). Inoculate mice with 25 µL of DNA preparation bilaterally via each TA muscle.
   Allow 14 d for intramuscular protein expression from the DNA constructs prior to viral challenge (**Fig. 1**, *see* **Note 8**).

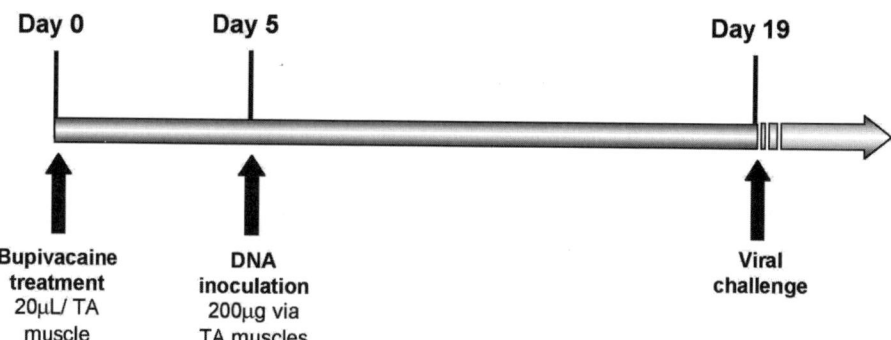

Fig. 1. Standard DNA inoculation schedule for in vivo expression of *IFN* transgenes. BALB/c mice at 4 wk of age were treated bilaterally with 20 μL of 0.5% bupivacaine intramuscularly via the TA muscle. At d 5, mice were inoculated with 200 μg of plasmid DNA diluted in pyrogen-free saline delivered bilaterally via the TA muscles. After 14 d of expression of the transgenes, mice were virus challenged and subsequently examined for antiviral and immunological responses.

3.3. IFN Bioassay

1. Thaw individual tissue homogenates and sera from mice and subject to pH 2.0 to remove acid-labile IFNs. Add 1 μL of 5.8 M HCl sequentially to samples until pH 2.0 is reached.
2. Incubate samples at –20°C for 1 h and microfuge at 13,000g for 5 min.
3. Transfer the supernatant to a fresh tube and add equivalent volume of 5 M NaOH and HCl to neutralize. Microfuge at 13,000g for 15 min. Aliquot and store at –80°C until use.
4. Add serial dilutions of above acid-treated samples in sterile DMEM containing 2% FCS to 70% confluent L929 cells in a 96-well plate. Include standard IFN samples on every plate and control cells without the addition of IFN.
5. Incubate at 37°C, 5% CO_2 overnight.
6. Remove samples and wash cells in sterile phosphate-buffered saline.
7. Add 100 μL of EMCV (diluted in DMEM/2% FCS appropriately from prior titration to give 100% cytopathic effect (CPE) in 18 h) per well (*see* **Note 9**). Leave half of the control cells free of virus. Incubate at 37°C, 5% CO_2, overnight.
8. Visualize CPE using light microscopy and score dilutions of samples giving 50% protection from virus-induced CPE of L929 cell monolayers. May use methylene blue stain overnight to assist in visualising endpoint titration.
9. Express titers as mean IU/g of tissue or IU/mL sera ± standard error (SE).

3.4. Virus Challenge and Quantitation

At 14 d after DNA treatment, inoculate mice with 100 μL of 1×10^4 pfu MCMV, diluted in pyrogen-free 0.09% saline, by the intraperitoneal (i.p.) route

IFN Gene Therapy

using a 25-gage needle (five mice per group). Collect tissues for virus quantitation by plaque assay (*see* **Note 10**).

1. Anaesthetize animal and then euthanize it by sodium pentobarbitone overdose followed by cervical dislocation.
2. Remove tissues aseptically and immediately place on ice.
3. Prepare 20% homogenates using RPMI and an electronic Ultra Turrax homogeniser (IKA T25, Staufen, Germany), clarify by centrifugation at 2000g at 4°C for 10 min. Keep on ice until ready to aliquot and store frozen at –80°C until use.
4. Titrate thawed mouse homogenates by adding serial dilutions to confluent washed monolayers of M2-10B4 stromal cells (ATTC, Rockville, MD) in 24-well microtiter plates.
5. Incubate for 1 h at 37°C in 5% CO_2 and then remove and replace with prewarmed 0.5 mL of methyl cellulose/RPMI/1%FCS overlay. Because the overlay is viscous, a blunt-ended 25-mL pipet is preferred for delivery.
6. Incubate 3 d at 37°C in 5% CO_2 followed by addition of 1 mL of methylene blue/formaldehyde solution to fix and stain the monolayers.
7. Wash away overlay using running water from tap and air dry plates for light microscopic examination and enumeration of plaques, visualised as clearings in the blue-stained monolayers.
8. Virus titers expressed as mean plaque-forming units (pfu)/g tissue ± SE (at least five mice per group).

3.5. Assessment of Myocarditis

1. Anaesthetize animal and euthanize by sodium pentobarbitone overdose followed by cervical dislocation.
2. Cut through the skin and rib cage to expose the thoracic cavity.
3. Aseptically remove hearts from infected mice.
4. Transect along the midline using a scalpel and blot with tissue paper.
5. Fix for 4 h in 5 mL of Bouin's fluid.
6. Transfer hearts to 70% ethanol overnight and then process into paraffin-embedded blocks.
7. Stain 5-μm sections with haematoxylin and eosin (H&E) and evaluate for evidence of cellular inflammation and necrosis (*see* **Note 11**). Express myocarditis severity as the mean number of inflammatory foci per heart section ± SE (at least five mice per group; **Fig. 2**).

4. Notes

1. To prepare the DNA constructs, subclone the full length murine *IFNA1*, *A2*, *A4*, *A5*, *A6*, *A9,* and *B* genes into the pkCMVint.polyLi expression vector via gene amplification using specific primers in the PCR (*[16]* **Fig. 3**). Fragments incorporated are IFNA1 –21 to +525bp, IFNA2 –21 to +596bp, IFNA4 –21 to +584bp, IFNA5 –18 to +593bp, IFNA6 –24 to +590bp, IFNA9 –25 to +595bp, and IFNB –10 to +599bp. These trimmed genes allow for improved consistency in stability and expression levels. The MCMV *gB* gene cassette is also cloned into the previous expression vector (**Fig. 3**).

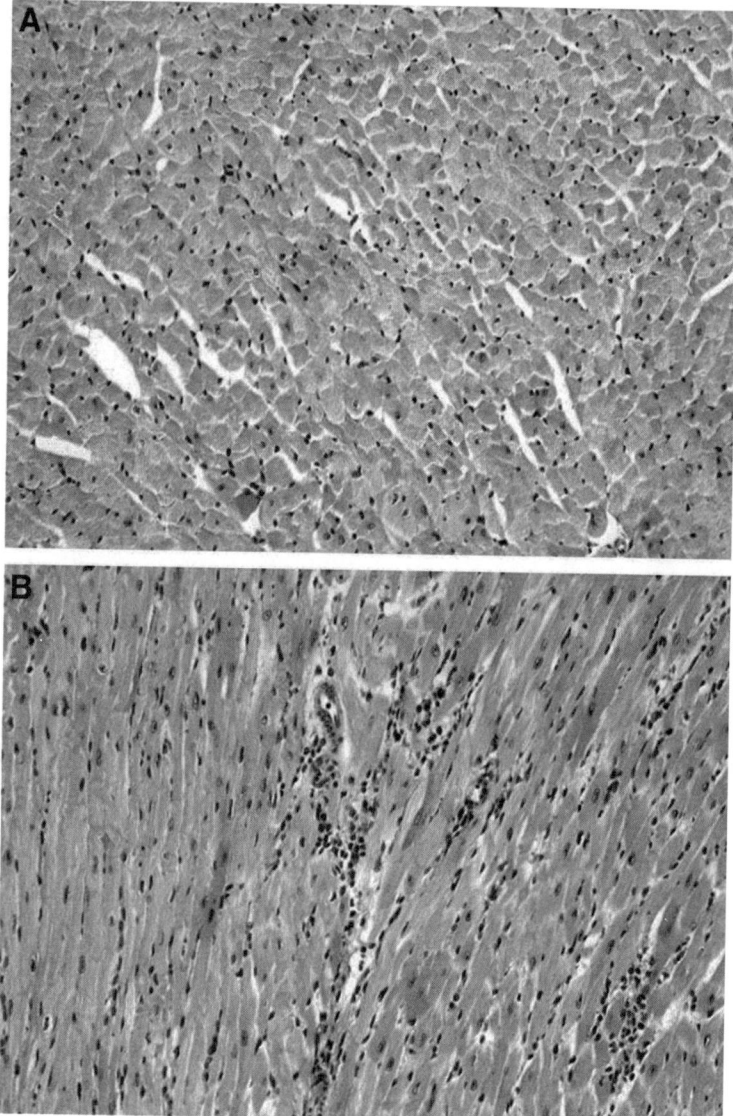

Fig. 2. MCMV-induced myocarditis in BALB/c mice. Myocarditis was determined by counting the foci of infiltrating cells in the myocardium of H&E-stained hearts. Hearts were transected down the midline, fixed in Bouin's fixative, and stained with H&E. Hearts shown for (**A**) normal, uninfected BALB/c mice and (**B**) BALB/c mice inoculated with Blank vector DNA (200 μg) and challenged 14 d later with 1×10^4 pfu MCMV at d 7 after infection demonstrate foci of inflammatory cells within the myocardium characteristic of acute stage MCMV-induced myocarditis.

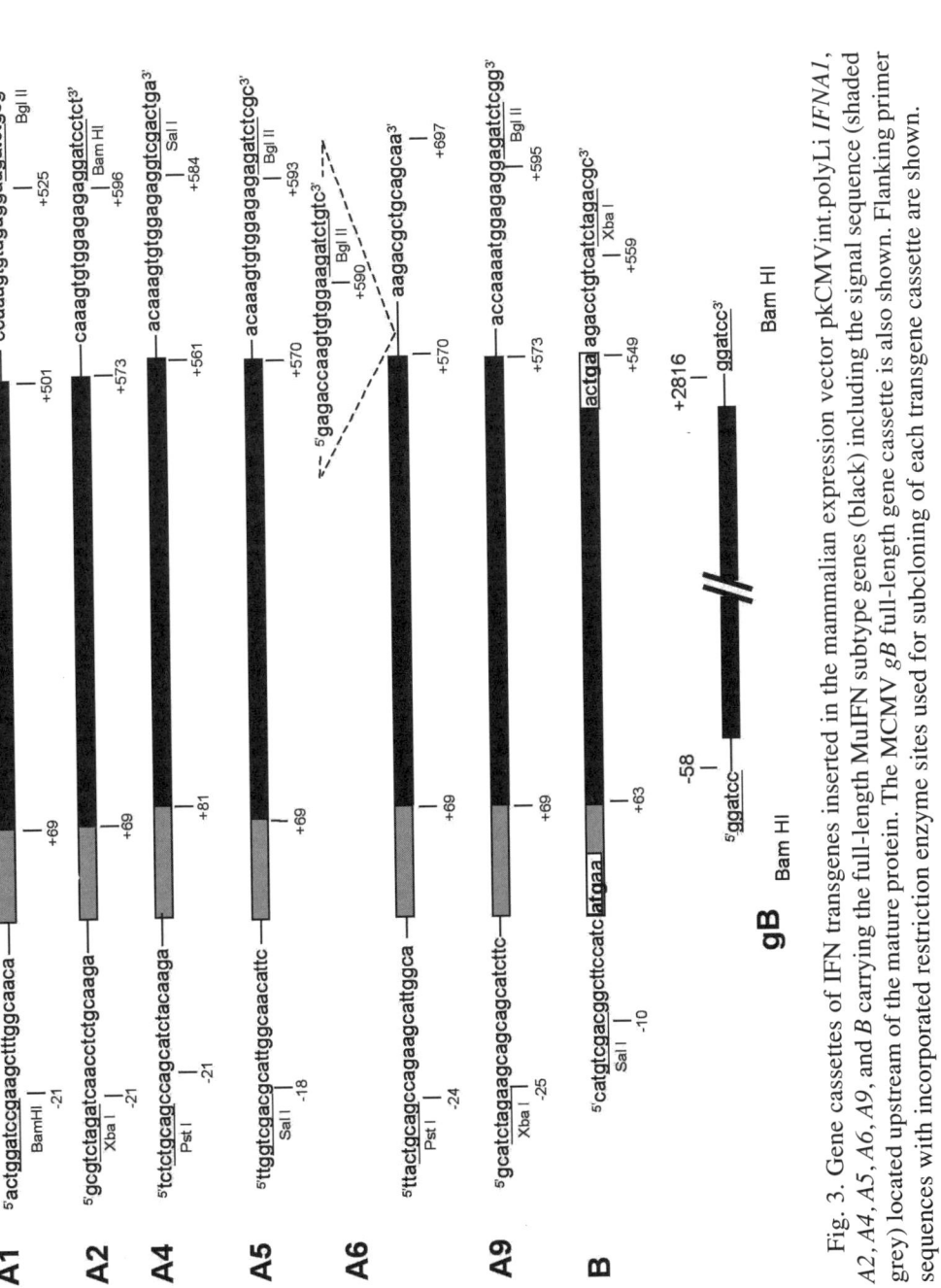

Fig. 3. Gene cassettes of IFN transgenes inserted in the mammalian expression vector pkCMVint.polyLi *IFNA1*, *A2*, *A4*, *A5*, *A6*, *A9*, and *B* carrying the full-length MuIFN subtype genes (black) including the signal sequence (shaded grey) located upstream of the mature protein. The MCMV *gB* full-length gene cassette is also shown. Flanking primer sequences with incorporated restriction enzyme sites used for subcloning of each transgene cassette are shown.

215

2. Measurement of biological activity of IFN by the bioassay establishes the expression of IFN transgene at both localized and systemic sites. Expression levels of the IFN transgene in immunised mice typically lie within the range of 10 to 40 IU/mL of sera at d 3. In the inoculated TA muscles, higher levels of expression of IFN can be detected in mice ranging threefold from 13,000 to 40,000 IU/g muscle at d 7 after infection after an additional 14 d of expression before virus infection. In uninfected mice, systemic IFN expression peaks at d 28 after *IFN* treatment and then declines to undetectable levels by d 84 after DNA inoculation *(8)*. Levels of transgene expression in the TA muscles peak earlier at d 21 post-DNA inoculation in uninfected mice *(8)*.
3. Bupivacaine induces rapid degeneration followed by regeneration of skeletal muscle and myogenesis, allowing improved uptake and expression of DNA *(19,20)*. In our hands, IFN transgene efficacy is improved when pretreating with bupivacaine. Viral titers in the liver were 9.4-fold greater in the group not treated with bupivacaine compared with the bupivacaine-treated group inoculated with efficacious *IFNA6*. Similarly, viral titers after *IFNA6* inoculation without bupivacaine treatment increased 7.8-fold and 2.8-fold in the spleen and salivary gland, respectively, compared with the bupivacaine treated group. Furthermore, myocarditis increased 3.5-fold without bupivacaine treatment compared with bupivacaine treatment following *IFNA6* treatment.
4. We obtain typical yields of DNA, approx 35 mg/L broth culture, using this method. The purity of the DNA is calculated by dividing A260 by A280. A value greater than or equal to 1.8 is considered suitable for DNA immunization of mice. Plasmid integrity and MW is assessed by electrophoresis using uncut and cut plasmid preparations run on a 1% agarose gel in TAE buffer. Both the gel and buffer contain ethidium bromide (10 mg/mL) for visualization of DNA on an ultraviolet (UV) transilluminator. Various forms of the uncut DNA may be apparent; supercoiled, coiled, and relaxed open circular. Endotoxin levels assessed by the limulus amebocyte lysate test are usually less than 1 endotoxin unit per 100 µg DNA.
5. We have examined the efficacies of a panel of seven individual IFN subtypes in the CMV model and have found differential efficacies amongst the subtypes *(16)*. Inflammation in the heart during MCMV infection was maximally reduced with *IFNA6* subtype treatment. In addition, *IFNA6* caused significant reductions of 5.7- and 19-fold in virus titers in the spleen and liver, respectively. The relationship between myocarditis and virus persistence has been characterised in our previous report *(21)*. Note that viral load in target organs does not affect the severity of acute phase myocarditis but that virus is a trigger for post-viral chronic inflammatory heart disease in the CMV model.
6. Because ranges from 25 to 200 µg of DNA have been used for immunotherapeutic gene transfer *(22)*, we tested other DNA concentrations. Lower concentrations of DNA, 50 µg and 100 µg, or higher concentrations of 400 µg inoculated into the TA muscles were not as effective in reducing virus titers and cardiac inflammatory foci as the optimal 200 µg per mouse dosage using the CMV model.
7. Combinations of select individual IFN subtypes show synergy. 100 µg of each DNA construct (optimal dose; 200 µg DNA per mouse) is injected via TA

muscles for optimal efficacy. Specifically, in the spleen, 200 µg of *IFNA6/A9* reduced virus titers 3-fold and *IFNA6/B* reduced virus titers 50-fold. Similarly, in the liver, 200 µg of *IFNA6/B* reduced virus titers 3.2-fold and *IFNA9/B* reduced virus titers 2.7-fold. *IFN* combinations had no detectable antiviral effects in the salivary glands in our CMV model.

For IFN adjuvant therapy with viral vaccines, a combination of *IFNA6* and *IFNB* with *gB* DNA vaccine was more efficacious than the *gB* vaccine alone in protecting mice from a subsequent live infectious virus challenge; reducing viral titers and myocarditis. Mice received the combination *gB/IFNA6/IFNB* as 100 µg, 50 µg, and 50 µg of DNA constructs, respectively. Mice that had been given the viral vaccine (MCMV *gB* DNA) and coimmunized with either IFN subtype *IFNA9*, or *IFNB* showed reduced acute myocarditis. However, *IFNA6, IFNA9*, and *IFNB* individual subtypes all reduced chronic myocarditis in mice coimmunized with *gB* DNA vaccine.

8. The timing of DNA inoculation also contributes to therapeutic efficacy of the IFN. Optimal efficacy is achieved when mice are treated with *IFN* DNA 14 d before viral challenge. Treatment with *IFNA6* and *IFNB* 2 d before and 2 d after viral infection proved ineffective during the acute phase of viral infection and disease. However, *IFN* DNA treatment 2 d before viral infection reduced the chronic autoimmune phase of myocarditis. Postviral *IFNA6* treatment at 14 d p.i. also significantly reduced chronic myocarditis observed at day 56 p.i.

9. Encephalomyocarditis virus originally was obtained from ATCC (Rockville, MD) and was prepared as a tissue-culture passaged virus stock using L929 fibroblast monolayers. Briefly, the L929 cells were overlayed with encephalomyocarditis virus in DMEM and incubated until 90% CPE was observed, the supernatant was then clarified by centrifugation and aliquots stored at –80°C.

10. Spleen, liver, and salivary glands are taken at d 3, 7, 10, and 56 after infection for kinetic analysis of virus dissemination and MCMV titer in target organs.

11. At least two heart sections are scored for each animal. Foci consisting of at least five mononuclear lymphocytes are counted. Hearts from control groups of uninfected mice inoculated with the blank expression vector do not show inflammation (**Fig. 2A**). Hearts taken from mice at d 7 after infection typically characterize acute phase myocarditis (usually 15–20 foci/heart section; **Fig. 2B**) and hearts taken at d 30 or 56 after infection (10–15 foci/heart section) typically characterize the chronic autoimmune phase of myocarditis after infection with 10^4 pfu MCMV by the intraperitoneal route.

References

1. Woodruff, J. F. (1980) Viral myocarditis, a review. *Am J. Pathol.* **101**, 427–479.
2. Endresz, V., Burian, K., Berencsi, K., Gyulai, Z., Kari, L., Horton, H., et al. (2001) Optimizsation of DNA immunization against human cytomegalovirus. *Vaccine* **19**, 3972–3980.
3. Danko I. and Wolff J. A. (1994) Direct gene transfer into muscle. *Vaccine* **12**, 1499–1502.
4. Rhodes, G. H., Dwarki, V. J., Abai, A. M., Felgner, J., Felgner, P. L., Gromkowski, S. H., et al. (1993) Injection of expression vectors containing viral

genes induces cellular, humoral, and protective immunity, in *Vaccines 93* (Channock, R. M., Brown, F., Ginsberg, H. S., Norby, E., eds.), Cold Spring Harbor Laboratory Press, Cold Spring Harbor, NY, pp. 137.

5. Biron, C. A. (1998) Role of early cytokines, including alpha and beta interferons (IFN-α/β), in innate and adaptive immune responses to viral infections. *Semin. Immunol.* **10**, 383–390.
6. Foster, G. and Finter, N. B. (1998) Are all type I human interferons equivalent? *J. Viral Hepatitis* **5**, 143–152.
7. Bartlett, E. J., Cull, V. S., Mowe, E. N., Mansfield, J. P. and James, C. M. (2003) Optimisation of naked DNA delivery for interferon subtype immunotherapy in cytomegalovirus infection. *Biol. Proced. Online* **5**, 43–52.
8. Bartlett, E. J., Cull, V. S., Brekalo, N. L., Lenzo, J. C., and James, C. M. (2002) Synergy of type I interferon-A6 and interferon-B naked DNA immunotherapy for cytomegalovirus infections. *Immunol. Cell Biol.* **80**, 425–435.
9. Cull, V. S., Broomfield, S., Bartlett, E. J., Brekalo, N. L., and James, C. M. (2002) Coimmunisation with type I IFN genes enhances protective immunity against cytomegalovirus and myocarditis in gB DNA-vaccinated mice. *Gene Ther.* **9**, 1369–1378.
10. Yeow, W. S., Lawson, C. M., and Beilharz, M. W. (1998) Antiviral activities of interferon-α subtypes *in vivo*. *J. Immunol.* **160**, 2932–2939.
11. Carr, D. J. J., Al-Khatib, K., James, C. M., and Silverman, R. (2003) Interferon beta suppresses herpes simplex virus type I replication in trigeminal ganglion cells through a RNase L-dependent pathway. *J. Neuroimmunol.* **141**, 40–46.
12. Harle, P., Cull, V., Agbaga, M.-P., Silverman, R., Williams, B. R., James, C., et al. (2002) Differential effect of murine type I IFN transgenes in antagonizing HSV-1 replication. *J. Virol.* **76**, 6558–6567.
13. Harle, P., Cull, V., Guo, L., Papin, J., Lawson, C., and Carr, D. (2002) Transient transfection of mouse fibroblasts with type I interferon transgenes provides various degrees of protection against herpes simplex virus infection. *Antiviral Res.* **56**, 39–49.
14. Cull, V. S., Tilbrook, P. T., Bartlett, E. J., Brekalo, N. L., and James, C. M. (2003) Type I interferon differential therapy for erythroleukemia: specificity of STAT activation. *Blood* **101**, 2727–2735.
15. Bartlett, E. J., Lenzo, J. C., Sivamoorthy, S., Mansfield, J. P., Cull, V. S., and James, C. M. (2004) Type I IFN-β gene therapy suppresses cardiac CD8$^+$ T-cell infiltration during autoimmune myocarditis. *Immunol. Cell Biol.* **82**, 119–126.
16. Cull, V. S., Bartlett, E. J., and James, C. M. (2002) Type I interferon gene therapy protects against cytomegalovirus-induced myocarditis. *Immunol.* **106**, 428–437.
17. Lenzo, J. C., Mansfield, J. P., Sivamoorthy, S., Cull, V. S., and James, C. M. (2003) Cytokine expression in murine cytomegalovirus-induced myocarditis: modulation with interferon-α therapy. *Cell. Immunol.* **223**, 77–86.
18. Hilkens, C. M., Schlaak, J. F., and Kerr, I. M. (2002) Molecular analysis of responses to interferon-alpha subtypes in human T cells and dendritic cells. *J. Interferon Cytokine Res.* **22**, S56.

19. Vitadello, M., Schiaffino, M. V., Picard, A., Scarpa, M., and Schiaffino, S. (1994) Gene transfer in regenerating muscle. *Human Gene Ther.* **5,** 11–18.
20. Danko, I. and Wolff, J. A. (1994) Direct gene transfer into muscle. *Vaccine* **12,** 1499–1502.
21. Lenzo, J. C., Fairweather, D., Cull, V., Shellam, G. R., and Lawson, C. M. (2002) Characterisation of murine cytomegalovirus myocarditis: cellular infiltration of the heart and virus persistence. *J Mol. Cell. Cardiol.* **34,** 629–640.
22. Prud'homme, G. J., Lawson, B. R., Chang, Y., and Theofilopoulos, A. N. (2001) Immunotherapeutic gene transfer into muscle. *Trends Immunol.* **22,** 149–155.

15

Transfection of Müller Cells With Type I Interferon Transgenes

Resistance to HSV-1 Infection

Benitta John-Philip and Daniel J. J. Carr

Summary

Gene transfer is a widely used experimental approach to determine the value of specific genes under a variety of conditions. This chapter focuses on the expression of two human antiviral genes, interferon (IFN)-α2 and IFN-β, driven by a cytomegalovirus immediate-early promoter in a human Müller cell line. The anti-viral efficacy of these two transgenes is determined by measuring resistant to herpes simplex virus type 1 infection assessing viral antigen expression and viral titers recovered from control and IFN transgene-transfected cells. Furthermore, comparing the antiviral efficacy of these two transgenes suggest the anti-viral environment elicited by the human IFN-α2 transgene is superior to that of the human IFN-β, which may be related to the amount of biologically active IFN secreted by these cells.

Key Words: Interferon; gene therapy; herpes simplex virus type 1; Müller cell; Western blot; transfection.

1. Introduction

Herpes simplex virus type 1 (HSV-1) is a highly successful deoxyribonucleic acid (DNA) virus that elicits an impressive immune response during acute infection in mice involving natural killer (NK) cells *(1)*, neutrophils *(2)*, and T lymphocytes *(3,4)*. After corneal infection, the virus spreads to the sensory ganglia (i.e., trigeminal ganglia) via retrograde transport, infecting Schwann cells *(5)* and establishing a latent infection in neurons *(6)*. The virus has been reported to infect the contralateral retina after anterior chamber inoculation via two temporally separated waves *(7)*. The ipsilateral retina is apparently spared from HSV-1 infection by NK cells and T lymphocytes *(8,9)*. In addition to retinal infection via the anterior chamber route of inoculation, it has also been reported that HSV-1 can infect the retina following the introduction of virus onto scarified cornea *(10,11)*.

HSV-1 infection of the retina can lead to acute retinal necrosis syndrome, a rare-but-serious disease associated with frank retinal inflammation that can lead to blindness in the afflicted eye(s) *(12–14)*. Although astrocytes and microglia are found within the retina, Müller cells are the predominant cell type, comprising 90% of the glial element with processes interdigitating the perikarya, axons, and dendrites of neurons within the retina *(15)*. Targeting these cells as factories for interferon (IFN) production may reduce the local inflammatory response by enhancing resistance to viral replication and spread. As a means to enhance local IFN production, the introduction of an expression platform that provides continuous production of type I IFN to the surrounding milieu via the Müller cells could serve such a purpose. In addition, the multiple species of type I IFNs with various anti-viral efficacies require the identification of the appropriate type most appropriate to counter HSV-1. The present study focused on the sensitivity of a Müller cell line to HSV-1 before or after transfection with type I IFN transgenes. This evaluation includes viral replication measuring viral protein expression and viral titer as well as type I IFN production in control and type I IFN transgene-transfected cells.

2. Materials

2.1. Plasmid Isolation

1. The human IFN-α2 (797-bp fragment) and IFN-β (607-bp fragment) genes were generously provided by Dr. Paula Pitha-Rowe (John Hopkins University, Baltimore, MD). The human IFN-α2 gene was cloned into the *PstI* and *XhoI* sites and the IFN-β gene was cloned into the *KpnI* and *XhoI* sites of the FDA approved pVAX vector (*[16]*, see **Note 1**).
2. Plasmid Maxiprep Kit: Bio-Rad, cat. no. 732-6130 (*see* **Note 2**).
3. Terrific Broth; Solution A: 1.3% w/v Bacto Tryptone (BDH), 2.7% w/v yeast extract, 0.4% v/v glycerol; Solution B: 719 mM K_2HPO_4 and 169 mM KH_2PO_4. Autoclave Solution A and Solution B separately. Combine the two solutions at a ratio of 9:1, respectively. Add the antibiotic ampicillin at 50 µg/mL.

2.2. Transfection of Cells

1. Human MIO-M1 (Moorfields-Institute of Opthalmology-Müller 1).
2. Fetal bovine serum (FBS).
3. Antibiotic/antimycotic (AB/AM) solution.
4. Gentamicin Reagent Solution.
5. Dulbecco's Modified Essential Medium (DMEM): Add 50 mL of FBS, 10 mL of AB/AM, and 1 mL of gentamicin in 450 mL of DMEM to prepare the DMEM complete medium. Prepare the serum-free DMEM by adding only AB/AM and gentamicin.
6. SuperFect Transfection Reagent, Qiagen, cat. no. 301305.

7. 1X phosphate-buffered saline (PBS) to make 8 L; 64 g of NaCl, 1.6 g of KCl, 11.5 g of Na_2HPO_4, 1.92 g of KH_2PO_4, add 6 L of dH_2O, pH to 7.4, and v/v volume up to 8 L.

2.3. Western Blot Analysis

1. Cell lysis buffer: 1% Triton X-100, 2 mM ethylene diamine tetraacetic acid, 1% protease inhibitor cocktail (Calbiochem cat. no. 539131), 1 mM Na_3VO_4 in 1X PBS, pH 7.4.
2. Protein Assay Kit: BCA Protein Assay Kit.
3. 3X sample buffer; 3.8 mL diH_2O, 1.0 mL of 0.5 M Tris-HCl, pH 6.8, 0.8 mL of glycerol, 1.6 mL of 10% sodium dodecyl sulfate (SDS), 0.4 mL of 2-mercaptoethanol, and 0.4 mL of 1% bromophenol blue.
4. 10X running buffer: 30.2 g of Tris-base, 144 g of glycine, 10 g of SDS; add up to 1000 mL of diH_2O.
5. Pre-cast polyacrylamide gels (7.5%) along with gel chamber and power supply.
6. Prestained molecular weight markers.
7. 10X Transfer Buffer: 30.0 g of Tris base, 144.0 g of glycine, 1.0 g of SDS; add up to 1000 mL of diH_2O.
8. Polyvinylidene difluoride (PVDF) membrane.
9. Blotting paper.
10. Semi-dry transfer cell.
11. 5X TTBS: 120 g of NaCl; 0.5% Tween-20, 100 mL of 1 M Tris-HCl, pH 7.4, add up to 1000 mL diH_2O.
12. Blocking Solution: 5% dry milk in 1X TTBS.
13. Hyper Cassette: Amersham, cat. no. RPN 12642, 18 × 24 cm.
14. Exposure Cassette: Sigma, cat. no. E-8635.

2.4. Plaque Assay

1. Add 50 mL of FBS, 10 mL of AB/AM and 1 mL of gentamicin into 500 mL of Rosewell Park Memorial Institute (RPMI) medium 1640 to prepare RPMI complete medium.
2. Methyl cellulose overlay: Autoclave 5% w/v methyl cellulose in PBS, pH 7.4, containing a sterile magnetic bar. After autoclaving, place the methylcellulose solution on a stirring platform and stir overnight (12 h). After overnight stir, add 400 mL of RPMI complete medium.
3. Vero Cells (maintained in RPMI complete medium; see **Note 3**).
4. 96-well sterile, flat-bottomed microtiter plates.
5. Inverted microscope.
6. Laminar flow hood.
7. Latex gloves.
8. Pipettmen (multichannel and p200) with autoclaved tips.
9. Sterile trough.
10. Pipet-aid and sterile plastic pipet (with cotton plugs).

3. Methods
3.1. Plasmid Isolation (see Note 4)

1. Dissolve 36 g of part A in 980mL diH$_2$O, autoclave, and let it cool before inoculating. Add 20 mL of part B and 1mL of 50mg ampicillin stock (maintained in –20°C freezer) to the broth under hood.
2. Inoculate 500 to 1000 mL terrific broth prepared the day before in **step 1** with a loopful of bacteria. Incubate overnight (approx 16–18 h) at 37°C with shaking.
3. The cells are harvested by centrifugation at 5000g for 5 min. The supernatant is discarded.
4. Resuspend the cells in 30 mL of the cell resuspension solution provided by manufacturer (Bio-Rad).
5. Vortex or pipet the cells to completely resuspend (*see* **Note 5**).
6. Add 46 mL of lysis buffer provided by the manufacturer (Bio-Rad).
7. After adding cell lysis solution, shake the bottle very well to ensure the lysis of cells. The solution will become viscous.
8. Upon adding the neutralization solution provided by the manufacturer (Bio-Rad) within 5 min upon adding the lysis buffer.
9. Next, swirl the bottle (0.5–2.0 min) to mix the solution which will become cloudy and develop a flocculent creamy precipitate.
10. Centrifuge for 30 min at 10,000g. Filter the supernatant through 3M paper.
11. Resuspend the quantum prep matrix provided by the manufacturer (Bio-Rad) vigorously shaking the bottle. Add 10 mL of matrix mix to the cleared, filtered lysate and swirl gently for 15 s.
12. Centrifuge for 5 min at 3000g to pellet DNA with matrix andthen pour off the supernatant.
13. Resuspend the matrix with 25 mL of wash buffer supplied by the manufacturer and centrifuge (3000g, 5 min).
14. Pour off the supernatant and resuspend matrix in 15 mL of wash buffer. Immediately transfer into the spin basket provided by manufacturer fitted into a 50-mL conical centrifuge tube.
15. Wash the pelleted matrix 2X with 15mL and then 10mL of wash buffer (3000g, 5 min) provided by the manufacturer (Bio-Rad).
16. Remove the spin basket from the original wash tube and place on a fresh 50-mL tube (*see* **Note 6**).
17. Elute DNA using 5-mL sterile diH$_2$O (*see* **Note 7**).
18. Precipitate the DNA by adding 278 µL of 5 M NaCl (provided by manufacturer) and 2 volumes of 95 to 100% ethanol (molecular biology grade) (*see* **Note 8**).
19. The DNA is pelleted by centrifugation at 4000g for 20 min.
20. The pellet is resuspended in 1 mL of 70% ethanol and transferred into a 1.5-mL microcentrifuge tube. The DNA is centrifuged for 1 min at 10,000g, the supernatant is discarded, and the pellet is washed again with 1 mL of 70% ethanol 3-5X.
21. After the final wash, the supernatant is removed and the pellet is air-dried (typically in a speed vacuum without heat for 5–10 min).

22. The pellet is then resuspended in TE buffer, pH 8.3 (typically 200–300 µL) and allowed to stand overnight at 4° C.
23. The DNA is then quantified using a spectrophotometer (*see* **Note 9**).

3.2. Transfection of Cells

1. Plate MIO-M1 cells the day before (approx 4–6 PM) at 100,000 cell/well in a six-well microtiter plate.
2. The next morning (approx 8–9 AM) pre-warm approx 15 mL of DMEM complete medium and approx 15 mL of 1X PBS at 37°C in an atmosphere of 5% CO_2.
3. Transfections are conducted in triplicates: 300 µL of serum-free DMEM, 15 pg of DNA pVAX alone, pVAX –IFN-α2, or pVAX-IFN-β (5 pg/well) and 30 µL superfect (SF).
4. Mix by finger flicking and incubate for 10 min at 37°C.
5. Next, take the MIO-M1 cells from the incubator (plated the day before) and remove the RPMI complete medium using a 10-mL automatic pipet.
6. Add 600 µL of prewarmed DMEM complete medium into wells containing the MIO-M1 cells
7. Pipette SF 2X up and down with a p1000 pipetman, and add 100 µL of the mix onto cells while gently shaking the 6-well microtiter plate.
8. Incubate the plate in an incubator for 3 h at 37°C, 5% CO_2 atmosphere.
9. Following the incubation, gently remove the supernatant, wash the cells once with pre-warmed (37°C) 1X PBS without disturbing the cells and incubate in pre-warmed (37°C) DMEM complete medium for 24 h in a 5% CO_2 atmosphere at 37°C.
10. The following day, the supernatant can be collected and assessed for IFN content by ELISA (**Fig. 1**) or bioassay (*see* **Note 10**).

3.3. HSV-1 Infection of Transfected Cells

1. Infect transfected MOI-M1 cells with HSV-1 (McKrae strain, multiplicity of infection, 0.5) in 1.0 mL RPMI complete medium (*see* **Note 11**). Incubate cells for 1 h at 37°C in 5% CO_2.
2. After a 1-h incubation period, remove the supernatant and replace with 2.0 mL of RPMI complete medium. Cells are then incubated for 24 h at 37°C in 5% CO_2.
3. The cells are then freeze-thawed (in –80°C freezer) twice. The supernatant is collected, clarified by centrifugation (10,000*g*, 1 min), and assayed for viral content using Vero cell monolayers in 96-well microtiter plates. (*see* **Note 12**).
4. Following a 32 to 36 h period to allow plaques to develop on the monolayer, the plates are read. The titer is derived from the inverse dilution for each sample multiplied by the total volume in the 6-well plate (**Fig. 2**).

3.4. Western Blot Analysis

1. Twenty-four hour post-transfection (**Subheading 3.1.**), the MIO-M1 cells are infected with HSV-1 (multiplicity of infection, 0.5) in 1mL of complete medium.

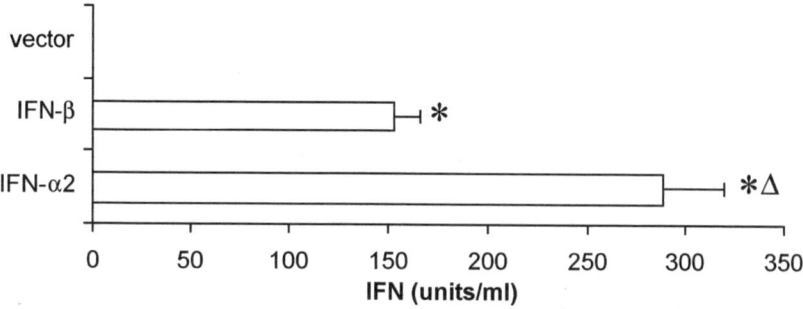

Fig. 1. Transfection of MI0-M1 cells with type IIFN transgenes leads to production of type IIFN. MI0-M1 cells (1×10^5 cells) were transfected with 5 µg of plasmid DNA (vector) alone or vector containing the IFN-α2 or IFN-β transgene. Twenty-four hours after transfection, the supernatant was collected and assayed for IFN-α or IFN-β content by ELISA. Cells transfected with the IFN-α2 transgene did not produce measurable IFN-β and cells transfected with the IFN-β did not produce measurable levels of IFN-α2. The figure is a summary of three experiments conducted in quadruplicate/experiment. $*p < 0.01$ comparing the type IIFN transgene-transfected cells to vector-transfected controls (no measurable type I IFN) $^\Delta p < 0.05$ comparing the IFN-α2 to IFN-β transgene-transfected cells as determined by ANOVA and Tukey's *post hoc* *t*-test.

2. Twenty-four hours after infection, the supernatant is removed and the cells are washed with 1X PBS.
3. Place the six-well microtiter plate containing cells on ice and add 250 µL of lysis buffer. Rock this plate on a rocker for 15 min (samples should be on ice at all times).
4. Using cell scrapers, gently scrape remaining adherent cells from the bottom of the plate and transfer the cells into a 1.5-mL centrifuge tube.
5. Centrifuge the sample at 12,000*g* for 10 min at 4°C to pellet the cellular debris.
6. Transfer supernatant to a sterile 0.5-mL centrifuge tube and proceed to perform protein assay on the samples (using a BCA protein determination kit).
7. Take 25 µg of protein and mix with 3X sample buffer (*see* **Note 13**).
8. Vortex the mixture gently and boil for 5 min (*see* **Note 14**).
9. Vortex again gently and pulse centrifuge (10,000*g*, 10 s).
10. While the sample is boiling, prepare 5X running buffer. Remove pre-cast 7.5% polyacrylamide gel from the refrigerator and insert it into the gel camber. Place the gel chamber in a bucket of ice. Fill the upper and lower gel chamber with 5X running buffer. Try to produce as little bubble as possible.
11. Load 15 µL of prestained marker in to the first and last well. Then load the samples, close the gel chamber and run the gel at 140 volts for 90 to 100 min (*see* **Note 15**).

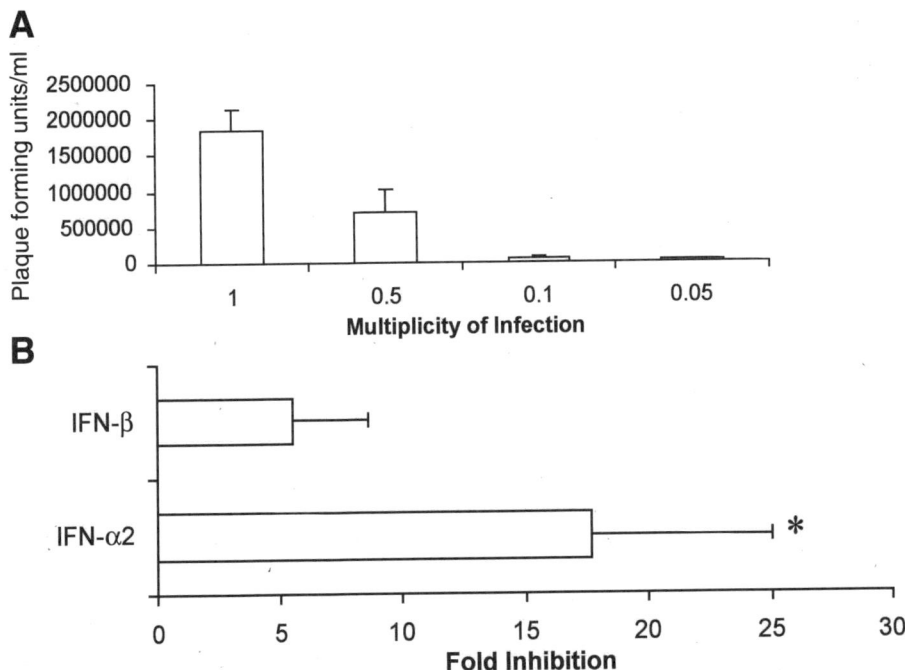

Fig. 2. **(A)** MI0-M1 Müller cells are sensitive to HSV-1 infection. MI0-M1 cells (1×10^5 cells) were infected with increasing amounts of HSV-1. Twenty-four hours after infection, the cells underwent a freeze–thaw cycle and the supernatant was collected, clarified (10,000g, 1 min), and assayed for infectious HSV-1 using Vero cells in a plaque assay. The results are a summary of three experiments each conducted in duplicate. Bars represent mean ± standard error of the mean. **(B)** Type, I. IFN transgene-transfected cells are resistant to HSV-1 infection. MI0-M1 cells (1×10^5) transfected with vector alone or vector containing the indicated type, I. IFN transgene were infected with, HSV-1 (multiplicity of infection = 0.5) 24 h after transfection. Twenty-four hours after infection, the cells underwent a freeze-thaw cycle and the clarified supernatant (10,000g, 1 min) was assayed for viral titer. The results are expressed as fold-inhibition of virus yield comparing the type IIFN transgene- to vector control-transfected, MI0-M1 cells. This figure is a summary of four experiments with each experiment conducted in duplicate. The bars represent mean ± standard deviation. *$p < 0.05$ comparing the IFN-α2 to IFN-β transgene-transfected groups as determined by ANOVA and Tukey's *post hoc* t-test.

12. Approximately 15 min before the end of the electrophoresis process is completed, prepare 20% MeOH in 10X transfer buffer (*see* **Note 16**).
13. Prepare the PVDF membrane. Place the membrane in a rectangular container and soak the membrane in 100% MeOH for 1 min while rocking. Dump MeOH, add

20% MeOH in 10X transfer buffer (enough to cover the membrane), and rock for at least 5 min. While rocking, flip the membrane upside down to be sure both surfaces are soaked well.
14. Next, prepare two blotting papers (e.g., 3M blotting paper) for each gel. Soak the blotting papers with 20% MeOH in 10X transfer buffer for 2 min. Be sure to eliminate air bubbles.
15. Upon resolution of the samples in the polyacrylamide gels, carefully remove the gel and break the plastic cast using forceps. The gel will be adhered to one side of the cast. Place one pre-soaked blotting paper on top of the gel gently. Place the blotting paper with gel (gel side up) onto a clean rectangular trough and add 20% MeOH in 10X transfer buffer enough to cover the gel and the paper. Rock this for 5 min (*see* **Note 17**).
16. Now place the PVDF membrane on top of the other presoaked blotting paper. Then make a sandwich using both the blotting papers, so that the gel and the PVDF membrane will be in the middle.
17. Place the sandwich in the center of the Semi-Dry Transfer Cell, close the apparatus and run for 32 min at 15 volts.
18. Once finished, take the sandwich apart and place the PVDF membrane in blocking solution and block for 2 hrs at room temp or overnight at 4°C (*see* **Note 18**).
19. Prepare 1X TTBS buffer. After adequate incubation in blocking solution, remove solution and transfer the blot to a clean trough and wash 2X using 1X PBS for 5 min.
20. Prepare primary antibody solution. Dilute rabbit anti-HSV-1 polyclonal antibody (1:1000) in 1X TTBS. You need about 20 mL of solution to cover the blot. After transferring the blot into a clean trough, add this solution on top of the blot and incubate by rocking for 2 h at room temp (25°C).
21. Transfer the blot to a clean trough and wash 3X with 1X TTBS for 5 min each.
22. During the last wash prepare secondary antibody solution. We used a polyclonal goat–anti-rabbit IgG conjugated to horseradish peroxidase (1:2000 dilution in 1X TTBS). You need 20 mL of solution to cover the blot. Incubate by rocking the blot in this solution for 1.5 h at room temp
23. Transfer the blot to a clean trough and wash 6X in 1X TTBS at 10 min each.
24. Prepare the chemiluminescence solution (requires 4 mL for 1 PVDF membrane) as per manufacturer's instructions. Take the blot from the wash buffer using forceps and place on top of plastic wrap and place the chemiluminescence on top of the blot (distribute evenly) and leave for 1 min.
25. Gently discard the chemiluminescence solution by blotting with clean paper towels. Cover blot with the end of the plastic wrap so that the blot will be sandwiched between the plastic wrap (make sure that no air bubbles get trapped in it). Cut the unwanted edges of the plastic wrap using scissors. Place this into the hypercassette and tape the sides (care should be taken to remove all creases from the plastic wrap).
26. Now take the cassette and film to the dark room and expose film to membrane for various times (e.g., 15 s, 30 s, 1 min, and 5 min (*see* **Note 19**).
27. Develop film (**Fig. 3**).

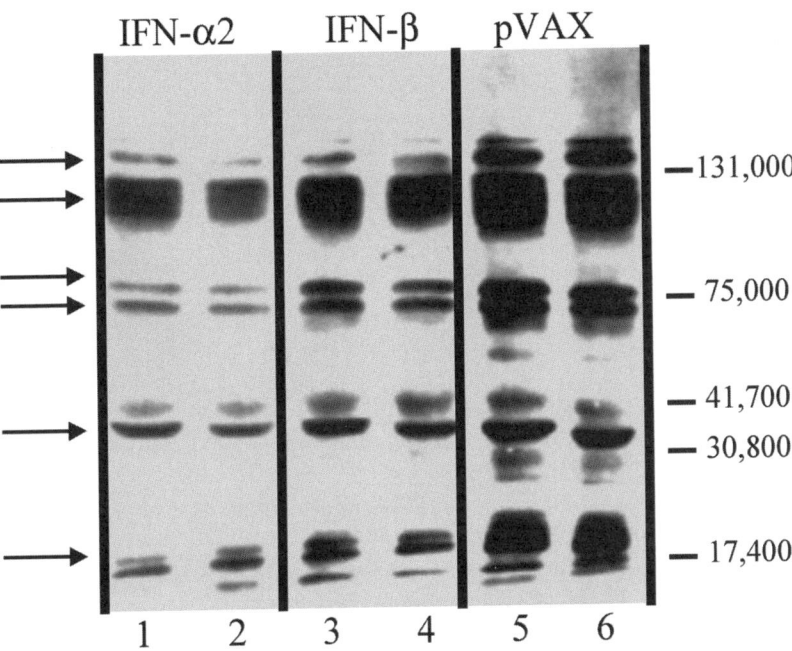

Fig. 3. Type I IFN transgenes antagonize HS-1 protein synthesis in transfected MIO-M1 cells. Total cell lysates (25 µg/lane) from transfected MIO-M1 cells (in duplicate previously infected with HSV-1 (multiplicity of infection = 0.5, 24 h earlier) were resolved on polyacrylamide gels, transferred onto PVDF membranes, and used for Western blot analysis with a polyclonal anti-HSV antibody. This figure is a representative of four experiments with identical outcomes. Molecular weight standards are shown to the right of the gel in daltons. Note the reduction in expression of HSV proteins indicated by the arrows. Such proteins were not detected in cell lysates from uninfected samples (data not shown). MIO-M1 cells were transfected with empty plasmid vector (pVAX) or plasmid vector containing the human IFN-α2 transgene (IFN-α2) or the human IFN-β transgene (IFN-β).

4. Notes

1. The vector contains a CMV immediate-early promoter, a bovine growth hormone polyadenylation signal, and a kanamycin- and ampicillin-resistance gene for selection when growing in *Escherichia coli*. The antibiotic resistance genes allow for a more diverse selection process if necessary. We noticed that although the CMV promoter offers a strong initiation signal, it is relatively short-lived and may be worth considering another promoter.
2. Plasmid isolation was conducted using manufacturer's instructions with minor changes mentioned in the methods section.

3. We chose to use Vero cells over another commonly used cell line, CV-1, because of Vero cells heightened sensitivity and plaque formation compared with CV-1 cells. It should be noted that Vero cells are discarded after 6 mo of continuous passage as the cells lose their sensitivity to HSV-1 infection.
4. We have attempted a number of different vendor's plasmid purification reagents and kits. We have found the Bio-Rad maxiprep kit for plasmid purification to be superior to any other maxiprep kit commercially available as measured by the consistency in the quantity and purity of product.
5. We recommend pipetting with a 10 mL disposable pipet. Vortexing a large quantity of cells is difficult and time-consuming.
6. We recommend polypropylene 50-mL tubes as this increases the DNA yield dramatically.
7. Although the manufacturer suggests either TE buffer or sterile water, we have found water to facilitate DNA precipitation better than TE buffer following the addition of 5 M NaCl and ethanol.
8. We have found that allowing the DNA to precipitate overnight (12 h) greatly increases the yield of DNA.
9. We typically recover between 0.5 and 3.0 mg of highly enriched plasmid DNA from a 500-mL Terrific Broth confluent culture.
10. The amount of IFN detected by enzyme-linked immunosorbent assay (PBL Biomedical Laboratories, Brunswick, NJ) has previously been found to coincide close to the amount predicted by bioassay using Hep-2 cells and EMCV *(16)*.
11. HSV-1 (McKrae strain) is propagated in Vero cells and aliquots are stored at –80°C at a concentration of 1.0 to 5.0×10^8 plaque-forming units/mL.
12. The supernatant is diluted in 1:5 increments in RPMI complete medium in the columns starting with no dilution and ending with 1:78,125. Depending on the cell type, transfections with the plasmid vector alone can lead to some resistance compared to nontransfected cells.
13. The maximum volume that can be added into the well of the gel employed is 45 μL. Therefore, if you have want to load 45 μL of sample, you should have 15 μL of 3X sample buffer and 30 μL of sample (containing 25 μg total protein). A maximum of 50 μg of protein can be added to wells. Increasing the protein concentration above this amount typically results in overloaded gels increasing the background and non-specific labeling of protein when probing with antibody.
14. We have found a heating block is superior to other forms of control (e.g., boiling water) owing to the lack of potential contamination (from lid popping open) and ease of use.
15. It is recommended that prestained molecular weight markers be used in the electrophoresis of samples because they serve a better guide when deciding the end of the "run." Typically, we stop our electrophoresis when the lowest weight prestained molecular weight standard is within 1 cm from the front of the gel.
16. One gel (enough to resolve 14 total samples) requires 200 mL of the transfer buffer. For 200 mL, you need 40 mL of MeOH, 20 mL of 10X transfer buffer, and 140 mL of dH_2O.

17. Transferring the gel from the cast to the blotting paper requires patience. It is relatively easy to tear the 1-mm thick gel so great care should be taken upon transferring the gel.
18. Dry milk is the most appropriate medium to block nonspecific sites on the PVDF membrane. Bovine serum albumin is not a good medium because we have found it to crossreact with HSV-1 antigen. Overnight incubation does not reduce the antigenicity of the resolved viral proteins and typically, reduces the background signal upon probing.
19. The film is exposed for different times to establish the highest quality result possible. Each antibody requires optimization.

References

1. Adler, H., Beland, J. L., Del-Pan, N. C., Kobzik, L., Sobel, R. A., and Rimm, I. J. (1999) In the absence of T cells, natural killer cells protect from mortality due to, H. S.V-1 encephalitis. *J. Neuroimmunol.* **93,** 208–213.
2. Tumpey, T. M., Chen, S., Oakes, J. E., and Lausch, R. N. (1996) Neutrophil-mediated suppression of virus replication after herpes simplex virus type 1 infection of the murine cornea. *J. Virol.* **70,** 898–904.
3. Niemialtowski, M. G. and Rouse, B. T. (1992) Predominance of, T.h1 cells in ocular tissues during herpetic stromal keratitis. *J. Immunol.* **149,** 3035–3039.
4. Liu, T., Tang, Q., and Hendricks, R. L. (1996) Inflammation infiltration of the trigeminal ganglion after herpes simplex virus type 1 corneal infection. *J. Virol.* **70,** 264–271.
5. Shimeld, C., Efstathiou, S., and Hill, T. (2001) Tracking the spread of a *lacZ*-tagged herpes simplex virus type 1 between the eye and the nervous system of the mouse: Comparison of primary and recurrent infection. *J. Virol.* **75,** 5252–5262.
6. Enquist, L. W., Husak, P. J., Banfield, B. W., and Smith, G. A. (1998) Infection and spread of alphaherpesviruses in the nervous system. *Adv. Virus Res.* **51,** 237–347.
7. Atherton, S. S. and Streilein, W. J. (1987) Two waves of virus following anterior chamber inoculation of, H. S.V-1. *Invest. Ophthalmol. Vis. Sci.* **28,** 571–579.
8. Azumi, A. and Atherton, S. S. (1994) Sparing of the ipsilateral retina after anterior chamber inoculation of, H. S.V-1: Requirement for either $CD4^+$ or $CD8^+$ T cells. *Invest. Ophthalmol. Vis. Sci.* **35,** 3251–3259.
9. Tanigawa, M., Bigger, J. E., Kanter, M. Y., and Atherton, S. S. (2000) Natural killer cells prevent direct anterior-to-posterior spread of herpes simplex virus type 1 in the eye. *Invest. Ophthalmol. Vis. Sci.* **41,** 132–137.
10. Spencer, B., Agarwala, S., Miskulin, M., Smith, M., and Brandt, C. R. (2000) Herpes simplex virus-mediated gene delivery to the rodent system. *Invest. Ophthalmol. Vis. Sci.* **41,** 1392–1401.
11. Carr, D. J. J, Chodosh, J., Ash, J., and Lane, T. E. (2003) Effect of anti-CXCL10 monoclonal antibody on herpes simplex virus type 1 keratitis and retinal infection. *J. Virol.* **77,** 10037–10046.
12. Lewis, M. L., Culbertson, W. W., Post, J. D., Miller, D., Kokame, G. T., and Dix, R. D. (1989) Herpes simplex virus type 1. A cause of the acute retinal necrosis syndrome. *Ophthalmology* **96,** 875–878.

13. Ezra, E., Pearson, R. V., Etchells, D. E., and Gregor, Z. J. (1995) Delayed fellow involvement in acute retinal necrosis syndrome. *Am. J. Ophthalmol.* **120,** 115–116.
14. Falcon, P. M. and Brockhurst, R. J. (1993) Delayed onset of bilateral acute retinal necrosis syndrome; a 34-year interval. *Ann. Ophthalmol.* **25,** 373–374.
15. Sarthy, V. and Ripps, H. (2001) *The Retinal Müller Cell*,1st ed. New York, Plenum Publishers.
16. Härle, P., Lauret, E., Pitha, P. M., De, M.aeyer, E., and Carr, D. J. J. (2001) Expression of human and macaque type, I. IFN transgenes interferes with, H. S.V-1 replication at the transcriptional and translational levels: IFN-β is more potent than IFN-α2. *Virology* **290,** 237–248.

Index

A

Affinity chromatography, *see* Genomic DNA affinity chromatography
Angiogenesis, interferon inhibition, 13
Apoptosis,
  clinical significance, 11
  interferon effects,
    angiogenesis inhibition, 13
    cell cycle, 12
    gene induction, 12
    immunomodulation, 13
    mechanisms, 12

B

Basal cell carcinoma (BCC), interferon therapy, 14
BCC, *see* Basal cell carcinoma

C

Cancer, *see also* specific cancers,
  epidemiology, 151
  vaccines, *see* Tumor vaccines
Cassette mutagenesis, interferon-α, 76
Chronic myelogenous leukemia (CML), interferon therapy, 15, 16
CML, *see* Chronic myelogenous leukemia
CMV, *see* Cytomegalovirus
Cytomegalovirus (CMV),
  clinical features, 207
  interferon gene therapy,
    cytopathic effect assay for interferon, 212, 217
    DNA construct preparation, 210, 211, 216
    inoculation, 211, 216, 217
    interferon subtypes, 208
    materials, 209, 210, 213, 216
    murine myocarditis model, 208, 209
    myocarditis assessment, 213, 217
    virus challenge and plaque assay, 212, 213, 217

D

DC, *see* Dendritic cell
Dendritic cell (DC),
  characterization of monocyte-derived IFN-DCs,
    antigen response, 172, 173
    enzyme-linked immunospot assay, 173, 174, 178
    immune response generation in severe combined immunodeficient mice,
      CD8$^+$ T cell-response, 177, 178
      enzyme-linked immunosorbent assay for human immunoglobulins, 174, 176
      overview, 174
      Western blot of antibodies, 176
    migration assays, 178
    mixed lymphocyte reaction, 172
    proliferation assay, 173
  differentiation from monocytes assay,
    monocyte preparation and cytokine treatment, 170, 179
    overview, 169, 178, 179
    phenotypic characterization, 170, 171, 179, 180
  materials for assays, 168, 169, 178, 179
  overview of interferon regulation, 167, 168
  plasmacytoid dendritic cell,
    abundance, 184
    cytokine and chemokine production, 183, 184
    flow cytometry,
      fluorescence-activated cell sorting, 190, 191
      intracellular staining of interferon-α, 190
      materials, 187
      overview, 186, 187
      phenotyping, 189, 190
    isolation, 185, 186
    markers, 184, 185
DNA affinity chromatography, *see* Genomic DNA affinity chromatography
DNA microarray, functional genomics studies of viral response to interferons,
  animal models, 50
  compendium analysis, 49
  computing hardware, 42
  engineered virus studies, 47, 48
  Expression Array Manager, 38–40
  gene annotation resources, 42–44
  gene expression analysis software, 40, 41
  human clinical sample analysis, 50, 51
  interferon treatment of cells, 45, 46
  materials, 38
  overview, 37, 38
  Venn diagrams and bioset tools, 44
  viral gene expression profiling, 46
  virulence profiling, 47
DNA vaccine, *see* Gene therapy

E

EAM, *see* Expression Array Manager
ELISA, *see* Enzyme-linked immunosorbent assay
ELISPOT, *see* Enzyme-linked immunospot assay
Enzyme-linked immunosorbent assay (ELISA), human immunoglobulins in severe combined immunodeficient mice, 174, 176
Enzyme-linked immunospot assay (ELISPOT), monocyte-derived IFN–DC characterization, 173, 174, 178
Expression Array Manager (EAM), functional genomics studies of viral response to interferons, 38–40

233

F

Flow cytometry, plasmacytoid dendritic cells,
  fluorescence-activated cell sorting, 190, 191
  intracellular staining of interferon-α, 190
  materials, 187
  overview, 186, 187
  phenotyping, 189, 190
Fluorescence resonance energy transfer (FRET),
    RNase L activation assay,
  analog oligoadenylates, 108
  incubation conditions, 110, 111
  materials, 108, 109
  natural oligoadenylates, 107, 108, 111
  oligoadenylate preparation, 110
  overview, 104, 105
  probe preparation, 110
  RNase L expression and purification, 109–111
FRET, see Fluorescence resonance energy
    transfer

G

GDAC, see Genomic DNA affinity
    chromatography
Gene therapy,
  cytomegalovirus and interferon gene therapy,
    cytopathic effect assay for interferon, 212, 217
    DNA construct preparation, 210, 211, 216
    inoculation, 211, 216, 217
    interferon subtypes, 208
    materials, 209, 210, 213, 216
    murine myocarditis model, 208, 209
    myocarditis assessment, 213, 217
    virus challenge and plaque assay, 212,
      213, 217
  Müller cell transfection with type I interferon
      genes,
    infection of transfected cells, 225, 230
    materials, 222, 223, 229, 230
    plasmid isolation, 224, 225, 230
    rationale, 222
    transfection conditions, 225, 230
    Western blot analysis of viral protein
      inhibition, 225–229, 230, 231
Genomic DNA affinity chromatography (GDAC),
  chromatography and analysis, 62, 63, 65
  cytoplasmic protein extraction, 62, 64
  interferon treatment,
    adherent cells, 60, 64
    suspended cells, 60, 64
  interferon-inducible transcription factors,
      57, 58
  materials, 59, 60, 63, 64
  nuclear protein extraction, 61, 62, 64
  overview, 58

H

Hairy cell leukemia, interferon therapy, 15
HBV, see Hepatitis B virus
HCV, see Hepatitis C virus
Hepatitis B virus (HBV), interferon therapy, 10, 11
Hepatitis C virus (HCV), interferon therapy, 11
Herpes simplex virus-1 (HSV-1),
  ICP0 and interferon resistance assays and
      mechanisms,
    materials, 196, 197

Northern blot analysis of replication cycle,
      gel electrophoresis and blotting, 200,
        203, 204
      hybridization and detection, 200
      probe labeling, 200, 204
      RNA preparation, 199
    nuclear run-on assays of gene
      transcription regulation by ICP0,
      hybridization, 202–204
      nuclei regulation, 201, 202, 204
      slot blot preparation, 202, 204
    overview, 195, 196
    plaque reduction assay of mutant virus,
      198, 203
  Müller cell transfection with type I interferon
      genes,
    infection of transfected cells, 225, 230
    materials, 222, 223, 229, 230
    plasmid isolation, 224, 225, 230
    rationale, 222
    transfection conditions, 225, 230
    Western blot analysis of viral protein
      inhibition, 225–229, 230, 231
  retinal infection, 221, 222
Historical perspective, interferon research,
  clinical applications, 30, 31
  discovery, 25
  genes,
    identification and cloning, 26, 27
    regulation, 27–29
  purification and characterization, 26
  receptors, 29
  stimulated genes, 29, 30
HSV-1, see Herpes simplex virus-1
ICP0, see Herpes simplex virus-1

I

IFN-α, see Interferon-α
IFN-β, see Interferon-β
IFN-γ, see Interferon-γ
Imiquinoid, interferon-α induction, 14, 18
Interferon-α (IFN-α),
  dendritic cell modulation, see Dendritic cell
  engineering for structure-function studies,
    cassette mutagenesis, 76
    expression of recombinant proteins,
      cell induction and growth, 78
      chromatography, 78–80
      competent bacteria preparation and
        transformation, 77, 78
      vector preparation and insert ligation,
        77, 79
    hybrid HY-2 construction, 75, 76, 79
    materials, 70–74, 79
    overview, 69, 70
    site-directed mutagenesis, 76, 79
  gene identification and cloning, 26, 27
  gene therapy, see Gene therapy
  inducers, 3
  subtypes, 208
  therapy,
    indications, 3, 4, 14–16
    toxicity, 16, 17
  viral defense, see Viruses, interferon defense,

Index

Interferon-β (IFN-β),
  inducers, 3
  gene therapy, *see* Gene therapy,
  dendritic cell modulation, *see* Dendritic cell,
  therapy,
    indications, 3, 4, 14–16
    toxicity, 16, 17
  viral defense, *see* Viruses, interferon defense
  gene identification and cloning, 26, 27
Interferon-γ (IFN-γ),
  gene identification and cloning, 27
  inducers, 3
  therapy,
    indications, 3, 4, 14–16
    toxicity, 16, 17
  viral defense, *see* Viruses, interferon defense
Interferon-inducible transcription factors,
  chromatin immunoprecipitation, 58
  electrophoretic mobility shift assay, 58
  genomic DNA affinity chromatography,
    chromatography and analysis, 62, 63, 65
    cytoplasmic protein extraction, 62, 64
    interferon treatment,
      adherent cells, 60, 64
      suspended cells, 60, 64
    materials, 59, 60, 63, 64
    nuclear protein extraction, 61, 62, 64
    overview, 58
  history of study, 29, 30
  STATs, 57
Interferon receptors,
  signaling, *see also* Interferon-inducible transcription factors; Mitogen-activated protein kinase,
    overview, 29, 135
  types, 29
Interferon regulatory factors (IRFs),
  activation, 27, 28
  antiviral response, 28, 29, 115, 116
  interferon induction mechanisms, 27, 28
  RNase protection assay of mouse central nervous system expression,
    cytokine transgenic mouse studies, 127, 129, 130
    hybridization conditions, 125–127, 131, 132
    labeling of probe, 125, 131
    materials, 117, 118
    principles, 116, 117
    probe set construction,
      chloroform extraction, 121
      dilution and storage, 124, 130
      first-strand cDNA synthesis, 120
      gel purification of insert and vector, 122
      insert cloning into vector, 122, 123, 130
      ligation and digestion, 121, 122
      linearization of cloned constructs, 123
      polymerase chain reaction, 119–121, 130
      sense target RNA preparation, 124, 125, 130, 131
    probe set design, 118, 119
    virus challenge studies, 127
  types, 27
IRFs, *see* Interferon regulatory factors

K

Kaposi's sarcoma, interferon therapy, 15

M

MAPK, *see* Mitogen-activated protein kinase
Melanoma, interferon therapy, 14, 15
Methylcellulose colony-forming assay, p38 MAPK effects on hematopoiesis, 139, 146, 147
Mixed lymphocyte reaction, monocyte-derived IFN-DCs, 172
Mitogen-activated protein kinase (MAPK),
  activation in type I interferon signaling, 136
  MAPKAP kinase-2/3 assays, 137, 138, 141, 142, 148
  methylcellulose colony-forming assays of p38 MAPK effects on hematopoiesis, 139, 146, 147
  p38 MAPK activity assay,
    immunoprecipitation, 140, 141, 148
    materials, 137, 140
    protein G-Sepharose preparation, 140, 148
  Rac1 activation assay,
    materials, 138
    glutathione-Sepharose preparation, 142, 143, 148
    glutathione S-transferase fusion protein preparation, 142, 148
    fusion protein purification, 143, 144, 148
  reporter assays of interferon-regulated gene transcription, p38 MAPK effects,
    β-galactosidase assay, 146, 149
    luciferase assay, 145
    materials, 138, 139
    overview, 144, 148, 149
    transfection, 144, 145, 149
  Western blot of p38 MAPK phosphorylation,
    erasing immunoblots, 140
    incubation conditions and blotting, 139, 140, 148
    materials, 136, 137
Müller cell, transfection with type I interferon genes,
  infection of transfected cells, 225, 230
  materials, 222, 223, 229, 230
  plasmid isolation, 224, 225, 230
  rationale, 222
  transfection conditions, 225, 230
  Western blot analysis of viral protein inhibition, 225–229, 230, 231

N

Northern blot, analysis of herpes simplex virus replication cycle and ICP0 role in interferon resistance,
  gel electrophoresis and blotting, 200, 203, 204
  hybridization and detection, 200
  probe labeling, 200, 204
  RNA preparation, 199
Nuclear run-on assays, gene transcription regulation by herpes simplex virus ICP0
  hybridization, 202–204
  nuclei regulation, 201, 202, 204
  slot blot preparation, 202, 204

Index

O

OAS, *see* 2′-5′ Oligoadenylate synthase
2′-5′ Oligoadenylate synthase (OAS),
  2′-5′ (A) binding and crosslinking, 93, 94, 98
  antiviral activity, 81–83, 103, 104
  assays,
    kinetic parameter determination, 91, 92
    polyacrylamide gel electrophoresis, 91
    RNA-binding assays, 92, 93, 98
    thin-layer chromatography, 89
  genes and homology between species, 82, 83
  isozymes, 83
  prospects for study, 96, 97
  purification from baculovirus-insect cell system,
    expression vector preparation, 86, 97
    FLAG-tagged protein purification, 88
    histidine-tagged protein purification, 89, 98
    infection and cell growth, 87, 97, 98
    materials, 84, 85
    transfection, 86
  reaction, 81
  RNase L activation, *see* RNase L
  structure, 83

P

p38 MAPK, *see* Mitogen-activated protein kinase
Plaque reduction assay, herpes simplex virus ICP0 mutant virus studies, 198, 203
Plasmacytoid dendritic cell, *see* Dendritic cell
Proteomics,
  global, 51, 52
  targeted, 52

R

Rac1, activation assay,
  fusion protein purification, 143, 144, 148
  glutathione-Sepharose preparation, 142, 143, 148
  glutathione *S*-transferase fusion protein preparation, 142, 148
  materials, 138
RNase L,
  2′-5′ (A) activation,
    binding stoichiometry, 104
    fluorescence resonance energy transfer assay,
      analog oligoadenylates, 108
      incubation conditions, 110, 111
      materials, 108, 109
      natural oligoadenylates, 107, 108, 111
      oligoadenylate preparation, 110
      overview, 104, 105
      probe preparation, 110
      RNase L expression and purification, 109–111
    antiviral activity, 103, 104
RNase protection assay, *see* Interferon regulatory factors

S

SCC, *see* Squamous cell carcinoma
Site-directed mutagenesis, interferon-α, 76, 79
Squamous cell carcinoma (SCC), interferon therapy, 14

T

TLRs, *see* Toll-like receptors
Toll-like receptors (TLRs), interferon regulatory factor activation, 28
Tumor vaccines,
  clinical prospects, 152
  protocol development with murine tumor models,
    cell preparation for injection,
      growth, 160, 161
      injection, 161–164
      ultraviolet exposure, 161
    efficacy of cancer vaccine cells, 156, 158, 162
    interferon concentration and efficacy, 156, 163
    materials, 153, 154
    models, 152
    nonimmunogenic tumor cell selection, 154–156, 162, 163
    overview, 152–154
    ultraviolet sensitivity of cancer cells, 158, 159
Type I interferons, *see* Interferon-α; Interferon-β
Type II interferon, *see* Interferon-γ

V

Viruses, interferon defense,
  enzyme mediation, *see* 2′-5′ Oligoadenylate synthase; RNase L
  evasion, 7, 8
  evidence, 4, 5
  functional genomics studies,
    animal models, 50
    compendium analysis, 49
    computing hardware, 42
    engineered virus studies, 47, 48
    Expression Array Manager, 38–40
    gene annotation resources, 42–44
    gene expression analysis software, 40, 41
    human clinical sample analysis, 50, 51
    interferon treatment of cells, 45, 46
    materials, 38
    overview, 37, 38
    proteomics,
      global, 51, 52
      targeted, 52
    Venn diagrams and bioset tools, 44
    viral gene expression profiling, 46
    virulence profiling, 47
  hepatitis B virus treatment, 10, 11
  hepatitis C virus treatment, 11
  host response, 6, 7
  interferon regulatory factors, 28, 29
  interferon regulatory factors, *see* Interferon regulatory factors

W

Western blot,
  antibodies from severe combined immunodeficient mice after monocyte-derived IFN-DC introduction, 176
  herpes simplex virus-1 protein inhibition by interferons in Müller cells, 225–229, 230, 231
  p38 MAPK phosphorylation,
    erasing immunoblots, 140
    incubation conditions and blotting, 139, 140, 148
    materials, 136, 137